The Genetics of Cancer

Genes Associated with Cancer Invasion, Metastasis and Cell Proliferation

The Genetics of Cancer

Genes Associated with Cancer Invasion, Metastasis and Cell Proliferation

G. V. Sherbet and M. S. Lakshmi

Cancer Research Unit,
The Medical School,
University of Newcastle upon Tyne,
Newcastle upon Tyne, UK

ACADEMIC PRESS

San Diego London Boston New York
Sydney Tokyo Toronto

Copyright © 1997 by ACADEMIC PRESS

Academic Press
525 B Street, Suite 1900, San Diego, California 92101-4495, USA
http://www.apnet.com

Academic Press Limited
24–28 Oval Road, London NW1 7DX, UK
http://www.hbuk.co.uk/ap/

ISBN 0-12-639875-5

Library of Congress Cataloging-in-Publication Data
Sherbet, G. V. (Gajanan V.)
   The genetics of cancer: genes associated with cancer invasion, metastasis, and
cell proliferation/by G. V. Sherbet and M. S. Lakshmi.
      p.   cm.
   Includes bibliographical references and index.
   ISBN 0-12-639875-5 (alk. paper)
   1. Cancer–Genetic aspects.   2. Metastasis.   3. Cancer invasiveness.
I. Lakshmi, M. S.   II. Title.
   [DNLM: 1. Neoplasm Metastasis–genetics.   2. Neoplasm Invasiveness–
genetics.   3. Cell Transformation, Neoplastic–genetics.   4. Neovascularization.
Pathologic–genetics.   5. Oncogenes–genetics.   QZ 202 S551g 1997]
RC268.4.S47   1997
616.99'4042–dc21
DNLM/DLC
for Library of Congress   97-11843
                                                                                     CIP

A catalogue record for this book is available from the British Library

Typeset by Paston Press Ltd, Loddon, Norfolk
Printed in Great Britain by WBC Book Manufacturers, Bridgend, Mid Glamorgan

97   98   99   00   01   02   EB   9   8   7   6   5   4   3   2   1

Contents

Preface

அருவினை என்ப உளவோ கருவியான்
காலம் அறிந்து செயின்

Nothing seems hard when the time is right and the means are right

Thiru Valluvar

(Tamil Poet, second century, India)

Thirukkural, chapter 48, verse 483

The scientific inquiry into tumour biology over the past few decades has occurred in three definable phases. One can regard the first five decades of this century as a classical phase of growth of the discipline and comprised the definition of tumour growth, histogenesis and the structure and comparative behaviour of tumours. The prodigious advances in our knowledge of tumour biology in the subsequent decades has in some ways tended to eclipse the significance of these achievements, which culminated in classical works like Willis' *Pathology of Tumours*[1] and *The spread of tumours in the human body*[2] and the comprehensive series *Cancer* edited by Raven[3]. Most of the latter day concepts and understanding have their basis in fundamental work on the definition of the anomalous growth characteristic of tumours, the criteria for assessing their degree of differentiation, and their application of these criteria in tumour grading and as markers of malignancy. Some of these tumour attributes are still used in the clinical setting and make an important contribution to patient management.

The second phase of emergence of tumour biology can be regarded as a phase of conceptual consolidation characterised by the formulation of concepts such as two-stage carcinogenesis by Berenblum and Shubik, and that of tumour progression by Foulds. The latter incorporated incisive analyses and identification of discrete stages in tumour development and secondary spread, often described as the metastatic cascade. The emergence of the notion that a cascade of events is associated with metastatic spread of tumour has enabled a dissection of the biological processes and the associated mechanisms. This phase also saw the emergence of the postulate of tumour suppressor concept of Harris and Klein, which has over the years unfolded into a generalised principle applicable in several areas of cancer research and has led to the isolation of genes such as the *p53, rb, p16/ink* genes, the several tumour suppressor genes associated with the pathogenesis of colonic cancer, as well as the putative metastasis-suppressor *nm23* gene. Thus the concept of Harris and Klein has had far-reaching implications in the understanding of tumorigenesis, and led to the advocacy and demonstration of the two-hit hypothesis by Knudson in the pathogenesis of retinoblastoma.

The third phase encompassing the past two decades have witnessed a phenomenal growth of literature relating to pathogenesis and progression of cancer. One of us has argued previously[4] that the growth of science is a reflection of the growth of technology, and that peaks of scientific activity have nearly always accompanied the invention and development of new technology. The unfolding of some of the intricate mechanisms of cell proliferation and cancer invasion and metastasis has been enabled by rapid advances in biochemical and molecular biological techniques. Their influence on the advance of scientific thought through these three phases, is amply illustrated in two books *The biology of tumour malignancy*[5], and *The metastatic spread of cancer*[6] written by one us (GVS) and by the present volume. The present phase of expansion of our knowledge of cancer biology, to which this volume addresses itself, is to a large extent a legacy of advances in the intricate methods of molecular biology, but scientists may well not regard the means as an end in itself. There are several aspects of the evolution of the invasive and metastatic phenotype not easily amenable to scrutiny by the run of the mill molecular biological techniques. Yet, nothing is hard when the means are right and the time is right. And the time is right for scientific advance on the apparently intractable question of cancer.

The writing of this book was undertaken after much deliberation, consultation and review, and as consequence, it has been a pleasurable experience. Several colleagues gave their time to reading and commenting on different sections of this book, to whom we owe a considerable debt of gratitude. We wish to express our gratitude especially to Dr M. Edward (University of Glasgow), Dr G. Pilkington (Institute of Psychiatry, University of London), Dr C. Parker (M.D. Anderson Cancer Centre, Houston) and Professor P.A. Riley (University College School of Medicine, London). Their comments and suggestions, as well those of other reviewers, for improving the presentation and expanding the scope of the book have been invaluable and were invariably taken on board; yet the overall treatment of the subject and any lapses and omissions in it are our responsibility. No less valuable was the assistance provided by Miss Paula Rutter of the Audio-Visual Centre of the Medical School, who prepared the figures with great skill, enthusiasm and enormous patience, for which we thank her profusely. The work in the authors' laboratory was supported by the North of England Cancer Research Campaign, The Gunnar Nilsson Cancer Research Trust and the Tom Berry Memorial Fund.

G.V. Sherbet
M.S. Lakshmi
The Medical School
Newcastle upon Tyne

1. Willis RA (1967). *Pathology of tumours*, Butterworth, London.
2. Willis RA (1934). *The spread of tumours in the human body*, Butterworth, London.
3. Raven RW (1956-1959). *Cancer*, Butterworth, London.
4. Sherbet GV (1978). *The biophysical characterisation of the cell surface*, Academic Press, London.
5. Sherbet GV (1982). *The biology of tumour malignancy*, Academic Press, London.
6. Sherbet GV (1987). *The metastatic spread of cancer*, Macmillan, Basingstoke.

Abbreviations

ALL	Acute lymphoblastic leukaemia
AML	Acute myelocytic leukaemia
APC	Adenomatous polyposis coli
AT	Ataxia telangiectasia
ATL	Adult T-cell leukaemia/lymphoma
ATPase	Adenosine triphosphatase
BALF	Bronchoalveolar lavage fluid
BCAM	Basal cell adhesion molecule
BWS	Beckwith–Wiedemann syndrome
CAK	cdk-activating kinase
CAM	Cell adhesion molecule
cdk	Cyclin-dependent kinase
CIN	Cervical intraepithelial neoplasia
CIS	Carcinoma *in situ*
CML	Chronic myeloid leukaemia
DAG	Diacylglycerol
DCC	[Gene] Deleted in colon carcinoma
DHFR	Dihydrofolate reductase
DM	Double minute chromosome
DPC	[Gene] Deleted in pancreatic carcinoma
ECM	Extracellular matrix
EGFr	Epidermal growth factor receptor
ELAM	Endothelial leukocyte adhesion molecule
EMS	Ethylmethane sulphonate
ER	Oestrogen receptor
FAP	Familial adenomatous polyposis
FGF	Fibroblast growth factor
GADD	Growth arrest and DNA damage-inducible gene
GAP	GTPase activating protein
HGF	Hepatocyte growth factor
HPRT	Hypoxanthine phosphoribosyl transferase

HPV	Human papilloma virus
IISC	Heat shock cognate protein
HSE	Heat-shock element
HSP	Heat-shock protein
HSV	Herpes simplex virus
ICAM	Intercellular adhesion molecule
IF	Intermediate filaments
IGF	Insulin-like growth factor
IL	Interleukin
IP$_3$	Phosphatidyl 1,4,5-trisphosphate
IR	Ionising radiation
kb	Kilobases
kDa	Kilodalton
KTS	Lysine-threonine-serine region (in Wilms' gene protein)
LFA	Lymphocyte function-associated antigen
LOH	Loss of heterozygosity
LPS	Lipopolysaccharide
LTR	Long terminal repeat
MI	Microsatellite instability
MAP	Microtubule-associated protein
MAP (kinase)	Mitogen induced protein (kinase)
MCC	[Gene] Mutated in colon carcinoma
MMP	Matrix metalloproteinase
MSH	Melanocyte stimulating hormone
NCAM	Neural cell adhesion molecule
NDP (kinase)	Nucleoside diphosphate (kinase)
NGF	Neurite growth factor
ORF	Open reading frame
PAI	Plasminogen activator inhibitor
PALA	N-(phosphonacetyl)-L-aspartic acid
PAR	Plasminogen activator receptor
PCNA	Proliferating cell nuclear antigen
PDGF	Platelet-derived growth factor
PgR	Progesterone receptor
PKA	Protein kinase A
PKC	Protein kinase C
PLC	Phospholipase C
PMA	Phorbol 12-myristate 13-acetate
RA	Retinoic acid
RAR	Retinoic acid receptor
RER (phenotype)	Replication error phenotype

SCC	Squamous cell carcinoma of the lung
SCE	Sister chromatid exchange
SCLC	Small cell lung carcinoma
SH (domains)	*src* homology domains
TBP	TATA binding protein
TGF	Transforming growth factor
TIMP	Tissue inhibitor of metalloproteinase
TP	Thymidine phosphorylase
TNM	Tumour-node-metastasis (staging)
TPA	12-*O*-tetradecanoyl phorbol 13-acetate
tPA	Tissue-type plasminogen activator
TLN	Telencephalin
TNF	Tumour necrosis factor
TSP	Thrombospondin
uPA	Urokinase-type plasminogen activator
VCAM	Vascular cell adhesion molecule
VEGF	Vascular endothelial growth factor
WAGR (syndrome)	Wilms'-aniridia-genitourinary-mental retardation (syndrome)
XHATM	Xanthine hypoxanthine adenine thymidine mycophenolic acid culture medium
XP	Xeroderma pigmentosum

1

Introduction

Metastatic disease is the cause of death in two-thirds of cancer patients. An understanding of the means by which tumour cells achieve metastatic dissemination is obviously of crucial importance for successful treatment of the disease and for evolving possible strategies for the prevention of secondary spread. Although in the clinical context the events associated with the generation of metastatic and drug resistant phenotypes within the tumour contribute significantly to failure of treatment, these events are still poorly understood at the biochemical and molecular biological level. An essential ingredient in the development of successful modes of cancer treatment and management is understanding of the mechanisms by which cancer cells disseminate from the primary site into distant target sites where they can develop into secondary tumours. The main objective of this book is to review these mechanisms and to examine whether genetic abnormalities or alterations can provide an insight into the progression of cancers.

Cancer metastasis is a highly complex process that often follows a deregulated phase of growth and can be described as a cascade divisible into physically and physiologically definable stages of dissemination (Figure 1). Thus, tumour cell dissemination is aided by: (a) adequate vascularisation of the tumour; (b) release of the cells from the primary tumour mediated by proteolytic enzymes produced and often secreted by the tumour into the extracellular environment; (c) adhesion of tumour cells to the basement membrane components prior to invasion of blood vessels and following a direct successful entry into the vascular system or indirectly via the lymphatic system, the cells which are carried to distant parts of the body extravasate from the vascular system into the parenchyma of target organs.

The Genetics of Cancer

PATHOGENESIS OF METASTASIS

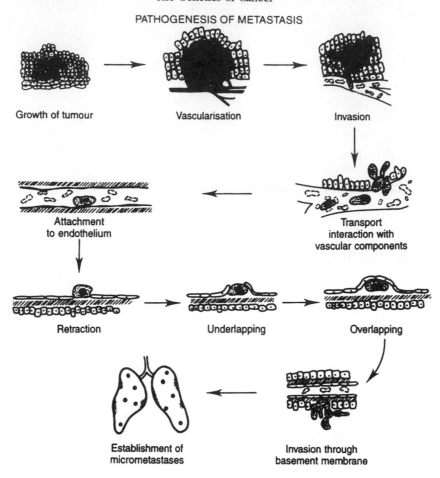

Figure 1. A diagrammatic representation of the processes occurring in the metastatic spread of cancers. Reproduced with permission from Welch (1984).

The targeting of the metastatic cells involves interactions between the tumour cell and the target organs, which are mediated by cell membrane components and aided by the ability of the disseminated cells to produce growth factors in an autocrine mode or to respond to factors in a paracrine fashion; here they grow autonomously into clonal metastatic tumours. Metastatic tumours have themselves the potential to metastasise to tertiary sites (Sugarbaker, 1979; Sherbet, 1982, 1987; Nicolson, 1988).

Malignant tumours are known to be heterogeneous with respect to the expression of biochemical markers, ploidy, degree of differentiation, immunogenicity, etc. It is now generally also accepted that they are not composed of cells of equal metastatic potential but contain a variety of subpopulations with widely differing invasive and metastatic capabilities (Sherbet, 1982, 1987; Nicolson, 1988; Welch, 1989). Foulds (1949, 1969) proposed that tumour development involved traverse through different stages where the neoplasm could be seen to acquire cellular and functional features that could be used to define its progression. Thus, there will exist subpopulations with diverse biological properties, including metastatic potential, depending on the degree of progression undergone by the tumour. The inevitable question, which is posed consistently and which forms the nucleus of discussion here, is whether any or some of these features can be identified with specific genetic determinants.

2

Clonal evolution of the metastatic phenotype

The evolution of cellular diversity within tumours is a significant feature of the development and progression of neoplasms. Not only is this phenomenon scientifically most challenging and conceptually most intractable, but it also has deep connotations for the treatment of cancer. Therefore, the generation of drug-resistant variants and variants with different degrees and patterns of metastatic ability is an area of tumour biology that is currently receiving considerable attention. It seems that the appearance of drug-resistant variants and metastatic phenotypes may be linked closely enough to make attempts at understanding the mechanisms involved a highly worthwhile objective in cancer research. Indeed, it may be fortunate that they may be linked since our ability to deal with drug-resistant variants and metastatic phenotypes is arguably the single most important factor that will determine success in the efforts to contain and cure the disease. These variants are genetically stable phenotypes, although phenotypic drift can and does occur in metastatic phenotypes under certain conditions. Interactions which might take place between different subpopulations within a tumour have often been credited with the maintenance of the stability of the metastatic phenotype (Poste *et al.*, 1981; Miller, 1983).

Tumours are thought to be monoclonal in origin to conform with the mutational concept of tumorigenesis proposed by Knudson (1971, 1973). Tumours of the lymphatic and haematopoietic system have been regarded as monoclonal in origin (Atkin and Baker, 1966; Preud'homme and Seligman, 1972; Fialkow, 1976). Conversely, there are many reports which may be construed as supporting the opposite view which attributes a polyclonal origin to human neoplasms (Beutler *et al.*, 1967; Fialkow *et al.*, 1977; Hsu *et al.*, 1983). Metastatic lesions are also believed to be monoclonal in origin (Poste *et al.*, 1982; Talmadge *et al.*, 1984) but cellular diversity also occurs with time in these secondary deposits (Poste *et al.*, 1982), presumably by the same mechanisms as those which operate in primary tumours.

A great deal is known about the genetic switching mechanisms that operate in diverse biological phenomena such as differentiation, antigenic expression, etc. Genetic instability, which can be viewed as an inherent property of a dynamic system, may be a primary source of this genetic diversity. Therefore, studying the role of genetic instability for understanding the basis of the evolution of the metastatic phenotype has been a logical step forward.

Manifestation of genetic instability

Genetic instability may be indicated by a variety of cellular features at the chromosomal and at the DNA level. At the chromosomal level, the incidence of aneuploidy, deletions, translocations, sister-chromatid exchanges, etc., are evidence of the instability of the genome. Instability of the genome is also manifested at the DNA level as altered DNA repair properties, gene amplification and deletion and point mutations (Table 1). Much evidence can be cited where genetic

Table 1.   Manifestations of genetic instability

At the chromosomal level
- (a)   aneuploidy
- (b)   translocations
- (c)   deletions
- (d)   sister chromatid recombinations
- (e)   fragile sites
- (f)   homogeneously stained regions (HSRs)
- (g)   Double minute chromosomes

At the DNA level
- (a)   Point mutations
- (b)   deletions
- (c)   insertions
- (d)   DNA damage/repair
- (e)   recombination
- (f)   gene amplification
- (g)   microsatellite instability

instability has paralleled the generation of diverse cell subpopulations, including subpopulations with metastasising ability, within the tumour. Genetic instability can be a source of variability and this has been regarded as a driving force in the generation of variants with increased invasive and metastatic potential (Nowell, 1976).

Chromosomal abnormalities in cancer

The abnormal nature of chromosomes of cancer cells was recognised many years ago, but the potential significance of chromosomal aberrations was realised only after the discovery by Nowell and Hungerford (1960) of the Philadelphia chromosome in patients with chronic myeloid leukaemia. The virtual invariability of the association of this abnormal chromosome with a form of human cancer served to emphasise the significance of chromosomal aberrations in the pathogenesis of cancer. The importance of cytogenetics as a major discipline of cancer biology has been strengthened by the non-random nature of chromosomal changes. Most of the abnormalities are restricted to a few sites of the human genome (Heim and Mitelman, 1987). Sutherland (1979) showed the presence of non-staining gaps in both chromatids, which are inherited in a Mendelian fashion. These have been called the fragile sites. These fragile sites appear to be the major targets of mutagens and carcinogens (Yunis et al., 1987). In some tumour cell lines, the incidence of sister chromatid recombination shows marked association with certain chromosomes and it is also predominantly associated with these fragile sites (Lakshmi and Sherbet, 1990). Reciprocal chromosomal translocations as well as sister chromatid recombination are now known to involve specific oncogenes, suggesting a mechanism by which the rearrangement of chromosome might bring these oncogenes into play. Transposition of genes by chromosomal rearrangement can result in inappropriate gene activation which can initiate and mediate pathogenesis. Sister chromatid recombination is strongly associated with the presence of double minute chromosomes, and has therefore been implicated in the process of gene amplification (Lakshmi and Sherbet, 1989; see pages 11–13).

Chromosomal and DNA ploidy is an important parameter which has served as a marker of prognosis in breast cancer (Hedley et al., 1987; Clark et al., 1989; Ferno et al., 1992; Grant et al., 1992; Wenger et al., 1993), as well as in other forms of cancer such as pancreatic adenocarcinoma (Porschen et al., 1993), melanoma (Karlsson et al., 1993), endometrial cancer (Rosenberg et al., 1989), and gastric leiomyosarcoma (Suzuki and Sugihira, 1993). An image cytometric study carried out in the authors' laboratory on breast cancer aspirate cells has also revealed a highly significant relationship between ploidy and prognosis (see Table 2) (G. V. Sherbet et al., unpublished data). Nevertheless, it should be noted that a dissenting view has been expressed with regard to the significance of aneuploidy as a prognostic indicator (Lanigan et al., 1992; Lipponen et al., 1992). Aneuploidy may be a consequence of cells entering the S-phase of the cell cycle prematurely. This can be inferred from the close association often observed between aneuploidy and the size of the S-phase fraction in tumours. Aneuploid

Table 2. Relationship between DNA aneuploidy in breast cancer aspirate cells[1] and tumour progression

DNA ploidy[2]	Number of samples	Non-malignant	M−	M+[3]
$2n-4n$	22	17	5	0
$4n-8n$	15	0	13	2
$8n-12n$	17	0	7	10

[1] Source: Sherbet GV, Lakshmi, MS, Wadehra V, and Lennard TWJ (unpublished data).
[2] DNA content was measured by image cytometry as described in Parker et al. (1994a).
[3] M−, node negative (no distant metastases); M+, node positive (with/without distant metastases). The relationship of degree of DNA ploidy to nodal/distant metastasis was statistically significant at $P < 0.009$ in Fisher exact probability test.

tumours have been reported to show a virtual doubling of the S-phase fraction (Wenger et al., 1993); in that study no information is available about the S-phase fractions of hypodiploid tumours. In contrast, Balslev et al. (1994) found that hypodiploidy correlated with a high S-phase fraction. D'Agnano et al. (1996) reported that 68% of aneuploid breast cancers and only 25% of diploid tumours contained >8.2% cells in the S-phase. The cut-off of 8.2% used in that analysis is somewhat arbitrary and one can conceivably obtain a totally different distribution using another cut-off level. However, in some tumour systems the prognostic value of S-phase fraction could be dissociated from DNA aneuploidy (Sigurdsson et al., 1990; Lipponen et al., 1991, 1992; Arnerlov et al., 1992; Suzuki and Sugihara, 1993). Some data obtained in our study of human breast cancer aspirate cells have revealed no correlation between the size of the S-phase fraction and the degree of ploidy (Figure 2) (G. V. Sherbet et al., unpublished data). Thus, there is not only a serious conflict in the views concerning both the value of DNA ploidy and S-phase fraction as markers of prognosis, but also about the possible relationship between degree of DNA aneuploidy and the size of the S-phase fraction. Despite this, one ought to take into account the observations from several quarters that DNA ploidy is associated with expression of growth factor and hormone receptors (Coulson et al., 1984; Stal et al., 1991; Visscher et al., 1991; Schimmelpenning et al., 1992). The increase in S-phase fraction could be a consequence of events such as gene amplification. Amplification of genes such as c-erbB2, myc, mdm2 but not p53 has been reported in adenocarcinoma of the breast (Latham et al., 1996). Schimmelpenning et al. (1992) also make the interesting statement that mammary carcinomas in situ that express c-erbB2 (encoding a growth factor receptor with similarities to the epidermal growth factor receptor, see page 148) proto-oncogene and possess anueploid DNA show a significantly greater predilection to develop into infiltrating mammary carcinoma. The clonogenic ability of cells derived from certain human tumours has been found to correlate with DNA aneuploidy (Verheijen et al., 1985), but this might represent an adaptive phenomenon determined by the properties relating to the adhesion of cells to the substratum. However, clonal expansion of

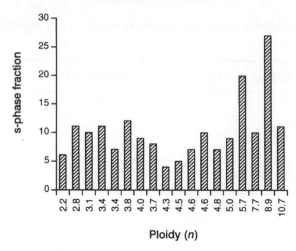

Ploidy (n)

Figure 2.   Relationship between ploidy and the size of the S-phase fraction in human breast cancer aspirate cells. The ploidy and S-phase fractions were measured by using image cytometric methods. DNA profiles were constructed and ploidy was calculated from the DNA levels of G_0G_1 cells, and the size of the S-phase fraction by integrating cell numbers in the region between G_0G_1 and G_2M peaks. No relationship has emerged from this study between DNA ploidy and the size of the S-phase fraction. (From Sherbet GV, Lakshmi MS, Wadehra V, and Lennard TWJ, unpublished observations.)

tumour subpopulations may be an authentic phenomenon, dependent upon how the component cells of a tumour respond to paracrine signals. Thus, even in the face of a degree of scepticism, DNA aneuploidy may be deemed to have some bearing on the progression of cancer.

Clonal expansion of tumour cell subpopulations

The diverse phenotypes generated during the expansion of tumours do not continue to proliferate and expand *ad infinitum*. They are subjected to a process of selective evolution. For instance, they are exposed to external pressures such as those imposed by immunological defence mechanisms, growth factor requirements and the ability of the variants to respond to these. From these selective pressures emerge variants which are better adapted to the ambient growth conditions and display more aggressive growth characteristics and metastatic capability. The proliferative expansion is counter-balanced by selective elimination by switching of cells into the pathway of apoptosis or programmed cell death. It is not inevitable that metastatic variants disseminated to distant target organs will develop into overt metastases. If appropriate growth stimuli are not received by the metastatic cell, a state of dormancy may be encountered (Alexander, 1984). Similarly, distant tumour deposits will remain dormant if a homeostasis is achieved by apoptotic cell death. Heterogeneity of the potential to proliferate, or the clonal expansion of the highly adapted variants is an essential ingredient of progression to the metastatic state and in the development of overt metastases. It follows, therefore, that progression may be accompanied by the expression of growth factor receptors or genes which confer such proliferative potential upon the variants. The *p53* is a gene, which, as we will discuss at length in a later section (page 27) controls cell cycle progression, and also shows marked abnormalities in a majority of human tumours. Abnormalities of this gene may appear early in tumour development or in late stages of progression of certain cancers. Alterations of ploidy and chromosomal aberrations may also occur, in parallel with these changes (Sun *et al.*, 1993; Yahanda *et al.*, 1995), suggesting that the loss of p53 function allows the cells to enter the S-phase prematurely and a consequence of this would be the appearance of cells with an abnormal karyotype and ploidy. A further implication would be that *p53* abnormalities promote genetic instability.

The progression of premalignant head and neck lesions has been shown not only to involve an increase in p53 expression but also a differential expression within the tumour (Shin *et al.*, 1994). These changes can be a result of accumulation of genetic damage or to the expansion of clones carrying *p53* abnormalities. In gliomas, *p53* mutations occur in primary tumours and recurrent tumours as well as in metastases (Sidransky *et al.*, 1992; DeLarco *et al.*, 1993; Kraus *et al.*, 1994). That clones carrying specific *p53* abnormalities may expand with progression is indicated by the finding that often the same mutations occur in low-grade tumours as well as in high-grade recurrent tumours (Sidransky *et al.*, 1992; Kraus *et al.*, 1994). In addition, critical alterations might occur in this gene in metastatic tumours. DeLarco *et al.* (1993) found that three out of eight metastatic tumours contained a mutant allele together with the loss of the second allele. One can then envisage a situation where a clonal population suffers a further genetic alteration which might carry the clone along the path of progression leading to metastasis. The pathway by which this is achieved may be merely by abdication by mutant p53 phosphoprotein of its control over cell cycle progression, but other pathways such as the regulation of genes coding for growth factors (Ueba *et al.*, 1994) can also be open for progression.

Genetic instability and the generation of metastatic variants

Nowell (1976) postulated that tumour progression was attributable to the generation of variant clones within a tumour by genetic instability and that these clones are then subjected to a variety of selective pressures leading to the emergence of aggressive and malignant sublines. Therefore, one would expect that the progression of tumours to the metastatic state will be accompanied by increased genetic instability and that this should be reflected by rates of spontaneous and induced mutations. The methodology followed in many of these studies is to employ ouabain or 6-thiopurine to select for resistant mutants. Resistance to these agents results from a point mutation in the gene which codes for the plasma membrane associated Na^+/K-ATPase (Baker *et al.*, 1974). Cifone and Fidler (1981) found that the rates of mutation to ouabain and 6-thiopurine resistance were three to sevenfold greater in cells with high metastatic potential than in cells with low metastatic potential. This study also contained two clones, differing markedly in metastatic ability, derived from the same tumour. The rate of generation of ouabain resistant mutants in the metastatic clone was 4.6-fold greater than in the low metastasis clone, suggesting that the highly metastatic clone was more unstable than the clone with low metastatic ability. These data have been supported by the rates of generation of drug-resistant mutants in B16 murine melanoma cell lines with different metastatic potential. The high metastasis variant, F10, has been reported to show a fourfold greater rate of generation of methrotrexate- and PALA-resistant mutations than the low metastasis variant F1 (Cillo *et al.*, 1987). The rate of generation of EMS (ethylmethane sulphonate)-induced ouabain-resistant mutants have been determined in mammary carcinoma cell lines. Three cell lines isolated from the same tumour were found to differ markedly in mutation rates for ouabain and 6-thioguanine resistance, but mutation rates did not correlate with metastatic potential (Yamashina and Heppner, 1985). However, the frequency of EMS-induced mutation for ouabain and 6-thioguanine resistance, did correlate with high metastatic potential. Usmani *et al.* (1993) studied both spontaneous mutation frequency for ouabain resistance and EMS-induced mutation for ouabain resistance, using the B16 murine melanoma model. Induction of ouabain-resistant colonies upon EMS exposure of F1 (low metastasis), and BL6 and ML8 (both with high metastatic potential) was $5.5–6.0 \times 10^{-5}$ in BL6 and ML8 cells compared with 2.9×10^{-5} in F1, consistent with the differences in their metastatic potential (Usmani, 1993; Usmani *et al.*, 1993). Bailly *et al.* (1993) found that spontaneous mutation rates of metastatic cell lines derived from melanomas were 10–50-fold greater than those of poorly metastatic cells. Seshadri *et al.* (1987) estimated that mutation rates for 6-thioguanine resistance in human leukaemic cells to be 100-fold greater than in phyto-haemagglutinin-activated normal lymphocytes.

Chambers *et al.* (1988) approached the problem by using temperature sensitive *ts-src* oncogene transformation system. They used a normal kidney cell line carrying the *ts-src* mutant and this cell line exhibits *in vitro* features of a typical transformed phenotype at the permissive temperature of 36°C but behaves like normal cells at the non-permissive temperature of 39°C. *In vivo*, upon intravenous injection into chorioallantoic membrane of 11-day chick embryos, these cells survived in the circulation, arrested and grew in the liver only at the permissive temperature (Chambers and Wilson, 1985). However, no differences have been found in the rates of generation of methotrexate-resistant variant at 36°C and at 39°C. Kaden *et al.* (1989) measured the spontaneous mutation rates at the hypoxanthine-guanine phospho-ribosyl transferase (HPRT) locus of tumorigenic and non-tumorigenic Chinese hamster embryo fibroblasts (CHEF). The tumorigenic CHEF/16 showed generally higher rates of spontaneous mutation than the non-tumorigenic CHEF/18. They then generated and tested three cell lines from CHEF/18 and two from CHEF/16, but found no correlation between tumorigenicity and spontaneous mutation rates.

The rates of appearance of drug resistant mutants in cells with high metastatic potential is in the range $0.5–1.10^{-5}$ per cell per generation and this is similar to the rate of generation of metastatic variants (Harris *et al.*, 1982), although Usmani (1993) and Usmani *et al.* (1993) have described somewhat higher rates of mutation in the B16 melanoma system. Chambers *et al.* (1988) suggest that these rates may be consistent with point mutations and regard the rates of spontaneous generation of metastatic variants as compatible with gene amplification, although others have reported far higher rates of gene amplification (10^{-3}) (Tlsty *et al.*, 1989; Tlsty, 1990). It is difficult to resolve the question of whether the appearance of metastastic variants occurs by a mechanism involving point mutations or gene amplification by the meagre experimental data available to date. However, genetic instability is measurable using yard sticks other than mutation rates. Much recent work has applied these alternative modes of measuring genetic instability.

DNA repair and repair fidelity in metastatic variants

The recognition and repair of DNA damage occurs before the cells enter the S-phase of the cell cycle and cells are held in the G_1 phase until the repair process is completed. This checkpoint control is exercised by the nuclear phosphoprotein p53 whose levels increase when any damage to the DNA is sustained (see page 28). Defects in DNA damage repair are often encountered, e.g. as seen in the human autosomal recessive disorder xeroderma pigmentosum (XP), which are defective in their ability to repair u.v.-induced DNA damage (Lehmann and Norris, 1989). Ataxia telangiectasia (AT) is another example of an autosomal recessive syndrome comprising progressive cerebellar degeneration, oculocutaneous telangiectasias and immune deficiencies. AT patients show high cancer incidence (Swift *et al.*, 1991). Cell lines isolated from AT patients show hypersensitivity to ionising radiation and to radiomimetic agents; this is believed to be due to defective DNA repair (Painter and Young, 1980). All the features of the AT phenotype could be corrected by introducing extraneous DNA by means of cell fusion (Lohrer *et al.*, 1994). Bloom's syndrome is a further example of an autosomal recessive disorder that is characterised by chromosomal fragility as reflected, for instance, in the enhanced incidence of sister chromatid exchange (SCE) in cells derived from patients with Bloom's syndrome (Kohn, 1983; Kihlman and Andersson, 1985). This fragility appears to result from deficiency of the repair enzyme DNA ligase I (Willis and Lindahl, 1987). Chromosomal fragility detectable in the form of SCE has been found to correlate with metastatic potential in the B16 murine melanoma system (Lakshmi *et al.*, 1988). The incidence of SCE has often been linked with defective DNA repair properties (Sherbet, 1987). However, no increases in SCE are found in XP, AT or in Fanconi's anaemia. Usmani *et al.* (1993) studied the DNA repair and the fidelity of DNA repair in metastatic variants of B16 murine melanoma that display marked differences in SCE incidence. No differences were noticeable in the repair of strand breaks induced by exposure to X-rays or bleomycin, but they differed markedly in the fidelity of repair. In this study the fidelity of repair was measured by transfecting the cells with the plasmid PMH16 which carries the *gpt* gene (Usmani *et al.*, 1993). A break was introduced into the gene before transfection, and the ability

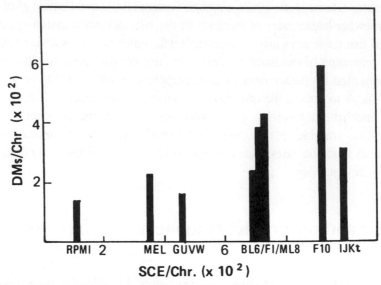

Figure 3.   This illustrates the direct relationship which appears to exist between the incidence of sister chromatid recombination (SCE) and double minute chromosomes in tumour cell lines grown in tissue culture. RPMI and MEL are human melanoma cell lines, BL6, ML8 and F1 are murine melanoma cell lines, and GUVW and IJKt are human astrocytoma cell lines. (From Lakshmi and Sherbet (1989).)

of the cell to re-ligate the gene correctly was measured by their ability to grow in medium containing xanthine, hypoxanthine, adenine and thymidine (XHATM). The high metastasis clones ML8 and BL6 re-ligated the *gpt* gene with repair fidelities of 98% and 64%, respectively, but repair fidelity was low (24%) in the low metastasis F1 clone. Thus, although metastatic

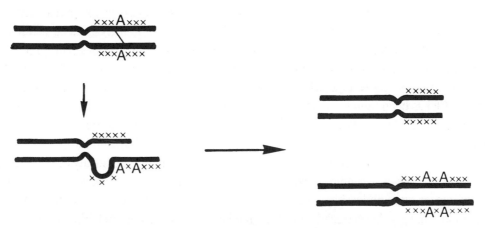

Figure 4.   A schematic representation of a postulated mechanism by which homologous but unequal sister chromatid exchanges can result in gene amplification.

variants of the B16 melanoma do not differ in their ability to re-ligate DNA strand breaks, they do differ markedly in fidelity of repair. With due recognition that these studies are manifestations of the DNA repair properties of tumour cells in culture, it would be desirable to examine whether primary cloned subpopulations derived from tumours also show such differences in repair fidelity, because the higher DNA re-ligation fidelity could be an important mechanism for the maintenance of the metastatic properties of tumour subpopulations.

Genetic recombination in the generation of metastatic variants

Aberrant recombination processes occurring at chromosomal level have been often thought of as a process leading to chromosomal abnormalities associated with cancer. Reciprocal translocation are found in several forms of leukaemia and lymphoma, carcinomas and sarcomas. Chromosomal translocations are found also in a murine plasmacytoma and rat immunocytomas (see Heim and Mitelman, 1987). Inappropriate activation of oncogenes can occur as a consequence of these chromosomal rearrangements (see Sherbet, 1987). As stated previously, chromosomal recombination in the form of SCE occurs at a higher level in Bloom's syndrome which is characterised by chromosomal fragility. SCE break points appear to occur at chromosomal fragile sites (Lakshmi and Sherbet, 1990) and, significantly, some of these sites also harbour certain oncogenes and genes coding for growth factors. Furthermore, the degree of sister chromatid exchange correlates positively with the incidence of double minute chromosomes (DMs) (Lakshmi and Sherbet, 1989) (Figure 3). Double minute chromosomes are thought to represent gene amplification. Homologous, but unequal, recombinations involving repetitive elements are known to result in deletion or duplication of exons (Alberts et al., 1983; Lehrman et al., 1987). Lakshmi and Sherbet (1989) therefore suggest that the association between incidence of SCE and double minute chromosomes could be a result of homologous but unequal exchange of chromatid segments (Figure 4). Sager et al. (1985) found that tumorigenic CHEF cells can amplify the dihydrofolate reductase (DHFR) gene more rapidly than non-tumorigenic cells. The ability to amplify DNA has been reported to correlate with metastatic ability (Cillo et al., 1987). As pointed out previously, it would be of interest to recall that the rate of generation of metastatic variants is on a par with that of mutation to methotrexate resistance and DHFR gene amplification. Thus, it is possible that a gene amplification mechanism may be involved in the progression of tumours to the metastatic state. Although gene amplification has been demonstrated in models of established tumour cell lines, it is uncertain whether subpopulations within tumours show a heterogeneity with respect to their ability for gene amplification.

Homologous recombination of transfected plasmid DNA, at extrachromosomal location, i.e. before integration and recombination after integration into chromosomes (chromosomal recombination), has been used as a marker for genetic variability and instability. Usmani and Sherbet (1996) used the pDR plasmid to study both chromosomal and extra-chromosomal recombination ability of metastatic variants of the B16 melanoma. The pDR plasmid contains a selectable marker (*gpt* gene) and the *neo* (neomycin resistance) gene. The latter is present as two truncated, non-tandem but overlapping segments. The plasmid was transfected into the cells and transfectants were selected by growing the cells in XHATM culture medium, indicating *gpt* function. The transfectant clones were then expanded and subjected to selection for the presence of functional *neo* gene. Only those transfectants carrying stably integrated plasmid DNA, that have successfully recombined the *neo* gene fragments into a functional gene, will come through this selection procedure. This procedure allows one to determine the chromosomal recombination events occurring in these cells. Surprisingly, the ability of the low metastasis variant F1 to carry out chromosomal recombination was three orders of magnitude greater than the high metastasis variants BL6 and ML8. Extrachromosomal recombination was measured by introducing pDR DNA into cells and selecting them for neomycin resistance by growth in G418-containing culture medium. In contrast to chromosomal recombination, the ability to carry out extra-chromosomal recombination, i.e. prior to integration of the plasmid DNA, was higher in the high metastasis variants BL6 and ML8 than in the low metastasis variant F1. Previously, Finn *et al.* (1989) found a higher frequency of extrachromosomal recombination of plasmid DNA in immortalised transformed cells. The recombination events occurring in the genomic DNA will depend on the sites of integration of the plasmid. Some integration sites are believed to be inherently unstable (Murnane and Young, 1989).

Genetic recombination may occur in association with defective DNA repair and reduced DNA repair can be seen as a condition conducive to recombination at the DNA and at the

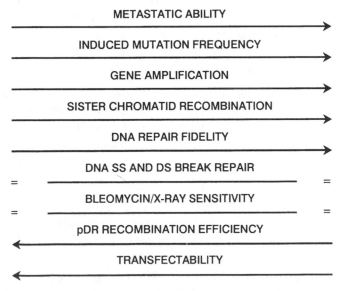

Figure 5.   This diagram shows the relationship between metastatic ability and some cellular features that are related to or are reflections of genetic instability and cellular metabolism. Reproduced with permission from Usmani (1993).

chromosomal level. Decreased extrachromosomal recombination has been reported by Wahls and Moore (1990) in repair deficient cell lines. The observations of Usmani and Sherbet (1996) are compatible with this view and demonstrate that cells which are more proficient in DNA repair also show high extra-chromosomal recombination. The complex relationship between specific cellular attributes related to genetic instability and metastatic potential is summarised in Figure 5. This partial picture may indeed reflect to some degree the existence of dynamic heterogeneity in tumours.

Microsatellite instability in cancer progression

The mutator *phenotype and cancer*

The progression of cancer to the metastatic stage is identifiable, as the above discussion implies, with genomic instability. This conceivably could lead to genetic alterations, primary as well as cumulative secondary changes, that might confer selective proliferative advantage on variants generated by this genomic flux. Therefore, clonal expansion of these variants may be considered to be a major force in tumour progression. The rate of generation of metastatic variants and the rate of spontaneous mutation of drug-resistant variants in tumours are several orders of magnitude greater than the rate of background mutations. Loeb (1991, 1994) therefore proposed the concept of the mutator phenotype in order to account for the high mutation rates occurring in cancer. This concept is based on the inherent instability associated with microsatellite loci occurring in the genome. Microsatellites are repetitive nucleotide sequences of varying lengths which occur in the human genome, between and within genes. The microsatellite sequences have been found to be unstable in the sense that variations can occur in repetitive sequence units within the microsatellites, resulting in the expansion or shortening of microsatellites. The instability of microsatellites can affect non-repetitive sequences of the genome. Eshleman *et al.* (1995), for instance, found that a 100- to 1000-fold increase in mutation rates in the HPRT gene in the RKO colon cancer cell line and, subsequently, that >10% of the HPRT mutants indeed carried a single 3 bp deletion outside the microsatellite repeats. Furthermore, one-third of the mutations were transitions or transversions, suggesting a wide range of features associated with the mutator phenotype (Eshleman *et al.*, 1996). A majority of microsatellite repeats occur outside the coding regions of genes, and therefore microsatellite instability (MI) may not directly lead to carcinogenesis, but could destabilise DNA sequences inside as well as outside the microsatellite repeats and make the genome hypermutable (Eshleman *et al.*, 1996). As a corollary, one should consider the possibility that microsatellite instability might be engendered by exposure to carcinogens. Although no direct evidence for this can be adduced, it would be worthwhile referring to the observation made by Boyd *et al.* (1996) that microsatellite instability was an invariable attribute of tumours of the vagina and the uterine cervix arising in association with exposure to diethylstilboestrol, but not of those where exposure to the hormone had not occurred.

Incidence of microsatellite instability in cancer

Microsatellite instability has been encountered in several forms of human cancer, e.g. in colonic (Aaltonen *et al.*, 1993; Ionov *et al.*, 1993; Thibodeau *et al.*, 1993; Patel *et al.*, 1994), endometrial (Risinger *et al.*, 1993; Burks *et al.*, 1994), gastric (Han *et al.*, 1993; Peltomaki *et al.*, 1993; Seruca *et al.*, 1995; Dossantos *et al.*, 1996), pancreatic (Han *et al.*, 1993), and oesophageal cancers (Meltzer *et al.*, 1994). This abnormality was not found in cancers of the breast, lung or testis (Peltomaki *et al.*, 1993), but recent reports do cite microsatellite instability in these tumours. MI may occur infrequently in sporadic and in familial breast cancer (Jonsson *et al.*, 1995) and at a high frequency in invasive lobular breast carcinoma (Aldaz *et al.*, 1995). Merlo *et al.* (1994) has stated that it occurs frequently in small cell lung carcinoma. Adachi *et al.* (1995) found no MI in small cell lung carcinoma, but did find MI in about one-third of non-small cell lung cancers. Instability of microsatellite repeats has been seen in a small proportion of cervical carcinomas and in cell lines derived from them (Larson *et al.*, 1996). The overall incidence of MI in ovarian carcinomas was 17% of 47 tumours, but it was far higher at 50% in endometrioid type of tumours (Fujita *et al.*, 1995). MI is apparently not generally involved in leukaemias and lymphomas (Volpe *et al.*, 1996), although it has been described in follicle centre cell lymphoma (Randerson *et al.*, 1996). It would be safe overall, to conclude that microsatellite instability is fairly widespread in human neoplasms and it would certainly be profitable to review the potential mechanisms by which MI can affect genetic function.

Microsatellite instability and genetic alterations in cancer

Microsatellite instability is associated with mutations in the genes, *MLH1*, *MSH2*, *PMS1*, *PMS2*, which are human homologues of mismatch repair genes of *Escherichia coli* (Fishel *et al.*, 1993; Leach *et al* 1993; Lindblom *et al.*, 1993; Bronner *et al.*, 1994; Nicolaides *et al.*, 1994; Papadopoulos *et al.*, 1994). Although not yet extensively studied, preliminary evidence suggests that one or more of these mismatch repair genes may be mutated in cancer (Umar *et al.*, 1994; Kobayashi *et al.*, 1996). From the concept of the 'mutator' phenotype and the involvement of the mismatch repair genes with MI follows the suggestion that there should be less efficient or reduced mismatch repair in cancer. Risinger *et al.* (1995) showed that cell extracts derived from cell lines exhibiting MI were unable to carry out mismatch repair, but cell lines showing no MI were quite proficient. This inability to carry out mismatch repair, they showed, was a consequence of a defect in the *MSH2* gene. However, proficiency of mismatch repair does not always correlate inversely with cell transformation or malignancy. Boyer *et al.* (1993) compared the fidelity of DNA replication in transformed cells with their normal diploid counterparts: no differences were found in their ability for mismatch repair.

If mutations of these genes are strewn across in cancer tissue, one can envisage how microsatellite instability, also known as the replication error positive (RER+) phenotype, can affect the expression of genes associated with cell proliferation, cell adhesion, invasion and metastasis. To date, a few studies are available that have examined the occurrence of MI at some chromosomal loci harbouring genes that are known to be closely involved in these biological processes. In this context one may cite the H-*ras* oncogene which has been identified with the pathogenesis of several forms of human cancer. In cancer of the head and neck, the loss of heterozygosity at the H-*ras* locus correlates with lymph node metastasis and, interestingly, some tumours also show instability of a microsatellite repeat which occurs in intron-1 of the gene (Kiaris *et al.*, 1994). Abnormalities of the Ki-*ras* homologue have been found in non-small cell lung cancer in association with MI (Fong *et al.*, 1995a). Conversely, no mutations in the *ras* oncogene homologues have been encountered in endometrial (Carduff *et al.*, 1996) and vaginal and cervical (Boyd *et al.*, 1996) cancers, even though they showed extensive microsatellite instability. The H-, Ki- and N-*ras* homologues have been screened for mutation in renal cell tumours with MI, but no mutations have been found (Uchida *et al.*, 1994). Another instance of a positive correlation between MI and an abnormality of a genetic locus is the association between loss of heterozygosity that occurs at *nm23*, a putative metastasis suppressor gene (see page 184), with MI, in sporadic colorectal tumours (Patel *et al.*, 1994).

Microsatellite instability and cell proliferation-related genes

There are several investigations pertaining to the association of MI with the suppressor gene *p53* which controls cell cycle progression (see page 28). In general, these have not found any alterations in *p53* in parallel with microsatellite instability. The *p53* locus is unaffected by MI in colorectal dysplasias and carcinomas (Suzuki *et al.*, 1994; Muta *et al.*, 1996). Abnormalities of *p53* such as loss of heterozygosity are not related to MI in gastric cancer (Semba *et al.*, 1996). Another study has shown that the expression of p53 protein is seen in 28% (12 out of 42) of gastric tumours, but this is not associated with MI (Lin *et al.*, 1995). Carduff *et al.* (1996) found no correlation between MI and p53 protein expression detected by immunohistochemical means in endometrial cancers. The low frequency of *p53* mutations and the high incidence of MI in renal cell carcinomas reported by Uchida *et al.* (1994) also suggests that the two phenomena may not be related. A further observation is that MI is not always present where p53 protein expression is detectable (Strickler *et al.*, 1994; Lothe *et al.*, 1995). However, molecular abnormalities in *p53* and *ras* oncogenes have been found in a small number of non-small cell lung cancers concomitantly with MI (Fong *et al.*, 1994). Clear-cell adenocarcinoma of the vagina and cervix also shows some relationship between MI and over-expression of p53 protein, as determined by immunohistochemistry (Boyd *et al.*, 1996). In these systems, obviously, one is looking at the aberrant or mutant form of p53; but, Boyd *et al.* (1996) found that the protein was over-expressed in the absence of any mutations of the gene. In so far as wild type p53 expression is concerned, it is elevated in response to DNA damage and therefore the RER+ phenotype cannot be expected and does not appear to be modified in such a transient fashion (Anthoney *et al.*, 1996). An important line of evidence of how p53 protein might yet prove to be important in the context of microsatellite instability has recently emerged. The promoter region of the mismatch repair gene *HMSH2* contains a site which bears homology to p53-binding consensus sequence. *In vitro* specific binding of p53 to the consensus sequence has been demonstrated (Scherer *et al.*, 1996). The mismatch repair genes might indeed prove to be another new target regulated by p53.

Transforming growth factor β (TGF-β) has been shown to be inhibitory to growth in several tumour models. The absence of the TGF-β receptor or mutation of the receptor may enable the cell to overcome the growth control exerted by TGF-β. Therefore, this has afforded a suitable model for examining the relationship between MI and the presence of inactivating mutation in TGF-β receptor II gene. Colon cancers with the RER+ phenotype have been shown to carry mutation in the TGF-β type II receptors (Eshleman and Markowitz, 1995; Markowitz *et al.*, 1995). RER+ gastric cancers similarly also contain mutations of the gene (Myeroff *et al.*, 1995). Thus, in these tumour models, the RER+ phenotype and the presence of inactivating mutations of the receptor gene, can confer upon the cells a proliferative advantage. Proliferative advantage may be conferred also by over-expression of other growth factor encoding genes such as the *erb*-B2. The expression of this gene has shown significant correlation with microsatellite instability in gastric carcinomas (Lin *et al.*, 1995).

Microsatellite instability and cancer progression

Although the evidence available at present is not sufficiently strong or persuasive to conclude that the RER+ phenotype is germane to cancer development, one should enquire whether changes in MI occur in the premalignant stage and whether any incremental changes take place or at one or more relevant loci during tumour progression. The initial studies on the significance of MI were carried out in colonic tumour where specific genetic alterations can be identified at definable stages of progression (Figure 18; see page 172). Microsatellite instability occurs frequently in hereditary non-polyposis coli adenomas (Aaltonen *et al.*, 1993). However, it is uncertain if the same genes are affected by microsatellite instability as those known to be associated with the progression of colorectal cancer. Allen (1995) appears to be suggesting that the progression of colorectal neoplasia may follow two distinct paths, namely, loss of heterozygosity of the genes as shown in Figure 18, or replication error pathway. If this was the case, one would not expect the same genetic changes in association with MI during tumour progression. The findings of Heinen *et al.* (1995) that the adenomatous polyposis coli (APC) protein is not affected by MI, suggest that the progression of colorectal carcinogenesis may follow two different pathways as Allen (1995) suggested.

Shibata *et al.* (1994) regarded the occurrence of this abnormality as an early event in sporadic colon cancer. Similar levels of MI incidence have been reported for colorectal dysplasias and also in more advanced lesions. There is no tendency for MI to occur at additional multiple loci detectable in advanced lesions (Suzuki *et al.*, 1994). Recent work has shown that the same proportion (20%) of primary as well as liver metastases display the RER+ phenotype. Furthermore, the RER+ phenotype was never encountered in liver secondaries when the corresponding primary tumours were RER negative (Ishimaru *et al.*, 1995), suggesting that MI is an event associated with early stages of tumorigenesis. Microsatellite instability appears to occur early in the progression of Barrett's-associated oesophageal adenocarcinoma, where MI is detectable in one in 14 cases of Barrett's metaplasia. Its incidence is far higher in adeno-carcinomas and in diploid nuclei derived from oesophageal adenocarcinomas. Adachi *et al.* (1995) have reported MI in 55% of metastatic compared with only 12% of primary non-small cell lung carcinoma. They also encountered identical RER+ phenotypes in four out of 10 pairs of primary and secondary tumours. Egawa *et al.* (1995) examined MI at several loci on chromo-some 5 in cancer of the prostate and found that the only clinical feature that correlated with MI was nodal and distant metastatic spread. Chong *et al.* (1994) found MI to be a late event in the progression of gastric cancers. MI occurred more frequently in advanced carcinomas than in early stages of the disease. This seems to suggest that MI may be responsible for altering gene function that propels the tumour along the metastatic pathway. Conversely, Dossantos *et al.* (1996) analysed six microsatellite loci of gastric carcinomas. Essentially, their data have suggested a reduced nodal involvement in tumours which had MI at >2 microsatellite loci. Furthermore, tumours with MI at >2 loci showed greater lymphoid infiltration, which indicates a less aggressive tumour behaviour; the RER+ phenotype also suggested a favourable prognosis in this study. A lack of correlation between MI and metastatic dissemination of gastric cancer is also supported by Nakashima *et al.* (1995) who reported that tumours with high MI showed no venous or lymphatic invasion. According to Carduff *et al.* (1996), the RER+ phenotype does not correlate with invasive behaviour of endometrial carcinomas. Investigation of possible micro-satellite alterations at several chromosomal loci including the suppressor gene *nm23*-H1 (see page 184) locus in colonic cancer has revealed no correlation between MI and metastasis (Patel *et al.*, 1994). In the light of these dissensions, a definitive conclusion must await further investigations.

There are indications that changes in MI may occur in a progressive fashion and that this may be reflected in the association of MI with tumour grade and the degree of differentiation. Poorly differentiated gastric (Seruca *et al.*, 1995) and endometrial (Kobayashi *et al.*, 1995) carcinomas have tended to present an RER+ phenotype. Surprisingly, the clinical stage of gastric cancers showed no relationship to MI (Seruca *et al.*, 1995). Relationship between MI and differentiation is also seen *in situ* and in invasive human breast cancer. A significant proportion (9/23) of invasive lobular breast cancers were RER+ compared with only 13% of 52 tumours showing ductal differentiation (Aldaz *et al.*, 1995). Muta *et al.* (1996) have stated that a high proportion of poorly differentiated colorectal cancer exhibited MI, but Schlegel *et al.* (1995) found no correlation between MI and tumour grade or stage. In contrast, Semba *et al.* (1996) reported that the RER+ phenotype is detectable in 33% (3/9) differentiated as opposed to 18% (2/11) poorly differentiated gastric cancers. However, the number of samples examined were far too small to warrant any serious credence to be attached to the inverse relationship between MI and the state of differentiation.

To summarise, it would be premature to form definitive views of the relevance of MI to the biological processes of cancer behaviour, but the evidence for the association of MI with biological features of proliferation, invasion, differentiation and metastasis, and for the involvement of genes that characterise these aspects of biological behaviour can be described as ambivalent. This does not diminish the potential value of microsatellite instability as a mechanism for the modulation of the structure and function of genes. Microsatellite instability appears to make genetic sequences of repeat motifs hypermutable (Eshleman *et al.*, 1995). Furthermore, the RER+ phenotype could represent a germ line mutation (Bergthorsson *et al.*, 1995). The critical experiments would be to test the Nowell hypothesis of genetic instability in generating the metastatic mosaic during progression and, in particular, it would be interesting to see whether clonal selection of variants that arise in the growing tumour population, by the acquisition of selective growth advantage, is related to microsatellite instability. In culture, invasive phenotypes can be defined and their invasive ability measured, together with experimental assays for metastatic potential. Realisation of the full potential of MI for the understanding of the basic biological processes related to behaviour of cells or assessing its value as a marker of progression, must begin with basic *in vitro* experimental strategies. The difficulty of interpreting any information on MI that might be currently available is solely a consequence of directly applying the technology to tumours *in vivo*. There is a great deal of ground work to be done before we can assess the utility and implications of the concept of microsatellite instability in cancer management.

Telomerase function, genetic instability, cell proliferation and cancer metastasis

Cellular transformation leading to the immortalisation of cells and to apoptotic death of cells is associated with characteristic chromosomal abnormalities. The chromosomal entities that are involved in the generation of these abnormalities have been identified in the past few years and there has been a significant advance in our understanding of the molecular mechanisms involved in the immortalisation of cells and limitation of the life span of cells by apoptotic processes. This area of study impinges also upon deregulation of cell proliferation and the appearance of variant cell populations characterised by deregulation of the cell cycle leading to tumorigenesis.

Telomeres are terminally located chromosomal regions which are essential in maintaining the function and integrity of the chromosome. These serve as caps at either end of the chromosome that stop its fragmentation. The cell loses some of the telomeric DNA at each round of replication. This progressive diminution of telomeres makes chromosomes unstable and leads to illegitimate recombinations and degradation of chromosomes (Counter et al., 1994a). For instance, the loss of telomeric DNA generates 'sticky' ends which can cause sister chromatids to fuse end–end or fuse with other chromosomes to produce chromosomal abnormalities such as dicentric or ring chromosomes. Telomeres are composed of highly conserved hexameric repeats of 5'-TTAGGG-3' nucleotide sequences and associated proteins (Moyzis et al., 1988; Meyne et al., 1989).

Telomeric diminution is a consequence of replication ineffeciency known as the end replication problem. DNA is synthesised by conventional DNA polymerases unidirectionally with a 5'–3' polarity and this requires an RNA primer and the lagging strand cannot be completed. This leaves a gap at the 5' end of the lagging strand (Watson, 1972; see also Olovnikov, 1996; Villeponteau, 1996). Failure to fill this gap results in a progressive loss of DNA and a consequent shortening of the chromosome. This loss has been postulated to be the reason why the replicative life of a cell is limited (Harley et al., 1990). An enzyme called telomerase has been identified in Tetrahymena thermophila (Greider and Blackburn, 1987). This enzyme solves the end-replication problem by adding repetitive telomeric sequences and maintains the integrity of the telomere. The telomerase is a ribonucleoprotein with an RNA component encoded by a single gene (Feng et al., 1995) and two proteins of 80 and 95 kDa (Collins et al., 1995). Telomere shortening has been observed in vitro and in vivo and, in parallel with this process, the replicative life span is also reduced (Harley et al., 1990; Hastie et al., 1990). Elongation of telomeres by experimental means extends the life span of cells (Wright et al., 1996a). Senescent cells are known to show chromosomal changes such as telomere–telomere association which are a characteristic feature of the loss of telomeric DNA. Telomeric association has been regarded as an early manifestation of apoptosis (Pathak et al., 1994). Telomerase protects cells from apoptotic death and promotes immortalisation and continued proliferation. Consistent with this, telomerase activity has been detected in the germ cells and embryonic cells of both Xenopus and human origin (Mantell and Greider, 1994; Wright et al., 1996b). It is also found in immortalised cells (Counter et al., 1992, 1994b) as well as in human cancers (Counter, 1994a; Nilsson et al., 1994; Hiyama E et al., 1995a,b), which as a result do not suffer losses of telomeric DNA sequences.

The active association of telomerase with the proliferative activity of cells is demonstrated by the cell cycle dependent expression of the polymerase. Asynchronous cultures and G_1-arrested cells show similar levels of the enzymes but an increase occurs as cells progress into the S-phase where the highest levels of the enzyme are detectable. Expression of the enzyme then diminishes and is virtually absent in G_2-M arrested cells (Zhu et al., 1996). Furthermore, differentiation-inducing agents inhibit telomerase activity in immortal cells (Sharma et al., 1995; Xu et al., 1996; Zhang et al., 1996), confirming by implication the involvement of telomerase in cell cycle progression and continued proliferation. This abrogation of cell cycle control may involve the cell cycle control genes, *p53* and *rb*. It has been postulated that diminution of the telomere beyond a critical length might activate *p53* leading to *M1* senescence. But telomerase-dependent immortalisation of cells, together with the inactivation of *p53* or *rb* genes by allelic loss or mutation, is postulated to lead to *M2* immortalisation. Furthermore, *M2* immortalisation is postulated to lead to progression of tumours to the metastatic state (Healy, 1995). This fits in with the picture of a late contribution by *p53* to the progression of colorectal cancers (see page 172 and Figure 18). The *M2* immortalisation concept is also compatible with the finding that telomerase activity is detected in colorectal carcinomas but not in adenomatous polyps (Chadeneau *et al.*, 1995). Eddington *et al.* (1995) believe that the activation of telomerase may be a late event in cancer progression and this may be associated also with loss of *p53* gene function by genetic alteration or allelic loss. K. Hiyama *et al.* (1995a) noticed changes in telomeric length in 16 primary lung cancers; of these 14 showed telomere diminution. Consistent with the *M2* postulate, they found 10 tumours out of 14 with telomere diminution contained allelic loss of both *p53* and *rb* genes. Telomerase activity is strongly associated with advanced gastric cancers and poor prognosis, but it is virtually undetectable in early stages of the disease (Hiyama E *et al.*, 1995a). The enzyme has been found to be expressed in a majority of prostate carcinomas compared with only approximately one in 10 benign prostatic hyperplasias. In addition, lymph nodes containing metastatic tumour have been found to be telomerase-positive (Sommerfield *et al.*, 1996). In carcinoma of the breast, 93% (of 130) of advanced stage cancers expressed telomerase but the incidence of telomerase positivity in early stage disease was far lower (20–30%). No telomerase was detected in normal breast tissue or non-malignant conditions, e.g. fibrocystic disease (Hiyama *et al.*, 1996). Virtually all advanced-stage bladder tumours were telomerase positive and telomerase activity also strongly correlated with deep muscle invasion by the tumours (Lin *et al.*, 1996). The telomere length itself has been found to diminish progressively with tumour progression and telomeres are said to be extremely short in metastatic cells (Counter *et al.*, 1994a). Conversely, there is a report that loss of the enzyme occurred in parallel with regression of some neuroblastomas (Hiyama E *et al.*, 1995b). Notwithstanding such a high degree of correlation between telomerase function and progression of tumours, reports have also begun to appear which do not support a significant role for the enzyme in tumour progression. Telomerase activity in non-malignant and malignant skin lesions shows no indication of any correlation with malignancy (Taylor *et al.*, 1996). According to Dahse *et al.* (1996) advanced stages of renal carcinomas do not show enhanced telomerase activity. Also intriguing is the frequent expression of the enzyme in small cell carcinomas of the lung, whereas it was highly variable in non-small cell cancers ranging from a total lack of it in some tumours to very high activity in others. Similarly, telomerase expression in metastatic disease was also not invariable (Hiyama K *et al.*, 1995b).

3

Inefficiency of the metastatic process

Metastatic dissemination of cancers has long been regarded as a somewhat inefficient process. Conceptually, one can envisage several reasons for this. Invasion of the vascular endothelium is an important step in tumour dissemination. The degree of efficiency with which the cancer cell can break through the endothelial barrier will have significant consequences for the overall success of metastatic spread. Invasive behaviour is in part due to the proliferative potential of the tumour. The spatial expansion of the tumour will exert mechanical pressures which naturally result in tumour spread via paths of least mechanical resistance. However, tumours will resort to actively breaching the basement membrane by secreting a spectrum of proteolytic enzymes. The diapedesis of tumour cells across the endothelium is also an active cellular process, but defects in the endothelium will aid this process. Systemic endothelia lack tight junctions between cells and often show intercellular discontinuities which can serve as ports of entry or exit. Weiss (1990) has argued, probably without successfully persuading everyone, that carcinomas *in situ* (CIS) of the uterine cervix do not penetrate the basement membrane nor invade the cervical stroma and do not normally metastasise, although untreated disease may become invasive. The considerable time lag often seen between the development of CIS and its progression into the invasive phase has been attributed to the requirement of evolution of cell types which have high motility and also the ability to adhere to and breach the basement membrane.

Loss of cells which have entered the vascular compartment is another major cause of metastatic inefficiency. Using experimental animal tumour models it has been demonstrated that although several million tumour cells may be released into the vascular system, only a small proportion of these will be able to survive the mechanical and immunological assaults mounted by the host and successfully form secondary tumours. The surviving fraction may be as small as about 0.01% of all cells released from the primary tumour. This surviving fraction has to cross the vascular barrier again into the parenchyma of metastatic target sites. Here, again, several constraints may operate, e.g. the enzymes associated with the luminal surface may affect interaction and adhesion to it. It should be borne in mind that the circulating tumour cells may have adapted in the first instance to adhesion and interaction with the basement membrane, but a totally different set of biological properties will be required for the exit of the cells from the vascular compartment. Furthermore, the tumour cell, having extravasated from the vascular compartment, will require optimal growth conditions in the parenchyma of the metastatic target organ and if these are unavailable the cancer cells which have arrested in the target organ may remain as dormant microscopic metastatic deposits.

4

Tumour growth and metastatic potential

The size of the primary tumour is an important parameter in clinical staging of cancers. It is uncertain, however, whether there is a direct correlation between primary tumour burden and the ability to metastasise. Tumour evolution may be associated with increased genetic instability which could lead to the emergence of aggressive phenotypes within the primary tumour. Thus, spontaneous mutation rates are known to be higher in cancer cells compared with corresponding non-malignant counterparts (see page 10). A more rapid growth rate associated with such higher rates of generation of aggressive malignant cells can lead to highly aggressive primary cancer.

Tumours also tend to be heterogeneous with regard to the distribution of the proliferative fraction. The infiltrative or invasive components of tumours in breast cancer, for instance, possess a higher proliferative index than the intraductal component (Verhoeven and Vanmarck, 1993). Human melanocytic tumours show a marked increase in proliferating cells from a benign condition to primary and metastatic melanoma (Smolle et al., 1991). However, proliferative pressure may only be one of the factors that lead to invasive behaviour. Benign pituitary adenomas with cavernous sinus invasion are larger in size than those showing no invasion but there is no relationship between proliferative capacity and invasive behaviour (Kawamoto et al., 1995). In the B16 murine melanoma a high expression of α-melanocyte stimulating hormone (MSH) has been demonstrated in the invasive peripheral regions of the tumour (Zubair et al., 1992). This hormone has been found to promote anchorage-independent growth of melanoma cells (Sheppard et al., 1984; Bregman et al., 1985; Parker et al., 1991) and highest levels of MSH immunoreactivity have been reported in the least differentiated and highly metastatic melanoma cell lines (Lunec *et al.*, 1990). In these cases the infiltrative behaviour may be attributable to other factors than proliferative pressure alone such as, for instance, the up-regulation of genes which promote metastatic spread (Parker *et al.*, 1991, 1994a,b). Nonetheless, on account of this possible relationship between tumour cell proliferation and metastasis, genes which are involved in controlling both cell proliferation and metastasis have been the targets of intensive investigation in recent years. The genetic deregulation of cell proliferation and the promotion of metastatic spread will therefore provide a point of focus here.

5

Cell cycle regulation and pathogenesis of cancer

Cancer has been described as a disease of the cell cycle (North, 1991). Genomic changes characterised by chromosomal aberrations, translocations and aneuploidy are associated with tumour progression and these arise by cumulative genetic changes resulting from loss of cell cycle control. There have been significant advances in our understanding of the mechanisms of the cell division cycle. Genetic analyses have revealed the involvement in this process of suppressor genes such as the *p53* and the retinoblastoma-susceptibility gene, *rb*. Mutation, allelic loss or inactivation of these genes have been demonstrated in a variety of tumours, leading to the suggestion that the protein products of these genes exert restraint on proliferation of the normal cell. The product of the retinoblastoma-susceptibility gene *rb* is differentially phosphorylated in relation to the stage of the cell cycle. The rb protein ($p110^{rb}$) is predominantly underphosphorylated in the G_1 phase and becomes hyperphosphorylated as cells enter the S-phase and this state of phosphorylation is maintained until they emerge from the metaphase (see page 52). Cell cycle progression is controlled by a variety of cyclins. Thus, progression in G_1 phase involves cyclins C, D and E and cyclins A and B in the S, G_2 and mitotic phases. The phase transition events appear to be triggered by cyclin-dependent kinases (cdks) which comprise a cyclin regulatory unit and *cdc2* kinase unit. The cdks require to be activated by phosphorylation by the cdk-activating kinase (CAK). The rb protein has been found to be a substrate for cdk-mediated phosphorylation. The hyperphosphorylation of rb protein appears to inactivate rb function and enables the cells to transit into the S-phase

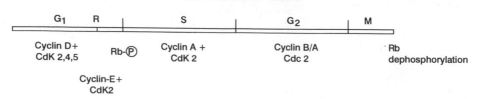

Figure 6. A representation of cyclin–cdk complexes with cell cycle progression, with reference to potential sites of their action. The phosphorylation of the rb protein releases it from its complex with transcription factors such as the E2F, so that the latter can activate the gene essential for the transition of cells into the S-phase (see also Figure 10, page 54).

(Figure 6). The suppressor gene *p53* has been found to induce the expression of certain inhibitors which block the activation of cdks by CAK. Thus, the *p53* gene is able to control the progression of the cell cycle (El-Deiry *et al.*, 1993; Harper *et al.*, 1993; Xiong *et al.*, 1993a; Noda *et al.*, 1994).

The regulatory role of p53 in G_1-S and G_2-M transition in cell cycle progression

The progression of the cell cycle is monitored for DNA damage at the G_1-S and G_2-M boundaries and cells with DNA damage are detained at either of these checkpoints pending appropriate DNA repair. Lane (1992) proposed the renowned 'guardian of the genome' role for *p53*, regulating the entry of cells into the S-phase following DNA repair and failing this the cells enter the apoptotic pathway. At the G_1-S checkpoint any damage sustained by cellular DNA is repaired with great fidelity. A normal functioning of p53 is required for the arrest of cells at the G_1 phase of the cell cycle following DNA damage. Mutated p53 does not appear to exert this cell cycle checkpoint control. A similar loss can also occur when wild-type p53 is sequestered by binding to cellular proteins such as mdm2 (Chen *et al.*, 1994). There are also indications that other genes such as *18A2/mts1*, a dominant metastasis-associated gene, may enable cells to enter S-phase by sequestering p53 and abrogating its control over the transition of cells past the G_1-S checkpoint (Parker *et al.*, 1994a,b). There is considerable evidence that viral oncoproteins affect p53 function in this way.

The second checkpoint occurs at the G_2-M boundary where cells are detained if they have sustained damage after entering into the S-phase. Recent evidence using temperature-sensitive mutants of p53 that exhibit conformation-dependent wild-type activity, shows that p53 may also control G_2-M transition of cells (Michalovitz *et al.*, 1990; Stewart *et al.*, 1995). Other investigators have failed to see G_2-M block by p53, which may be attributable to loss of G_2-M cells by apoptosis. Recently, Pellegata *et al.* (1996) employed two fibrosarcoma cell lines, namely, HT1080 which had wild-type *p53* and HT1080.6TG carrying a mutant *p53*.

Synchronised HT1080.6TG cells which had been irradiated showed no G_1 arrest but were arrested at the G_2-M checkpoint. But the cell lines carrying wild-type $p53$ that had passed through this checkpoint were not arrested in G_2 because the radiation damage had already been repaired. Furthermore, the HT1080 cells irradiated after they had entered the S-phase were arrested at the G_2-M checkpoint and, interestingly, they then showed no G_1 arrest. The pattern of arrest of the cell line with wild-type $p53$ does support the 'guardian of the genome' hypothesis of Lane (1992). Although our understanding of the mechanisms by which $p53$ appears to control the G_2-M checkpoint is still rather rudimentary, a substantial body of evidence has accumulated that a gene called stathmin, whose expression seems to be controlled by $p53$, may take part at this checkpoint.

The stathmin gene, discovered some years ago, is associated with cell cycle cycle progression. The stathmin gene product is a 19 kDa cytosolic phosphoprotein. It has recently been shown to interact with tubulin and may be involved in microtubule dynamics of the cells associated with the physical process of mitosis (Belmont and Mitchison, 1996). Stathmin is progressively phosphorylated by mitogen-induced protein (MAP) kinases (Leighton et al., 1993; Brattsand et al., 1994; Beretta et al., 1995) as well as kinases of the cyclin-dependent kinase family, in response to proliferative and differentiation signals. The significance of phosphorylation as a means of stathmin function is still unclear. Larsson N et al. (1995) found that the transition of cells past the G_2-M checkpoint involves phosphorylation of specific sites of stathmin, normally phosphorylated by cyclin-dependent kinases. The induction of differentiation of PC12 cells by nerve growth factor has been reported to be dependent upon the phosphorylation of stathmin by MAP kinases (DiPaolo et al., 1996). However, in some experimental models such as HL-60 cells, the induction of their differentiation into monocyte by 1α,25-dihyroxyvitamin D3 does not affect the phosphorylation of stathmin, but clearly leads to the down-regulation of its expression (Eustace et al., 1995). The transfection of anti-stathmin constructs blocks the cells expressing strathmin at the G_2-M boundary. Using inducible $p53$ constructs, it has been demonstrated that when $p53$ is switched on the stathmin gene is down-regulated together with G_2 arrest of the cells. The ability of $p53$ to down-regulate the stathmin promoter has been also demonstrated recently (E. J. Stanbridge, personal communication).

Genomic organisation of the $p53$ gene

The $p53$ gene is located on chromosome 17p13.1 (Benchimole et al., 1985; Umesh et al., 1988). The gene corresponds to c.20 kb of genomic DNA. The genomic structure is highly conserved in all species studied and the gene consists of 11 exons, of which the first exon is a non-coding exon. This is followed by a large 10 kb intron (Lamb and Crawford, 1986). The transcription of the gene is controlled by two regulatory sites. One 400 bp element occurs 5' upstream of exon 1 (P_1) and a second promoter element, P_2, occurs in intron 1, approximately 1 kb downstream of P_1 (Harlow et al., 1985; Reisman et al., 1988; Tuck and Crawford, 1989). The $p53$ transcript is

2.8 kb long. The product is a 53 kDa phosphoprotein containing 393 amino acids. Five highly conserved regions of the protein have been identified, termed regions I, II, III, IV and V, corresponding to codons 13-19, 120-143, 172-182, 238-259, and 271-290 (Nigro *et al.*, 1989; Levine *et al.*, 1991, 1994; Vogelstein and Kinzler, 1992) and these occur in exons 4, 5, 7 and 8. Mutations of p53 encountered in human neoplasms have been found to be clustered in hotspots in the conserved regions II-V (Nigro *et al.*, 1989) and therefore these are regarded as important functional domains and represent the sequence-specific DNA-binding domain of the protein extending from amino acid residue 90 to 290 (Bargonetti *et al.*, 1993; Halazonetis and Kandil, 1993; Pavletich *et al.*, 1993; Wang Y *et al.*, 1993). This core DNA binding domain contains 10 cysteine residues, suggesting the involvement of metal ions. Indeed, DNA binding is abolished by metal-chelating agents and the core domain contains zinc: therefore it has been suggested that p53 is zinc metalloprotein (Pavletich *et al.*, 1993). Oligomerisation is an important event for DNA binding, and p53 occurs predominantly in a tetrameric form (Stenger *et al.*, 1992; Friedman *et al.*, 1993). The p53 protein forms stable tetramers, mediated by a 53-amino acid *C*-terminal domain (Pavletich *et al.*, 1993) and the binding of the protein to DNA is allosterically regulated (Hupp *et al.*, 1992; Halazonetis and Kandil, 1993; Halazonetis *et al.*, 1993). The binding property is regulated by changes in the conformation of the tetramers between states of high and low affinity to DNA (Halazonetis and Kandil, 1993; Halazonetis *et al.*, 1993). The p53 binding DNA sequence contains four pentanucleotide repeats of the motif PuPuPuC(A/T)(A/T)GPyPyPy (Bargonetti *et al.*, 1991; El-Deiry *et al.*, 1992; Funk *et al.*, 1992; Kern *et al.*, 1992). Each DNA binding domain of the protein recognises one repeat motif (Halazonetis and Kandil, 1993; Cho YJ *et al.*, 1994) and it follows from this therefore that p53 tetramer would show greater DNA binding than the monomer protein. Tetramerisation is also important in controlling wild-type p53 function. It has been found that hetero-oligomers formed between mutant and wild-type p53 are unable to bind to DNA (Milner and Medcalf, 1991; Bargonetti *et al.*, 1992; Farmer *et al.*, 1992; Kern *et al.*, 1992; Shaulian *et al.*, 1992). Several other functional domains of the protein, e.g. heat shock proteins, E1B, mdm2, SV40 large T antigen-binding domains have also been identified (Figure 7).

p53 abnormalities and dysfunction

The dysfunction of the tumour suppressor *p53* gene has been regarded as a most significant event in the pathogenesis of cancer. This is known to occur as a consequence of mutation of *p53* resulting from allelic deletions, rearrangement, or base pair substitutions. These aberrant proteins will have lost their suppressor function and also gained new functions which alter the phenotypic features of tumour cells. Therefore, the status of *p53* abnormalities has been investigated in a wide spectrum of human malignancies with a view to correlating possible loss of its function with their development, progression and prognosis. Mutation of *p53* occurs in a wide variety of human cancers including breast, colon, stomach, bladder, ovary, endometrium,

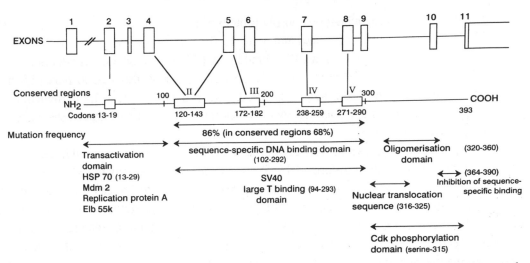

Figure 7.   The structural and functional domains of p53. Based on Lamb and Crawford (1986), Bischoff *et al.* (1990), Shaulsky *et al.* (1990), Soussi *et al.* (1990), Milner and Medcalf (1991), Lam and Calderwood (1992), Bargonetti *et al.* (1993), Halazonetis *et al.* (1993), Pavletich *et al.* (1993), Ruppert and Stillman (1993), Wang Y *et al.* (1993), Cho YJ *et al.* (1994), Levine *et al.* (1994), Bayle *et al.* (1995), and other references cited in the text.

testicular tumours, soft tissue sarcomas, melanomas and haematological malignancies (Nigro *et al.*, 1989; Bartek *et al.*, 1991; Hollstein *et al.*, 1991; Caron de Fromentel and Soussi, 1992; Toguchida *et al.*, 1992; Andreassen *et al.*, 1993; Berchuck *et al.*, 1994; Liu *et al.*, 1994). Levine *et al.* (1991) reported that approximately 60% of human cancers show *p53* mutations together with a loss of heterozygosity (LOH) which results in a complete loss of the wild type alleles. A majority (*c.*86%) of these are missense mutations; *c.*8% involve deletions or insertions and 5.5% non-sense mutations or frame shift mutations (Levine *et al.*, 1993). A definable pattern of location of these mutations has also emerged. Thus, the missense mutations occur predominantly between codons 120 and 290, whereas non-sense mutations tend to occur outside this region. Loss of suppressor function may be expected, however, to be associated with both types of mutation and therefore it is intriguing that there should be so marked a loss of uniformity in the incidence of these mutations in different regions of the gene.

Regulation of p53 function

The phosphoprotein product of *p53* is known to suppress cell transformation as well as cell proliferation (Eliyahu *et al.*, 1989; Finlay *et al.*, 1989; Michalowitz *et al.*, 1990). These functions of the p53 protein have come to light from its interaction with the products of certain tumour-promoting genes. The oncogenic proteins of DNA tumour viruses achieve cell transformation by forming complexes with the wild-type phosphoprotein p53 (Lane and Crawford, 1979; Linzer *et al.*, 1979; Sarnow *et al.*, 1982; Lin and Simmons, 1991). The simian virus 40 (SV40) large T antigen has since been shown to block DNA binding by p53 and its function as a transcription factor (Mietz *et al.*, 1992). The adenovirus E1B 55 kDa protein is also able to bind p53 and neutralise it (Sarnow *et al.*, 1982; Kao *et al.*, 1990; Berk and Yew, 1992). The introduction of wild-type p53 into transformed cells is known to block the growth of transformed cells (Baker *et al.*, 1990b; Diller *et al.*, 1990).

The p53 protein is expressed at very low levels in normal cells and tissues and it has a short half-life. However, in cells transformed by SV40 and adenoviruses, much higher levels are detected (Benchimole *et al.*, 1982) and this appears to be due to increased stability and a consequent enhancement of the half-life of the protein. Using a temperature-sensitive mutant of the large T antigen, Oren *et al.* (1981) showed that this depended upon the functioning of the T antigen. Interaction of p53 with other cellular proteins has also been demonstrated, which may lead to an inactivation and abrogation of its normal function.

It was demonstrated some years ago that human papilloma viruses (HPV), especially HPV 16, 18 and also some other types, are associated with high-grade cervical intraepithelial neoplasia (CIN) and invasive cervical squamous carcinomas. The integration of these viruses in the genome results in increased expression of the proteins known as E6 and E7, and these proteins have the ability to transform cells into the neoplastic state. Immunohistochemical studies have shown co-localisation of p53 phosphoprotein and E6, suggesting an association between them (Liang *et al.*, 1993). It would appear that the E6 protein binds the p53 phosphoprotein (Werness *et al.*, 1990). This requires another cellular factor called the E6-associated protein (E6-AP). This event leads to a rapid degradation of p53 protein, mediated by ubiquitin-dependent proteolysis (Huibregtse *et al.*, 1993). The introduction of a single HPV16-E6 gene causes the immortalisation of cells and sharply reduces p53 protein levels (Band *et al.*, 1991). The E6-E7 fusion proteins will also degrade the retinoblastoma protein (rb) (Scheffner *et al.*, 1991, 1992). Therefore, the concept has emerged that the sequestration of p53 protein by formation of complexes with oncoproteins such as E6 might lead to the development of cervical neoplasia. In HPV-negative carcinomas, inactivation of *p53* by mutation or allelic deletion, leading to the abrogation of its normal function of regulation of cell proliferation, can be postulated as a mechanism of tumorigenesis. But this has not been found to be the case. Park *et al.* (1994) found *p53* mutations only in 10% of HPV-negative tumours. There are also other reports that allelic or mutation of this gene is not a frequent event, irrespective of HPV status (Fujita *et al.*, 1992). In contrast, another study has reported that HPV-positive tumours contained *p53* mutation in only 8% of the tumours examined whereas four out of nine HPV-negative tumours contained point mutations (Lee *et al.*, 1994). This suggests that tumour development can occur either by mutation of p53 or by neutralisation of wild-type p53 by interaction with HPV proteins. A consensus view is that the formation of p53-E6 complex leads to a sequestration of p53 protein and this prevents it from exercising its normal suppressor function.

There is also the possibility that other oncogenes might be cooperating with HPV in tumour induction. Some experimental studies by DiPaolo *et al.* (1989) showed that although HPV types are associated with cervical malignancies, transfer of HPV16 or18 DNA into normal cervical cells caused their immortalisation but did not confer tumorigenicity on them. However, upon sequential transfection of the HPV-immortalised cells with the oncogene H-*ras*, these cells were able to produce cystic squamous cell carcinomas in immune-deficient mice.

p53, cancer progression and prognosis

The contribution of abnormal p53 to carcinogenesis has also suggested their potential use in determining cancer prognosis. This gene is located on chromosome 17p13.1 (Benchimole *et al.*, 1985; Umesh *et al.*, 1988). Loss of heterozygosity on several chromosomes including chromosome 17 frequently occurs in ovarian cancer. Okamoto *et al.* (1991a) reported allelic loss of *p53* in 16/20 cases. Allelic loss on chromosome 17 is also a common feature of endometrial carcinoma (Okamoto *et al.*, 1991b). Allelic loss at locus THH59 (17q23-ter) shows a more significant association with grade III than with grades I + II ovarian carcinomas. In contrast, association between loss of *p53* and tumour grade is poor (Lowry and Atkinson, 1993). Therefore, these authors suggested that there may be a putative suppressor gene on chromosome 17q23-ter whose deletion may be associated with anaplastic ovarian cancers.

Over-expression of p53 has been reported to occur in 40-50% of stages III and IV adenocarcinomas of the ovary and endometrium, but only in 10-15% of early stages of the disease (Kohler *et al.*, 1992; Berchuck *et al.*, 1994). A far higher (79%) incidence has been reported for ovarian cancers by Kupryjanczyk *et al.* (1993). An association of p53 immunoreactivity with high-grade epithelial ovarian cancer has also been reported by Hartman *et al.* (1994), but they found some immunoreactivity also in low-grade cancers. Furthermore, they found that *p53* expression was associated with decreased overall survival in a univariate analysis. The expression of *p53* is generally low in benign endometria, but high expression has been reported in 15% of atypical hyperplasias and in 23% of carcinomas. Although the frequency of over-expression is comparatively low, *p53* expression *per se* was consistent with spread of the disease outside the uterus (Ambros *et al.*, 1994). According to Berchuck *et al.* (1994) *p53* mutations are infrequent in cancers of the cervix, vulva or vagina. These findings seemingly contest the concept that *p53* is a tumour suppressor gene, or at least the universality of its suppressor function.

Whether mutations of *p53* reflect progression of the disease cannot yet be established. In order that this may be assessed it is important to determine whether these are temporal changes and whether they are progressive and cumulative. It is also necessary to examine whether there is also a topographical change in the pattern of expression of the p53 protein. In oesophageal and lung cancers, *p53* abnormalities arise early (Casson *et al.*, 1991; Bennett *et al.*, 1992; Sozzi *et al.*, 1992). A low frequency of point mutation may be found in one in 10 squamous cells and in one in 14 adenocarcinomas in oesophagus; mutations have also been found in four out of seven Barrett's epithelium adjacent to the adenocarcinomas, possibly related to pre-malignant changes

(Casson *et al.*, 1991). In head and neck squamous cell tumours, the abnormalities are progressive, i.e. measurements of p53 protein have revealed an increase concomitant with progressive tissue abnormalities. In the normal epithelium, p53 expression is limited to the basal layer but in hyperplastic or dysplastic tissue expression of the protein extended to the parabasal and superficial layers (Shin *et al.*, 1994).

Mazars *et al.* (1991) studied 30 primary ovarian cancers and four matched metastatic tumours for *p53* mutations. It was found that 36% of the tumours showed a mutated allele. The mutations were point mutations and were clustered in exons 5 and 7. Interestingly, the same mutations were found in the matched primary and metastatic tumours. Hyperplasia of the endometrium show no *p53* mutations, although these may show mutation of other oncogenes such as the K-*ras* (Sasaki *et al.*, 1993). As stated earlier, *p53* mutations occur frequently with extrauterine disease in invasive endometrial cancers. This suggests the possibility that these mutations might be a late event in tumour progression (Berchuck *et al.*, 1994). A recent study reports *p53* mutations in stage I ovarian carcinomas but not in true borderline tumours (Kupryjanczyk *et al.*, 1995). Nonetheless, when *p53* mutations are detected in primary ovarian cancers, identical mutations are invariably detectable in intra-peritoneal metastases (Jacobs *et al.*, 1992). This may lend weight to the suggestion that these could occur not only as a late event but that metastatic deposits may be clonal in nature, arising from cells which carry the mutation.

Mutations of *p53* occur in 75% of colonic tumours (Fearon and Jones, 1992). In a majority of these neoplasms mutation of one allele occurs together with the deletion of the second wild-type allele (Baker *et al.*, 1989; Nigro *et al.*, 1989; Rodrigues *et al.*, 1990). They seem to occur as a late event (Vogelstein *et al.*, 1988; Baker *et al.*, 1990a) and follow cumulative prior genetic changes that might be providing the appropriate genetic background for *p53* mutations to influence progression to the malignant state. However, much uncertainty is associated with *p53* mutation status or over-expression of p53 protein and their value in assessing prognosis in colorectal cancer. There have been claims that p53 over-expression correlates with poor patient survival (Remvikos *et al.*, 1992; Sun *et al.*, 1992; Starzynska *et al.*, 1992). Hamelin *et al.* (1994a) found *p53* mutations in 52% of 85 colorectal tumours investigated and that occurrence of a mutation correlated very strongly with poor survival; others (Scott *et al.*, 1991; Bell *et al.*, 1993) found no such correlation.

In chronic myeloid leukaemia (CML) p53 mutations occur in the acute phase or blast crisis (Ahuja *et al.*, 1989; Mashal *et al.*, 1990; Feinstein *et al.*, 1991). In B-cell lymphoma and multiple myeloma advanced stages of the disease are also characterised by the incidence of p53 mutations (Ichikawa A *et al.*, 1992; Neri *et al.*, 1993). Loss of heterozygosity involving the *p53* locus and mutations of the gene occur at the late stages in hepatocellular carcinogenesis (Teramoto *et al.*, 1994). Frank *et al.* (1994) studied p53 expression in squamous cell carcinoma of the hypopharynx and reported that although p53 abnormalities occur frequently in these tumours, there was no correlation of p53 expression with tumour grade, DNA ploidy, or S-phase fraction. However, all p53-positive patients had advanced-stage disease (stages III, IV) compared with 74% of the p53-negative group.

Over-expression of p53 protein was reported in >50% of breast cancers (Horak *et al.*, 1991). Mutations of the gene are also common (25–40% incidence) in sporadic breast cancer, with the frequency of G–T transversions generally higher than expected, and these occur predominantly in the conserved exons 5–8. In many cases mutation of one allele is also accompanied by deletion of the second allele. In summary, p53 mutation characterises a highly aggressive form of the disease, associated with poor prognosis in both node-positive and node-negative patients (Lemoine, 1994). But, in contrast to colon cancer, these tend to be early events. It may be that the distinction lies in the fact that in tumorigenesis in the colon results from mutations in a series of genes, including the DCC gene, which produce a progressive alteration in the phenotype and p53 may have a complementary role (see page 172). Abnormalities of *rb*, another suppressor gene that actively regulates cell cycle progression, are also significantly associated with breast cancer. It is difficult to dissociate the functions of these two genes. It might be worthwhile pointing out here that Ewing sarcomas, where the *EWS* gene is actively involved in tumorigenesis, *p53* mutations do not correlate with *EWS* activity (Hamelin *et al.*, 1994b). In primary prostate cancer mutation levels are low (Voeller *et al.*, 1994). The expression of p53 protein is also less marked, with the exception of metastatic tumours and stage D primary tumours which show higher p53-positivity, as judged by the proportion of cells with nuclear staining (Grizzle *et al.*, 1994).

In contrast, loss of heterozygosity with respect to *p53* has been reported in both low- and high-grade astrocytomas (El-Azouzi *et al.*, 1989; Fults *et al.*, 1989; James *et al.*, 1989; Bello *et al.*, 1994). Mutations of *p53* and abnormal expression of p53 protein occur commonly in different forms of brain tumour (Chung *et al.*, 1991; Mashiyama *et al.*, 1991; Frankel *et al.*, 1992; Fults *et al.*, 1992; Louis *et al.*, 1993; Newcomb *et al.*, 1993). Again, these have been found in both low-grade tumours as well as glioblastomas (von Deimling *et al.*, 1992). Transfection of glioma cell lines with wild-type p53 markedly inhibits cell proliferation irrespective of whether the cell lines are derived from low- or high-grade gliomas and in addition induces the expression of differentiated features in the cell cultures (Merzak *et al.*, 1994a). Similarly, when wild-type *p53* was transfected into a medulloblastoma cell line, there was a restoration of cell cycle control in the transfected cells (Rosenfeld *et al.*, 1995).

Mutation of *p53* may not be an obligatory step in neuroepithelial tumorigenesis. There can be p53 mutation-dependent and mutation-independent pathways to tumorigenesis (van Meir *et al.*, 1994a). A high frequency of p53 accumulation has been described in low-grade and anaplastic astrocytomas in the absence of mutations of the gene (Lang *et al.*, 1994). In these cases where tumorigenesis takes the mutation-independent pathway, wild-type p53 inactivation could conceivably occur through sequestration of the protein. Saxena *et al.* (1992) suggested the possibility of another suppressor gene located close to *p53* being responsible for tumour formation. As van Meir *et al.* (1994a) have pointed out, one does come across astrocytomas in which neither heterozygosity at the *p53* locus or mutations of the gene is found. They also examined 13 glioblastoma cell lines for *p53* mutation status and found that four of these had retained their wild-type phenotype. Indeed, if *p53* mutations were a significant cause for the genesis of these tumours, one would have expected that in familial gliomas germ line mutations of *p53* would be found but this does not appear to be the case and no mutations have been detected in exons 5–9 (van Meyel *et al.*, 1994a), but the authors do not exclude alterations outside these exons.

Germ line p53 mutations have been reported by Kyritsis *et al.* (1994) in six out of nine patients with multifocal glioma, of which two patients had familial history of cancer, one patient with another form of primary neoplasm and two with all three risk factors, namely multifocality, a different primary neoplasm and familial cancer. In contrast, no mutations were found in one patient with unifocal glioma plus another primary tumour and in twelve patients with unifocal glioma and without a second malignancy or familial cancer incidence.

There are some reports which suggest that the expression of p53 protein is related to tumour grade (Bruner *et al.*, 1991; Ellison *et al.*, 1992; Jaros *et al.*, 1992; Chozick *et al.*, 1994). But Kros *et al.* (1993) have reported a total absence of any correlation between *p53* mutation and tumour features such as grade, mitotic index and ploidy, in oligodendrogliomas. However, these authors observed that the presence of >75% p53 protein-positive cells within a tumour related strongly to a very unfavourable clinical outcome.

There is an interesting piece of evidence adduced by Sidransky *et al.* (1992) which suggests the association of *p53* mutations with disease progression. They studied seven pairs of gliomas which were high-grade tumours at both presentation and recurrence (group A), and another group of three gliomas which were low grade at presentation but had progressed to a higher grade at recurrence (group B). Three out of four recurrent tumours which had *p53* mutations had the same mutation at the primary stage. In group B tumour pairs, a small proportion of cells of the low-grade tumours contained the same *p53* mutation as the tumours which had progressed to the glioblastoma stage. Iuzzolino *et al.* (1994) found that median survival time of patients with low-grade glioma was similar irrespective of p53 protein expression status. But upon 5-year follow-up, there was a marked differentiation between p53-positive and p53-negative groups. The estimated survival for p53-negative group was 45.9% compared with 21.2% for the p53-positive group. These data may be interpreted as suggesting that the small subpopulation carrying the specific mutation may subsequently expand into recurrent tumour of a higher grade. However, contradictory views have also been expressed. Koga *et al.* (1994) have argued that low-grade gliomas not only carried *p53* mutations but that they took too long to recur and therefore mutation of the gene may not be relevant to their progression. The report by Kraus *et al.* (1994) supports this view; this report shows that mutations which characterised 17 out of 38 low-grade astrocytomas also occurred in six out of 10 high-grade recurrent tumours. However, in support of Sidransky *et al.* (1992) one must cite the work of van Meyel *et al.* (1994b) in which 15 astrocytic tumours were screened for mutations in exons 5–9, both at the low-grade primary stage and recurrent anaplastic stage. They found a highly significant correlation between mutation status of primary and recurrent gliomas, i.e. primary tumours with mutated *p53* are liable to recur as anaplastic gliomas. DeLarco *et al.* (1993) found that both low- and high-grade tumours contained mutations but noted a significant difference. The mutations in the low-grade tumours were heterozygous but in high-grade gliomas both alleles of the genes had mutated. This suggests operation of the familiar two-hit mechanism.

Taking a wider view of the situation, one may comfortably postulate that cell subpopulations carrying *p53* mutations may be at a selective advantage in that they are not subject to growth control normally exerted by this gene and this might enable them to progress to a more malignant stage. Nevertheless, one must bear in mind that one is considering only a facet of the process of progression, namely proliferative ability, and the possible relationship between the incidence of *p53* mutation and the acquisition of metastatic ability is yet to be demonstrated. Possibly, gliomas are not ideally suited as a model for this. These tumours are a remarkable group of tumours because they are intrinsically highly malignant and can be locally highly invasive, but they do not normally metastasise to extracranial sites (Sherbet, 1987). It would appear that enhanced p53 expression may be associated with malignancy but no attention seems to have been focused upon a possible relationship between invasive ability and p53 expression in gliomas. Such information would be valuable in the management of patients. A study of gastric carcinomas has revealed that in undifferentiated tumours p53 expression correlated with depth of tumour invasion (Kushima *et al.*, 1994). High levels of p53 protein have been detected in both pre-invasive and invasive squamous cell carcinomas of the oesophagus and mutation of *p53* may indeed precede the invasive stage (Bennett *et al.*, 1992). In some breast tumours greater nuclear staining for p53 protein has been reported in the invasive margins of the tumours (Friedrichs *et al.*, 1993). Laryngeal carcinomas that progress to the invasive stage tend to be more frequently p53-positive (Munck-Wikland *et al.*, 1994). Over-expression of the protein is also a feature of pre-invasive male germ cell tumours (Bartkova *et al.*, 1991).

Cutaneous melanomas show marked p53 immunoreactivity (Bartek *et al.*, 1991; Stretch *et al.*, 1991; Cristofolini *et al.*, 1993; McGregor *et al.*, 1993). Cristofolini *et al.* (1993) also examined a series of 75 benign skin naevi and described 15% of these specimens as p53-positive. It ought to be pointed out, however, that the criteria for declaring specimens as positive for p53 staining vary considerably. Cristofolini *et al.* (1993) found less than 1% of cells composing the naevi stained for p53, but the melanomas contained a far higher proportion of p53-staining cells; also six out of eight metastatic melanomas were p53-positive with up to 10% of cells staining for the p53 protein. McGregor *et al.* (1993) found malignant melanoma to be highly p53-positive with the majority of tumour cells (>75%) staining for p53. These authors regarded tumours with <10% cells staining for p53 as weakly positive. It seems reasonable therefore to regard the Cristofolini series of benign naevi as weakly staining or indeed p53-negative, as in the McGregor *et al.* (1993) series of benign naevi. However, other investigators, e.g. Campbell *et al.* (1993), believe that mutations of *p53* tend to be early events, preceding even the invasive stage.

Invasive bladder cancers appeared to be more immunoreactive than superficial tumours (Wright *et al.*, 1991). In this tumour type a strong association between tumour stage and grade and p53 protein expression has been reported also by Moch *et al.* (1993). Tumours belonging to stage pT1 and pT2-4 were more frequently p53 positive compared with pTa. Both pTa and pT1 are regarded as non-invasive stages. The differences in p53-positivity of these two stages might be of some clinical value. The association between p53 expression and incidence of metastatic lesions was also very strong. In a series of patients, metastases occurred in 77% of 48 patients with p53-positive tumours but only in 50% of 24 patients with p53-negative tumours. As noted previously, metastatic melanomas have been reported to be predominantly p53-positive compared with primary malignant tumours (Cristofolini *et al.*, 1993), which confirms the increased detection of mutant p53 protein in metastatic melanoma reported by Stretch *et al.* (1991).

It might be of some interest to note in this context that p53 is mutated in MDA-MB-231 breast cancer cells which are more invasive *in vitro* compared with MCF7 breast cancer cell line which show no p53 abnormality. This is compatible with the observation that the MDA cell lines expresses the S-100 family *18A2/mts1* gene very strongly. Expression of this gene is further closely associated with CD44 expression and greatly enhanced metastatic potential (Sherbet and Lakshmi, 1995). It would appear that the expression of the patriarch S-100 protein is related to the depth of invasion of transitional cell carcinoma of the bladder (Inoue *et al.*, 1993). Furthermore, p53 positive tumours tend to express epidermal growth factors and may respond positively to extracellular growth factor signals. Admittedly, most of this evidence is indirect and circumstantial, but it would be reasonable to assume that invasive potential and progression of tumours may be reflected in p53 expression status. Thus, the evidence for the involvement of *p53* mutations and interaction with other cellular proteins in relation to tumour development and progression may be described as overwhelming; however, one should not lose sight of the fact that some carcinogenic processes do not appear to involve any alteration of the gene at all. Tobacco-related oral carcinomas do not show *p53* aberrations. Thirty-eight oral squamous carcinomas, believed to be associated with tobacco chewing or smoking, have been reported to show low p53 expression by immunohistochemistry and in only five out of the 38 tumours in which over-expression occurred have mutations been detected in exons 5-9 (Ranasinghe *et al.*, 1993a,b). Unfortunately, the study does not include *p53* abnormalities in a comparable control sample. Similarly, Matthews *et al.* (1993) found no influence of tobacco smoking on p53 protein expression in lingual squamous cell carcinomas. However, earlier studies have supported a link between smoking and p53 positivity of oral and head and neck cancers (Field *et al.*, 1991, 1992; Ogden *et al.*, 1992). Point mutations in the conserved exons of the gene occur only at a very low frequency in chemically induced renal mesenchymal tumours of rat (Weghorst *et al.*, 1994). Human kidney epithelial cells exposed to and immortalised by nickel compounds, however, show a T → C transition in codon 238 (Maehle *et al.*, 1992).

It would be worthwhile also pointing out here that there are instances where low levels of mutations may occur or none may be encountered at all. For instance, mutations of *p53* are detected at very low levels also in myelodysplastic syndrome (Jonveaux *et al.*, 1991; Neubauer, 1993). None have been found in the exons 5-8 of the gene in benign parathyroid adenomas and carcinomas (Hakim and Levine, 1994). The Li–Fraumeni syndrome which carries germ line mutations of *p53* does not include parathyroidism as a feature (Frebourg and Friend, 1992). Furthermore, *p53*-deficient mice, in which a host of spontaneous tumours can arise, do not develop parathyroid tumours (Donehower *et al.*, 1992). It can be suggested therefore that *p53* modifications may not be associated with the development of parathyroid neoplasia. However, aberrations of the *rb* gene (Cryns *et al.*, 1993) and cyclin D1 (*PRAD1*) (Arnold *et al.*, 1992) are known to occur in these neoplasms. Both of these genes, like *p53*, are closely involved in the control of cell cycle progression.

Somewhat intriguing, but nonetheless relevant in this context, is the observation in some studies that patients who have gliomas with mutated *p53* have survived significantly longer than patients whose tumours contained no mutations (van Meyel, 1994b). According to Jones *et al.* (1995), patients with high-grade gliomas showing loss of heterozygosity for chromosomes 17 and 10 also survived considerably longer than patients with tumours that did not exhibit loss of heterozygosity. To add to the uncertainty, some investigators have claimed that the occurrence of *p53* mutations does not relate to prognosis at all (Danks *et al.*, 1995) while others claim that they indicate poor prognosis in high-grade gliomas (Soini *et al.*, 1994). Similarly, much uncertainty exists in the case of advanced stages of non-small cell lung cancer even though *p53* abnormalities have been significantly associated with poor prognosis (Mitsudomi *et al.*, 1993).

The conclusion is inescapable that relating *p53* abnormalities to state of tumour progression and using mutations status is fraught with difficulties on account of the existence of numerous factors which determine the course of the disease. In addition to the obvious pathways by which p53 might function, the point at which it might impinge upon tumour progression also appears to be variable. Whereas in some tumours its involvement might be in the early stages of development, in others such as colonic tumours, abnormalities of the gene occur as late events. This may be the reason why the influences of *p53* on the clinical course of the disease are so variable. Furthermore, although it is easy to envisage the impact of the loss of control on proliferation to tumour development, there are no testable hypotheses as to how *p53* might be involved in cell transformation. For example, mouse astrocyte cells lacking both alleles of the gene (*p53* $-/-$) have been found to grow faster in early passages than those which possess both alleles. These cells do not show transformation but upon repeated passaging in culture they do transform and exhibit changes in ploidy and karyotype (Yahanda *et al.*, 1995), possibly suggesting that some other gene, entering into the fray in a different time frame, might be leading the cells on to the path of transformation.

Subcellular localisation of p53 protein

The p53 phosphoprotein is a nuclear protein. The *C*-terminal region of the protein contains signals for nuclear localisation (Dang and Lee, 1989; Addison *et al.*, 1990; Shaulsky *et al.*, 1990). Mutant proteins with deletions in the *C*-terminal region show cytoplasmic localisation (Sturzbecher *et al.*, 1988). Similarly, mutations occurring in the proximity of the nuclear localisation signal domain can affect the localisation of the human p53 (Diller *et al.*, 1990). Consistent with this, the protein can show nuclear and/or cytoplasmic localisation. Moll *et al.* (1992) and Stenmark-Askmalm *et al.* (1994) found the protein in both locations. Staining for the protein can be exclusively nuclear or cytoplasmic, or a mixture of both (Faille *et al.*, 1994). Non-Hodgkin's lymphomas show virtually exclusive (90 out of 96 samples) nuclear staining (Pezzella *et al.*, 1993a). Its localisation in breast cancer was described as predominantly cytoplasmic (Horak *et al.*, 1991). Both the nucleus and the cytoplasm may be stained in melanomas (Weiss *et al.*, 1993; Parker *et al.*, 1994a).

In the light of the interactions of p53 with cellular proteins (see page 31), it seems likely that the subcellular localisation patterns seen in tumours might be suggestive of the pathways by which wild-type and mutant proteins might be functioning. Moll *et al.* (1992) carried out sequence analysis of *p53* cDNAs from breast cancers showing cytoplasmic staining and found wild-type alleles in six out of seven specimens. In contrast, where nuclear staining of p53 was encountered, missense and nonsense mutations were found. Furthermore, a sample of normal lactating breast tissue also showed cytoplasmic p53 staining. Cytoplasmic accumulation of p53 is encountered in non-neoplastic salivary gland but in neoplastic lesions the distribution is mainly nuclear (Li XW *et al.*, 1995). Kastrinakis *et al.* (1995) found that in some hepatic metastases of colorectal carcinomas nuclear staining for p53 was seen, but not in the corresponding primary tumours. They further showed that the metastatic tumours carried point mutations of the gene but no mutations were detectable in the primary tumours. Thus, the mutant protein might tend to localise predominantly in the nucleus. Parker *et al.* (1994a) showed that in B16 murine melanoma cells up-regulation of the metastasis-associated *18A2/ mts1* gene was accompanied by a parallel increase in the detection of p53 protein, in both nuclear and cytoplasmic locations and often with marked accumulation in the submembranous regions. They suggested that the 18A2/mts1 protein, which strongly associates with cytoskeletal proteins, might be sequestering the wild-type p53 and that this could account for the cytoplasmic location of p53.

On the basis of these observations, it may be suggested that the subcellular localisation of p53 protein might yield valuable information about the pathways of p53 functioning, especially in relation to its cooperation with other cellular proteins which might be involved with or impinge upon the processes of cellular transformation. It is conceivable, therefore, that the patterns of p53 protein staining may be related to tumour development and progression. There are several indicators in this direction. Nuclear p53 staining is far more predominant in aneuploid tumours than in diploid tumours (Sun *et al.*, 1993). In breast cancer where both nuclear and cytoplasmic staining is seen, p53 accumulation correlates strongly with DNA ploidy, among other variables (Stenmark-Askmalm *et al.*, 1994). There are also indications that p53 staining pattern might be related to cancer prognosis. p53 staining of both the nucleus and the cytoplasm of colorectal tumours was associated with poor survival of the patients compared with p53-negative tumours and patients with tumours that showed either nuclear or cytoplasmic staining showed intermediate survival (Sun *et al.*, 1993). Cytoplasmic staining in the absence of nuclear staining correlated with survival free from recurrent or distant metastatic disease (Stenmark-Askmalm *et al.*, 1994), whereas, in sharp contrast, nuclear p53 staining was found with advanced stages of prostate cancer and metastatic disease in the bone (Aprikian *et al.*, 1994). In a series of colorectal tumours investigated by Kastrinakis *et al.* (1995), nuclear localisation of p53 occurred together with point mutations of the gene in hepatic metastases but not in the corresponding primary colorectal tumours. Although not every study of p53 expression contains unequivocal information about the pattern of expression, from the data available to date it would be reasonable to suggest that this would be highly relevant in the prediction of the course of the disease.

p53 protein as a transcription factor

The biochemical basis for p53 function is the ability of the phosphoprotein to regulate transcription by binding to DNA. The region between residues 120 and 290 functions as a specific DNA-binding domain. The consensus nucleotide sequence for p53 binds to DNA is 5'-Pu-Pu-Pu-C-A/T-A/T-G-Py-Py-Py-3' (El-Deiry *et al.*, 1992; Funk *et al.*, 1992). p53 will enhance transcription of a gene that has a p53 responsive element (Farmer *et al.*, 1992; Zambetti *et al.*, 1992). There are five conserved regions in the p53 protein, namely I, II, III, IV and V. Regions II–V carry 68% of missense mutations and the corresponding codons 120–290 contain 86% of *p53* mutations. Therefore this section of the protein encompassing regions II–V might contain a domain essential for p53 function. Missense mutations of abnormal *p53* will result in a defective protein product which cannot bind to a target gene with a *p53* responsive element.

The wild-type p53 phosphoprotein can down-regulate a variety of promoters including β-actin, hsp 70, c-*jun*, c-*fos*, *mdr1* and PCNA (proliferating cell nuclear antigen) (Ginsberg *et al.*, 1991; Chin *et al.*, 1992; Deb *et al.*, 1992; Subler *et al.*, 1992; Zastawny *et al.*, 1993). Several promoters, which include SV40 early promoter-enhancer, herpes simplex virus type 1 (HSV-1) thymidine kinase and UL9, and LTR promoters of Rous sarcoma virus and human immunodeficiency virus, and human T-lymphoblastic virus type 1, are repressed by wild-type p53 (Subler *et al.*, 1992). A mutation of p53 at amino acid 143 resulted in a significant release of inhibition of transcription of reporter genes placed under the control of these cellular and viral promoters. Mutations at amino acid positions 143, 175, 248, 273 and 281 that are commonplace in cancer, were also associated with the release of inhibition of HSV-1 thymidine kinase promoter (Subler *et al.*, 1992). Furthermore, whereas wild-type p53 activates promoters with the appropriate binding sites, transcription is inhibited from promoters which lack these sites. Martin *et al.* (1993) have shown that the TATA-binding protein (TBP) interacts with wild-type and with mutant p53 and that the TBP-p53 complex then binds the TATA box; they suggest that the nature of the complex might determine the success of transcription. Funk *et al.* (1992) found that *in vitro* p53 binds only when it is used together with nuclear extracts and therefore suggest that either p53 may need to be post-translationally modified or may need to form complexes with other nuclear proteins.

Alternative splicing of the *p53* gene transcript

Genetic alterations of the *p53* gene and its dysfunction as a consequence leads, as the preceding pages have shown to a deregulation of cell proliferation and pathogenesis. Other modes of *p53* regulation involving post-transcriptional events such as the alternative splicing of pre-mRNA have been suggested. The generation of splice variants of pre-mRNAs of several genes, including *p53*, has been known for some years. In rat tissues, in which alternative splicing of the original *p53* transcript has not yet been found, *p53* pseudogenes have been identified which could result from the integration of spliced mRNAs into the genome of the germ line (Lin and Chan, 1995).

It has been postulated that *p53* splice variants may have a role in the regulation of the function of this gene. A specific pattern of expression of splice variants has been reported in mouse epidermal cells. The major form of splice variant of *p53* here is said to be expressed in the G_1 phase and a splice variant, with an additional 96 nucleotides resulting from alternative splicing of intron 10 sequences, is expressed mainly in the G_2 phase (Kulesz-Martin *et al.*, 1994). It is conceivable that this differential expression may have some bearing on the transition of cells at the G_1-S and G_2-M boundaries, but at present there is no experimental evidence to link individual *p53* transcripts to either checkpoint.

Alternative splicing may modulate the activation of *p53* transcription. According to Bayle *et al.* (1995), alternative splicing of the mouse *p53* pre-mRNA generates a variant in which the amino acid residues 364–390 are replaced by 17 different residues, which is in accord with the findings of Kulesz-Martin *et al.* (1994). The murine p53 has two DNA-binding domains – a domain spanning amino acid residues 102–290, constituting a sequence-specific binding site, and another site encompassing amino acid residues 364–390, which is a DNA-binding site without sequence specificity. Bayle *et al.* (1995) found that the alternatively spliced form (p53as) is constitutively a sequence-specific binding isoform that has lost its non-specific DNA binding ability. This is consistent with the findings of Wu *et al.* (1994) who described some differences in sequence-specific binding of isoform (p53as) generated by alternative splicing. They noted that p53as exhibited far greater sequence-specific DNA binding than the normal splice isoform (p53ns). Furthermore, p53as levels were far lower than p53ns and p53as occurred as a heterodimer with wild-type 53 protein (Wu *et al.*, 1994). Flaman *et al.* (1996) have shown that human lymphocytes express a splice isoform with reduced transcriptional activity that is expressed only in quiescent cells. Again, in this isoform, the *C*-terminal region is affected by alternative splicing. It is possible that p53 function could be regulated by the levels of expression of individual isoforms and that the sequence-independent DNA-binding site, which is lost in p53as, regulates sequence-specific binding of p53ns.

The occurrence of alternatively spliced *p53* transcripts have been found in many normal tissues and cell lines, including normal human lymphocytes. There has even been a suggestion that splice variants may be expressed in a tissue- or even a species-specific fashion (Will *et al.*, 1995). In analogy with the occurrence of alternatively spliced variants of other macromolecules, alternative splicing of p53 may represent a regulatory mechanism from which one can envision abnormal cell proliferation and aberrant behaviour.

The functions of p53 as a transcription factor may be impaired, as discussed above, not only by mutation and alternative splicing of the gene transcript, but also consequent to its interaction with transforming viral proteins. Several cellular proteins have been discovered which can also inactivate the transcription factor function of p53.

Regulation of *mdm2* by p53

The *mdm2* (murine double minute 2) was isolated from transformed mouse 3T3 cells and its expression was associated with high tumorigenic potential (Cahilly-Snyder *et al.*, 1987; Fakharzadeh *et al.*, 1991). This gene has been mapped to chromosome 12q13. The *mdm2* gene is amplified in a number of human malignancies. Multiple transcripts of *mdm2* have been detected in breast epithelial cells, with protein products ranging from 54–68 kDa to 90–100 kDa (Gudas *et al.*, 1995a). mdm2 has been shown to bind p53 protein and inactivate its function as a transcription factor (Momand *et al.*, 1992). Recently, Picksley *et al.* (1994) have established the mdm2 binding site to the sequence TFSGLW in mouse and TFSDLW in man (amino acids 18–23) at the *N*-terminal end of p53.

The oncogenic properties of *mdm2* have also been attributed to p53 inactivation (Momand *et al.*, 1992; Oliner *et al.*, 1992; Barak *et al.*, 1993; Finlay, 1993). *mdm2* expression is itself up-regulated by p53 (Barak *et al.*, 1993; Otto and Deppert 1993; Wu *et al.*, 1993). The mouse *mdm2* contains two promoters; one of these, P_1, is located upstream of the gene and the second promoter P_2 occurs within the first intron. Transcription from P_2 has been shown to be strongly p53-dependent, but the up-stream promoter P_1 is only mildly responsive (Barak *et al.*, 1994). The human *mdm2* also contains the highly p53-responsive intronic promoter (Zauberman *et al.*, 1995). This activation pattern results in two distinct transcripts which translate into mdm2 proteins with different p53 binding ability (Barak *et al.*, 1994). When there is a suboptimal induction of p53, as in ataxia telangiectasia (AT) cells, there is also a suboptimal induction of mdm2 and other proteins such as Gadd45 and p21 (waf1/cip1) (Canman *et al.*, 1994). Transfection of wild-type *p53* has been shown to restore wild-type p53 function and increase the levels of *mdm2* expression (Rosenfeld *et al.*, 1995).

mdm2 abnormalities in cancer

Amplification of *mdm2* and/or abnormal expression of mdm2 protein has been described in a variety of human neoplasms. Earlier studies reported an increase in tumorigenic potential in cells which exhibited amplified *mdm2*, often accompanied by mutations in *p53*. However, it is still unclear whether *mdm2* has an intrinsic tumorigenic ability and whether the degree of its expression is indicative of tumour progression. The amplification of *mdm2* has been reported in a number of human sarcomas, with approximately 10% of the tumours carrying both *mdm2* amplification and *p53* mutation (Oliner *et al.*, 1992; Cordon-Cardo *et al.*, 1994). In bladder cancer, high levels of mdm2 and p53 proteins have been described and in 18% of the tumours both the proteins were highly expressed (Lianes *et al.*, 1994). In Hodgkin's disease co-expression of these genes in the same cell is also quite common (Chilosi *et al.*, 1994). A significant association between *p53* mutations and over-expression of mdm2 protein, without *mdm2* gene amplification, has been described in a study of thyroid carcinomas (Zou *et al.*, 1995). However, *mdm2* abnormalities do not always occur wherever there are abnormalities of *p53*. Esteve *et al.* (1993) identified *p53* mutations in exons 5–8 in 12 out of 24 oesophageal carcinomas, but none of these had *mdm2* amplification. No amplification or over-expression of *mdm2* was detectable in ovarian carcinomas where 50% of the tumours contained p53 mutations (Foulkes *et al.*, 1995). Similarly, *p53* and *mdm2* abnormalities did not coincide in human melanomas (Florenes *et al.*, 1994), nor is inactivation of *p53* by HPV oncoprotein accompanied by *mdm2* amplification (Miwa *et al.*, 1995). Abnormalities of *mdm2* can occur with or without mutations of *p53*, e.g. in leukaemias (Quesnel *et al.*, 1994a; Schottelius *et al.*, 1994). In human malignant gliomas which had *mdm2* amplification no *p53* mutations were detectable (Reifenberger *et al.*, 1993). Watanabe *et al.* (1994) found low *mdm2* expression in normal B-cells but there was a 10-fold greater expression in 28% of chronic lymphocytic leukaemias and non-Hodgkin's lymphomas. The mdm2 protein is expressed at very low levels in non-small cell lung carcinoma, irrespective of *p53* status (Maxwell, 1994; Marchetti *et al.*, 1995a). Paediatric lymphoblastic cell lines which expressed wild-type p53 also invariably over-expressed mdm2 protein, although no amplification of the gene was encountered (Zhou *et al.*, 1995).

mdm2 binds to the *N*-terminal end of p53 and mutations in the DNA-binding domains (corresponding to conserved regions II–V) of p53 do not affect mdm2 binding to p53 (Marston *et al.*, 1994). Furthermore, not all mdm2 isoforms possess equivalent p53 binding ability, and a splice variant lacking the *N*-terminal region was found to be devoid of p53-binding capacity (Haines *et al.*, 1994). Nonetheless, it is possible that *mdm2* is regulated by wild-type p53 but may be expressed independently of mutated *p53*. As noted earlier, *mdm2* contains two promoters, P_1 and P_2, which are differentially responsive to p53 and this results in the generation of two transcripts which conceivably might have different biological functions. Interestingly, p53 and mdm2 appear to be functionally independent during cell proliferation and, whereas p53 synthesis parallels DNA synthesis, that of mdm2 does not (Mosner and Deppert, 1994). Furthermore, there is evidence that over-expression of wild-type p53 can occur without the involvement of mdm2 protein (Maestro *et al.*, 1995). Therefore, one might legitimately raise the question whether p53 sequestration by another gene product might play an important part in cell proliferation and also in tumorigenesis.

mdm2 has been regarded as a component of an autoregulatory feedback system relating to *p53*. A transcription regulatory role independent of *p53* has been suggested for mdm2 on the basis of its ability to interact with human TATA-binding protein *in vitro* and *in vivo* in the absence of p53 (Leng *et al.*, 1995). There are probably other proteins which have not yet been characterised that might interact with mdm2 proteins (Gudas *et al.*, 1995a). It would appear that *p53* and *mdm2* abnormalities might represent distinct but not mutually exclusive pathways of tumour development and progression. This conclusion is further supported by the observation that the suppressor retinoblastoma-susceptibility gene (*rb*), another major player in neoplastic progression and cell cycle regulation, is also known to be negatively regulated by mdm2 (Xiao *et al.*, 1995).

mdm2 and tumour progression

It would be premature to weigh the significance of over-expression of mdm2 and p53 in relation to cancer prognosis, although the studies discussed above have suggested a possible relationship between them. Cordon-Cardo *et al.* (1994) reported that high expression of both genes in the same tumour correlated with poor survival. In leiomyosarcomas, abnormalities of either *p53* or *mdm2* appeared to be associated with a more advanced clinical stage of the disease (Patterson *et al.*, 1994). Three cases of Ewing's sarcomas which had metastasised showed *mdm2* amplification, whereas only one of 15 *mdm2*-negative primary tumours had metastasised (Ladanyi *et al.*, 1995). However, the cyclin-dependent kinase CDK-4 gene was co-amplified in the tumours that had metastasised and therefore it is difficult to evaluate the significance of *mdm2* amplification alone in relation to the metastatic process, from this study. Nilbert *et al.* (1995) found *mdm2* amplified in five malignant fibrous histiocytomas, whereas in 11 other tumours, which included pleomorphic liposarcomas and atypical lipoma, 2-5 other genes were also amplified. Thus, although *mdm2* may be the major target of amplification, other genes in the 12q13-15 amplicon may also be co-amplified.

In breast cancer, no correlation is seen between clinico-pathological and biological parameters and mdm2 protein levels (Marchetti *et al.*, 1995b), where amplification of the gene may be a rare event (Quesnel *et al.*, 1994b; McCann AH *et al.*, 1995). Co-amplification of certain oncogenes, and of growth factor and oestrogen receptor genes has also been reported, e.g. *Wnt-2*, *myc*, *ras*, *erbB2*, etc. (Fontana *et al.*, 1994; Habuchi *et al.*, 1994; Marchetti *et al.*, 1995b). This only emphasises the importance of examining the significance or functions of the genes which are co-amplified with mdm2.

There is a suggestion that high mdm2 expression may be related to the degree of differentiation of liposarcomas (Nakayama *et al.*, 1995). Increase in p53 and mdm2 positivity seems to correlate with loss of differentiation in premalignant and malignant lesions of the oropharyngeal mucosa. In the late stage of this disease a far higher number of specimens have proved to be positive for both p53 and mdm2 (Girod *et al.*, 1995). As mentioned earlier, multiple transcripts of *mdm2* has been identified in breast epithelial cells and the low molecular weight form of mdm2 is expressed abundantly in normal epithelial cells, whereas in tumour cells the level of expression is highly variable (Gudas *et al.*, 1995a,b). Whether this has any biological significance with regard to tumour differentiation or behaviour has yet to be studied.

Transactivation of growth factor receptor genes by p53

Epidermal growth factor receptor (EGFr) expression has long been regarded as an indicator of malignancy in certain forms of human cancer. Therefore, it is of considerable interest that high EGFr expression has often been found to accompany p53 abnormalities. EGFr over-expression has shown significant correlation with *p53* mutation status in oesophageal carcinomas (Esteve *et al.*, 1993). p53 over-expression is strongly correlated with EGFr expression in breast cancer (Horak *et al.*, 1991). Wright *et al.* (1991) found that p53 and/or EGFr over-expression was strongly associated with invasive transitional cell carcinoma of the bladder, but there was no statistically significant association between p53 and EFGr expression. Amplification of c-*erbB2* was found together with *mdm2* amplification in breast cancer (Fontana *et al.*, 1994). Over-expression of *p53* and *erbB2* has been reported in breast cancer (Horak *et al.*, 1991; Tsuda *et al.*, 1993), in bladder cancer (Moch *et al.*, 1993), and in adenocarcinoma of the stomach (Sasano *et al.*, 1993). Although there appears to be a general association between growth factor receptors and p53 broadly in the same tumour, it is unclear whether the amplification of these markers occur concomitantly in the same cells within a tumour. Co-localisation of the proteins can occur in a proportion of cells within a tumour (Sasano *et al.*, 1993). Unfortunately, there are too few studies of this rather important feature of co-expression. Nevertheless, it should be pointed out that wild-type p53 can transactivate the human EGFr promoter (Deb *et al.*, 1994). It is therefore conceivable that wild-type p53 will induce EGFr expression in some cell types and possibly under specific conditions, e.g. post-G_1 delay for DNA repair. Since the EGFr induction effect is apparently dose-dependent (Deb *et al.*, 1994), it is feasible that this could provide a pathway for mutant p53 proteins, which accumulate in large amounts on account of their significantly long half-life, to participate in cell proliferation. Alternatively, EGFr and p53 signal transduction may follow independent paths, because EGFr expression can also occur where no concomitant increase in p53 expression occurs (Gilhus *et al.*, 1995).

GADD genes and their regulation by p53

Having discussed how p53 influences positive signals for proliferation imparted to the cell by growth factors, it would be appropriate to discuss the role of this suppressor protein in regulating genes which impart growth arrest signals. The *GADD* (Growth *A*rrest and *D*NA

*D*amage inducible) family of genes are induced by DNA damage and are associated with growth suppression. *GADD45* has a p53 responsive element in the third intron and p53 obtained from irradiated cells binds this to the p53 responsive element (Kastan *et al.*, 1992) and *GADD45* transcription increases upon the DNA being damaged (Fornace *et al.*, 1989). Using temperature-sensitive mutant p53 transfectants, it has been shown that activation of wild-type p53 function induces *GADD45*, *waf1/cip1* (see page 60) and *mdm2* (Guillouf *et al.*, 1995). Obviously, p53 is regulating its expression in order to inhibit the entry into the S-phase. Thus, p53 regulates two different sets of genes in order to fulfil its function of detaining DNA damaged cells at the G_1-S checkpoint and releasing the inhibition when DNA repair has been carried out.

The *MyD* genes are a group of genes involved with myeloid differentiation; *MyD116* is a murine homologue of the hamster *GADD34*. *MyD118* and *GADD45* encoded proteins from different species possess a high degree of homology (Carrier *et al.*, 1994; Yoshida *et al.*, 1994). *GADD34/MyD116*, *GADD45*, *GADD153* and *MyD118* code for certain acidic proteins and share this property and pattern of induction by p53 with *mdm2* (Zhan *et al.*, 1994). GADD45 is a nuclear protein and is expressed in normal tissues, especially in quiescent cell populations. Its expression is high in G_1 cells but it is reduced in S-phase cells (Kearsey *et al.*, 1995). Another feature shared with other p53 regulated genes such as *p21 (waf1/cip1)* is the ability of GADD45 to interact with proliferating cell nuclear antigen (PCNA) (Smith *et al.*, 1994), which is a component of DNA replication–repair complexes. GADD45 can also bind to p21 (waf1/cip1) protein (Kearsey *et al.*, 1995).

Zhan *et al.* (1995) compared the response of *GADD45*, *waf1/cip1* and *mdm2* to ionising radiation (IR) in a panel of human cell lines. All three genes showed similar levels of transcriptional response to IR and the response was p53-dependent; radiosensitisers enhanced and caffeine inhibited *GADD45* and *waf1/cip1* induction by IR. *GADD45* and *waf1/cip1* also showed similar growth suppressive effects. In ataxia telangiectasia cells, where p53 induction by exposure to radiation is delayed, the transcription of *GADD45* and *waf1/cip1* is also delayed (Artuso *et al.*, 1995). Wild-type p53 may also modify the expression of other negative growth regulators. The mitogenic signal provided by insulin-like growth factor-1 (IGF-1) is inhibited by IGF-binding protein 3 (IGF-BP3) and it would appear that wild-type, but not mutant, p53 can induce the expression of IGF-BP3 (Buckbinder *et al.*, 1995).

Investigations of the association of *GADD* family members with tumorigenesis have already begun. *GADD153*, which is apparently activated by a chromosomal translocation (t12,16) in human myxoid liposarcoma, has been found to be amplified in two sarcoma cell lines and tissues derived from human sarcomas. It is possible that the contribution of *GADD153* may be complementary to other genes such as *mdm2* which is also co-amplified with *GADD153* (Forus *et al.*, 1994).

Metastasis-associated *18A2/mts1* gene in cell cycle progression

The genes of the S-100 family encode a host of Ca^{2+} proteins which subserve several important physiological functions. The expression of these proteins is known to be closely associated with cell cycle progression. Several members, e.g. S-100β, calcyclin, etc., are expressed in specific stages of the cell cycle. In common with these other members of the S-100 family, the mouse homologue of *18A2/mts1* gene also shows cell cycle-related expression (Jackson-Grusby *et al.*, 1988). Its expression is also associated with microtubule depolymerisation (Lakshmi *et al.*, 1993). Both Lakshmi *et al.* (1993) and Parker *et al.* (1994a) have therefore examined whether the expression of *18A2/mts1* and p53 are related. In these studies, they have demonstrated that an experimental modulation of *18A2/mts1* expression also produces variations in p53 protein expression. The detection of p53 increased or decreased in parallel with increase or decrease in *18A2/mts1* expression. In B16-F10 murine melanoma variant cells carrying transfected *18A2/mts1* gene, switching on its expression markedly increases p53 detectability (Parker *et al.*, 1994b). It should be pointed out that Pedrocchi *et al.* (1994) found no correlation between p53 and *18A2/mts1* expression. It is difficult to assess this work, since they provided no data concerning p53 in the human cancers they studied. However, we would like to emphasise that we have consistently found a correlation between these two features in a variety of experiments, which included gene transfer studies.

The mutated forms of p53 have a longer half-life and are therefore detectable by immuno-histochemical staining. Increased levels of wild-type p53 can be detected when these proteins form complexes with other macromolecules and thus become stabilised (Reich *et al.*, 1983; Jenkins *et al.*, 1985). Baudier *et al.* (1992) have recently shown that the S-100β protein, which has a 55% sequence homology with the 18A2/mts1 protein in respect of the Ca^{2+}-binding domains (Ebralidze *et al.*, 1989) forms a complex with the p53 phosphoprotein. This has therefore led to the suggestion that the correlation between *18A2/mts1* expression and p53 phosphoprotein may be due to the formation of such a complex and the consequent stabilisation of p53, allowing its detection immunohistochemically (Parker *et al.*, 1994a) (see Figure 8).

The formation of the 18A2/mts1-p53 complex may effectively sequester p53 and thereby result in the loss of control of cell proliferation which is normally exercised by wild-type p53. We know that melanoma cells in which *18A2/mts1* is up-regulated show greater anchorage and localisation in the lung (Parker *et al.*, 1991, 1994b). Therefore it seems possible that p53 sequestration by 18A2/mts1 may conceivably be involved in the *18A2/mts1*-induced metastatic spread.

The S-100 proteins are known to inhibit phosphorylation of target proteins such as annexin II (Bianchi *et al.*, 1992). S-100 proteins also modulate tyrosine phosphorylation of a number of substrate proteins by pp60^{src}, but not by protein kinase C, which suggests that S-100 might interact with substrate-binding sites of tyrosine kinases and regulate tyrosine phosphorylation (Hagiwara *et al.*, 1988). However, Baudier *et al.* (1992) reported that S-100β binds to p53 in a

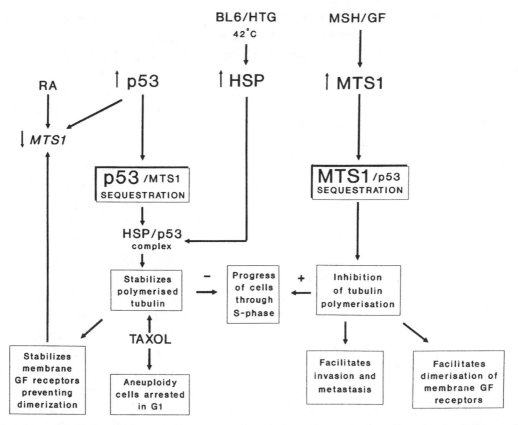

Figure 8. Possible pathways of function of the 18A2/mts1 protein in cell cycle regulation and cancer invasion. Induction of *18A2/mts1* expression drives the cells into the S-phase of the cell cycle and concomitantly causes an increase in the detectability of p53 protein. It is suggested that the 18A2/mts1 protein forms a complex with and stabilises p53. This complex formation also sequesters p53 and thereby prevents it from exercising its normal function of restraining the cells in the G_1 phase. Enhancement of *18A2/mts1* expression has also severe effects of depolymerisation of cytoskeletal structure, which has been regarded as a signal for G_1-S transition of cells. Furthermore, enhanced expression of *18A2/mts1* is also conducive for greater membrane deformability and therefore enhanced invasive propensity. This schematic presentation was constructed in consultation with Dr C. Parker.

calcium-dependent fashion and inhibits *in vitro* the phosphorylation of p53 by protein kinase C. Therefore, the further possibility that the *18A2/mts1* product might interfere with the phosphorylation of p53 and thereby regulate G_1/S transition of cells should also be considered.

We have recently drawn together the correlations demonstrable between *18A2/mts1* expression and p53 detection levels and their relationship to microtubule depolymerisation to postulate a model by which the 18A2/mts1 protein might control cell invasion and metastasis, as well as affect growth control (Figure 8). We have suggested that the 18A2/mts1 protein may have a dual function, namely sequestration of p53 leading to loss of growth control, and a second possible function being a direct inhibition of tubulin polymerisation in analogy with S-100β.

The depolymerisation of microtubules has been regarded as a regulatory signal for the transition of cells from the G_1 phase to the S phase. Crossin and Carney (1981a,b) have demonstrated that drug-induced depolymerisation of microtubules initiates DNA synthesis and, using taxol, which stabilises microtubules, they have shown that the depolymerisation of microtubules is an essential signal for the induction of DNA synthesis. Human cancer cell lines in which the *18A2/mts1* gene is constitutively highly expressed also contain a larger proportion of cells in the S-phase compared with cells that are low *18A2/mts1* expressors (Sherbet *et al.*, 1995). Furthermore, there is now evidence that enhanced *18A2/mts1* expression drives cells into the S-phase (Parker *et al.*, 1994b). The sequestration of p53 by 18A2/mts1 may compound the direct cell proliferation signal imparted by 18A2/mts1 by means of cytoskeletal depolymerisation.

We have proposed further that a state of equilibrium between p53 and 18A2/mts1 may regulate G_1-S transition. This proposal subsumes an equilibrium between the two proteins, but that when high levels of 18A2/mts1 exist, p53 is sequestered and 18A2/mts1 can promote tubulin depolymerisation, thus providing the signal for G_1-S transition. Alternatively, with p53 preponderance 18A2/mts1 can be deemed to have been sequestered leading to an inhibition of tubulin depolymerisation. In the absence of this regulatory signal the cells are arrested in the G_1 phase. Whether 18A2/mts1 protein can function independently of p53 has not been studied.

There is now a considerable body of evidence which supports the view that 18A2/mts1 is a novel p53-binding cellular protein and that *18A2/mts1* and *p53* genes function in a coordinated way in controlling tumour growth and also invasion by tumour cells as a prelude to metastatic deposition (see page 191).

Retinoblastoma susceptibility gene (*rb*) abnormalities in cancer

Retinoblastoma is a paediatric cancer arising in the retina of the eye. This disease occurs in both hereditary and sporadic forms. There are, however, marked differences in their patterns of development and incidence. In the hereditary form the disease is bilateral and multifocal but sporadic retinoblastoma is unilateral and unifocal. The incidence of the familial tumour is higher than the sporadic form. These features of retinoblastoma and statistical analyses of incidence led to the 'two-hit' hypothesis proposed by Knudson (1971). The suggestion was that one mutated *rb* allele was inherited and occurred in all cells, including germ cells, of the progeny and that a mutation of the second allele would lead to the development of the tumour. It was reported many years ago that retinoblastoma was induced by a bi-allelic inactivation and the retinoblastoma-susceptibility gene (*rb*) was identified and cloned (Friend *et al.*, 1986; Fung *et al.*, 1987; Lee *et al.*, 1987a).

The *rb* gene is expressed in all normal tissues and cell lines (Lee *et al.*, 1987b). It is expressed in a mutated form or absent in retinoblastomas (Lee *et al.*, 1987b, 1990; Horowitz *et al.*, 1990). Abnormalities of this gene have been described in several other human tumours, e.g. small cell lung cancer (SCLC) (Harbour *et al.*, 1988; Hensel *et al.*, 1990; Mori *et al.*, 1990). Harbour *et al.* (1988) found that 13% of primary SCLC and 18% of SCLC-derived cell lines showed structural abnormalities of *rb* and 60% of SCLC-derived cell lines showed a loss of the gene. Loss of gene expression has been reported in 30% of primary non-SCLCs (Xu *et al.*, 1991) and it appears also from this study that altered *rb* expression may be related to tumour stage. Inactivation of *rb* was reported in two bladder cancer cell lines and lack of expression without gross gene deletion in another cell line (Ishikawa *et al.*, 1991). Of considerable interest is the suggestion of rb inactivation with tumour progression. For these authors failed to detect rb alterations in 16 low-grade non-invasive bladders, whereas only two out of 14 high-grade invasive cancers showed rb protein expression. Wright *et al.* (1995) have confirmed the association of the absence of rb protein expression with invasive growth and high-grade tumours. In this latter study, tumour growth fraction, as indicated by Ki67 staining, was twice as large in p53+/rb− tumours as in p53−/rb+ tumours. Abnormalities of the gene are also associated with carcinomas of the breast (Lee *et al.*, 1988; T'Ang *et al.*, 1988; Varley *et al.*, 1989), where the gene has been found to be deleted or rearranged. The same abnormalities were detectable in primary breast carcinomas and in metastatic tumour where matching specimens had been examined (Varley *et al.*, 1989). Furthermore, expression of *rb* appears related to the stage of differentiation of human testicular tumours (Strohmeyer *et al.*, 1991). Mutations in exons 13-22 of the *rb* sequence have been found in 55% (27 out of 49) of thyroid carcinomas whereas no mutations in these exons were detected in benign tumours. Mutation of both *rb* and *p53* genes appeared to be more frequent in advanced disease (Zou *et al.*, 1994). These data suggest a possible involvement of the gene in tumour growth and progression rather than its initiation.

Loss of heterozygosity at the *rb* locus occurs frequently in oesophageal cancers (Boynton *et al.*, 1991). Structural changes of the gene are associated with human soft tissue tumours (Friend *et al.*, 1987; Stratton *et al.*, 1989). Other tumour types with *rb* involvement are cancer of the prostate (Bookstein *et al.*, 1990a), leukaemias (Cheng *et al.*, 1990; Furukawa *et al.*, 1991), and osteocarcinomas (Toguchida *et al.*, 1988; Shew *et al.*, 1989).

The *rb* gene is located on chromosome 13q14. Cytogenetic abnormalities of chromosome 13 and loss of heterozygosity at the *rb* locus have been reported in a variety of human cancers, e.g. lung, bladder, breast, osteosarcomas, etc. Allelic loss at the locus has been found also in ovarian cancers (Li *et al.*, 1991; Cliby *et al.*, 1993). Dodson *et al.* (1994) also found loss of heterozygosity at the *rb* locus in 25 out of 48 ovarian cancers, but found that functional rb protein was expressed in 23 out of 25 cancers where loss of heterozygosity had occurred. While loss of heterozygosity was associated with high-grade tumours, again functional rb protein was detectable in a majority of these cases (Kim *et al.*, 1994). This suggests that abnormalities associated with some other gene, but not *rb*, may be responsible for the aggressiveness of these tumours. Consistent with these thoughts is the observation by Wrede *et al.* (1991) that no abnormalities of *rb* or *p53* are detectable in human papilloma virus (HPV)-positive cervical carcinoma cell lines. The rb protein expressed in these cell lines was of the wild-type (Scheffner *et al.*, 1991), but evidence of abnormalities are found in HPV-negative cell lines. Riou *et al.* (1992) found that early-stage invasive cervical cancers which over-express the *myc* oncogene in the absence of HPV show a high risk of distant metastases, thus *myc* gene over-expression may be deemed as an independent prognostic indicator of metastasis.

Regulation of cell cycle progression by retinoblastoma-susceptibility gene product

When the normal *rb* gene is transferred into retinoblastoma cells and/or into cells which carry the inactivated *rb* gene, there is suppression of growth and tumorigenicity (Huang *et al.*, 1988; Bookstein *et al.*, 1990b); therefore, it has been regarded as a tumour suppressor gene (Figure 9). The function of tumour suppression appears to be mainly due to its ability to act as a negative regulator of cell cycle progression. It has been shown that the product of this gene is a 110 kDa (p110^{rb}) phosphoprotein. This protein is differentially phosphorylated in relation to the cell cycle (Buchkovich *et al.*, 1989; Chen *et al.*, 1989). The unphosphorylated rb protein is found predominantly in the G_1 phase of the cell cycle (Pardee, 1989). Stimulation of resting cells by mitogens is associated with phosphorylation of the rb protein and transition of cells from G_1 to S phase of the cell cycle (Chen *et al.*, 1989). Relatively higher levels of phosphorylated rb are found in the logarithmic phase of growth of cells compared with those arrested in the G_1 phase (Xu *et al.*, 1989). The unphosphorylated form has therefore been regarded as a suppressor of cell proliferation. The hyperphosphorylated status of rb protein is maintained throughout the remainder of the cell cycle and it is dephosphorylated upon the exit of the cells from mitosis. The cell cycle-dependent phosphorylation of the rb protein is mediated by cyclin D and CDK4/6 (Dowdy *et al.*, 1993; Ewen *et al.*, 1993a). The expression of cyclin E also can lead to rb phosphorylation (Hinds *et al.*, 1992) and it has been suggested that cyclin E/CDK2 complexes may mediate this process.

The sequestration of unphosphorylated rb protein will allow the cells to transit into the S-phase. It is known that functional rb protein forms stable complexes with transforming oncoproteins such as those encoded by the simian virus 40 (SV40) and human papilloma viruses (Templeton *et al.*, 1991). HPV E7 binds to rb protein and such binding is necessary for E7 protein to immortalise and transform cells (Dyson *et al.*, 1989; Munger *et al.*, 1989; Gage *et al.*, 1990). The SV40 T-antigen is known to bind preferentially to the underphosphorylated rb protein (Ludlow *et al.*, 1989). Although these studies suggest a close correlation between phosphorylation and the transition of cells from G_1 into the S-phase of the cell cycle, phosphorylation might be a progressive event and this may be reflected in the molecular heterogeneity found in rb proteins (Xu *et al.*, 1989). The process of rb phosphorylation may be an incremental process beginning in late G_1, several hours before transition into the S-phase

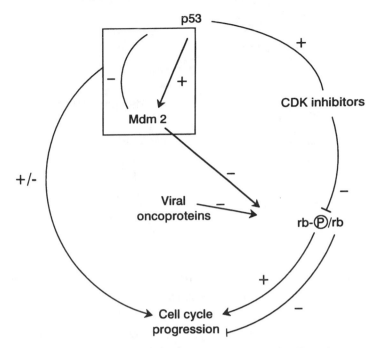

Figure 9. A schematic representation of cooperative control of cell cycle progression by p53 and rb proteins. The phosphorylation of rb is a major requirement for progression of the cell cycle beyond the restriction point. p53 may suppress rb phosphorylation by inducing the expression of CDK inhibitors. The phosphorylation of rb releases transcription factors such as E2F (see Figure 10) from their complexes with rb, and this allows the transcription of genes required for entry of cells into the S-phase. Viral oncoproteins may tether underphosphorylated rb and allow G_1-S transition of the cells. The figure also presents a postulate which implicates mdm2 with the function of both p53 and rb.

(Mittnacht et al., 1994). Furthermore, underphosphorylated rb binds to other cellular proteins such as the E2F transcription factor (Chellappan et al., 1991; Shirodkar et al., 1992) and cyclins D1 and D3 (Dowdy et al., 1993; Ewen et al., 1993a).

The rb protein needs to control transcription of genes which are essential for the progression of the cell through the cell cycle and this appears to be effected by rb interaction with the E2F transcription factors (Figure 10). The latter comprise a family of transcription factors. Five members of this family have been identified, namely E2F1, E2F2, etc. (Lam and La Thangue, 1994; Hijmans et al., 1995; Sardet et al., 1995). These transcription factors show sequence-specific binding as homodimers to DNA and this can be enhanced when E2Fs form heterodimers with the DP1 family of transcription factors (Bandara et al., 1993, 1994; Helin et al., 1993; Krek et al., 1993; Wu et al., 1995). Other rb-related proteins deemed as members of the rb family of proteins also interact with E2F in a manner similar to rb itself (Vairo et al., 1995).

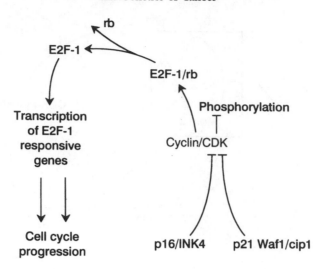

Figure 10.   The significance of the complex formation between rb protein and the transcription factor E2F-1 is depicted here. Phosphorylation of rb results in the release of E2F-1 from the complex and this transcription factor mediates the transcription of E2F-1 responsive genes necessary for the progression of the cell cycle. As shown also in Figure 9, a p53-mediated control mechanism might be the inhibition of cyclin-dependent kinases by p16/ink4 and waf1/cip1.

Johnson DG *et al.* (1993) found that if E2F-1 protein is introduced into a quiescent cell it enters the S-phase. But interaction between rb and E2F proteins produces a down-regulation of E2F-dependent transcription (Lam and La Thangue, 1994; Wu CL *et al.*, 1995). E2F binding occurs predominantly to the underphosphorylated form of the rb protein (Chellappan *et al.*, 1991; Helin *et al.*, 1992; Kaelin *et al.*, 1992; Shan *et al.*, 1992). The phosphorylation of rb releases it from its association with E2F, thus allowing E2F-dependent gene transcription. E2F-1 is itself differentially regulated. In the late G_1-early S phase, E2F-1 is bound by cyclin A/cdk2. The latter also phosphorylates the DP1 in the DP1/E2F complex. As a consequence E2F-1 loses its DNA-binding ability and is essentially negatively regulated (Dynlacht *et al.*, 1994; Krek *et al.*, 1994). This is believed to be the pathway by which the rb protein exerts a negative regulatory control on cell cycle progression (Figure 10).

The cell cycle regulatory function of rb may involve other transcription factors, such as the Ets family members which are involved in cell cycle progression in activated T cells. The Ets related transcription Elf-1 has been found to bind rb protein by a sequence motif which is related to rb-binding motifs carried by viral oncoproteins (Wang CY *et al.*, 1993). As with E2F, phosphorylation of rb results in the release of Elf-1. The rb protein is also known to bind to other transcription factors such as the ATF2, causing transcription of ATF2 target genes (Kim *et al.*, 1992).

The cooperation of rb *and* p53 *genes in cell cycle regulation*

Since both *rb* and *p53* genes are associated with the progression of cells into the S-phase of the cycle, one would expect a cooperative effect on tumour growth and progression, when both genes are expressed in the inactive form or undergo deletion. As stated previously, abnormalities in either or both of these genes result in a significantly higher proliferative index than when tumours do not carry abnormalities of either (Wright *et al.*, 1995) Also, abnormalities in both genes are more common in advanced stage tumours (Zou *et al.*, 1994).

It has been suggested that p53 exerts its negative regulatory control over cell cycle progression by the induction of a downstream target gene p21$^{waf1/cip1}$ which codes for a cyclin-dependent protein kinase (cdk) inhibitor (see page 59). Since these kinases are involved in the phosphorylation of rb, there are sufficient grounds for proposing a cooperation of rb and p53 in cell cycle regulation. For example, the cyclin–cdk complex phosphorylates rb protein and this allows E2F to be released from its complex with rb and E2F is then able to activate the transcription of genes such as the dihydrofolate reductase (DHFR) and thymidine synthase (TS) genes whose expression is essential for the entry of cells into the S-phase. The p53 protein may regulate rb phosphorylation. Exposure of cells carrying wild-type *p53* to ionising radiation produces an increase in waf1/cip1 protein and an accumulation of underphosphorylated rb. In contrast, when *p53* is abnormal or is functionally inactivated, neither of these changes are noticed (Slebos *et al.*, 1994). Furthermore, p53 represses transcription from the promoters of a number of genes such as thymidine kinase gene, c-*myc* and DNA polymerase α (Lin *et al.*, 1992; Moberg *et al.*, 1992; Yuan *et al.*, 1993) and these genes are also transactivated by E2F. As stated earlier, E2F involvement might be impaired by p53 by means of the p21$^{waf1/cip1}$ inhibitor protein. This would appear to be another area where rb and p53 control pathways overlap. Furthermore, by virtue of its properties as a transcription factor, p53 appears to be able to regulate the transcription of the *rb* gene itself and two regions of the gene have been identified: one of these can stimulate transcription from *rb* promoter and the second one represses *rb* transcription (Osifchin *et al.*, 1994). The *mdm2* gene offers another link in the cooperation between *p53* and *rb* genes. As discussed in an earlier section (see page 43), mdm2 protein can interact with and inactivate *p53*. Furthermore, p53 has been found to up-regulate the expression of *mdm2*. Xiao *et al.* (1995) found the mdm2 protein was also capable of interacting with rb protein and inhibit its negative regulatory control over cell cycle progression. Thus, p53 seems to be subject to a self-regulatory loop, but p53-mediated up-regulation of *mdm2* expression may provide the tumour cell a mechanism to override the control imposed upon cell proliferation by the rb protein (Figure 9).

Other mechanisms for control of cell proliferation may also be envisaged. For instance, we have discussed the role of E2F transcription factor as a possible positive regulator of G$_1$-S transition of cells. E2F, as we have noted before, may be under the regulatory control of *rb*. Recently, it has emerged that E2F might interact also with p53. When E2F1 and p53 are co-expressed the cells appear to undergo apoptosis (Wu and Levine, 1994), presumably upon being detained in the G_1 phase. Other genes, e.g. those encoding growth factors may be prone to regulation by rb protein, as in the case of *neu (erb-B2)* (Martin and Hung, 1994).

There is therefore an array of evidence suggesting a close cooperation, perhaps even link-up between *rb* and *p53* in the growth and progression of neoplasms.

Cyclins, cell cycle progression and cyclins as proto-oncogenes

The initiation of DNA synthesis and mitosis are controlled by two key elements: (a) the cyclin-dependent protein kinases (CDKs) containing a cyclin regulatory subunit and a cell division control (cdc2) family kinase subunit, and (b) CDK inhibitors. The cdc2 proteins are expressed uniformly during cell cycle progression, but another family of proteins, the cyclins, show variable expression. The formation of complexes between cdc2 and cyclins provide the regulatory signals required for cell cycle progression.

The cdc2 proteins do not possess protein kinase activity. However, they form a complex with cyclins which accumulate during various cell cycle phases. The complex known as the S-phase promoting factor is the best characterised $p34^{cdc2}$ kinase-cyclin complex. Cyclin B is synthesised during the S-phase. In the G_2 phase cdc2 proteins complex with cyclin B and this induces phosphorylation of threonine 161, which is required for the activation of the enzyme. In contrast, enzyme activation is controlled by phosphorylations at threonine-14 and tyrosine-15 in the ATP-binding site which inactivate the kinase during the G_2-S phase. When these inhibitory phosphates are removed from the $p34^{cdc2}$-cyclin B complex, the $p34^{cdc2}$ kinase is activated and this triggers the cells at the G_2/M boundary into mitosis. The cells exit from mitosis on degradation of cyclin B by ubiquitin which results in the inactivation of $p34^{cdc2}$ (summarised by Baguley, 1991; Murray, 1992; Sherr, 1993).

There are several cyclins associated with the G_1 phase. These G_1 cyclins form complexes and activate the $p34^{cdc2}$ kinase. This activation provides the signal for transition of cells from G_1 to the S-phase, by inducing DNA replication. The molecular aspects of regulation of the S-phase promoting factor, which is in many ways analogous to the maturation promoting factor MPF, are well understood in yeast but our understanding of the processes in mammalian cells is rather scanty. In mammalian cells, the association of D type cyclin with CDK2, CDK4 or CDK5 and the association of cyclin E with CDK2 are required for G_1-S transition (reviewed by Hunter, 1993; Sherr, 1993).

As discussed in previous sections, G_1-S transition is negatively regulated by the p53 phosphoprotein. How p53 might abrogate the 'Start' signal imparted by the S-phase promoting factor is still unresolved, but this may be mediated by the induction by *p53* of waf1/cip1 protein which associates with and inhibits cyclin-cdk function. Another protein with M_r 16 K has been shown to associate with CDK4 and inhibit the activity of cyclin D-CDK complex (Serrano *et al.*, 1993) and may be involved in the negative regulation of cell proliferation. Alternatively, the abrogation of p53 function may also be achieved by the sequestration of the protein by cellular target proteins as discussed previously (see pages 31 and 48). The 18A2/mts1 protein alluded to before is one of these downstream target proteins which appears to be able to trigger G_1-S transition. If, as postulated earlier, the 18A2/mts1 protein were to sequester wild-type p53 phosphoprotein, one could envisage a situation in which p53-mediated induction of the CDK inhibitor is prevented and this would have the effect of continual activation of the cyclin–CDK complexes and a continual G_1-S transition of cells and consequent deregulation of tumour growth. In this context, one should bear in mind that although the induction of waf1 protein was initially believed to be a p53-dependent event, there have been several reports that its expression may be triggered by a mechanism independent of p53 expression (Jiang et al., 1994; Steinman et al., 1994). Indeed, even with p53/p21-waf1 activation, constitutive expression of B-myb can rescue cells from p53-mediated G_1 arrest (Lin et al., 1994).

It is known that p53 interacts with $p34^{cdc2}$ in vivo (Sturzbecher et al., 1990) and that the serine-315 residue of p53 is phosphorylated by cdc2 kinase (Bischoff et al., 1990). In an analogous fashion, the rb gene product is also a substrate for cdc2 kinase (Lin et al., 1991). Therefore, it is also conceivable that sequestration of p53 by 18A2/mts1 protein can happen only when p53 is in the unphosphorylated state. Both p53 and rb proteins share the property of binding to several DNA tumour virus proteins (Green, 1989; Lane and Benchimol, 1990; Lee et al., 1990). We also know from Ludlow et al. (1989) that the SV-40 large T antigen binds preferentially to an underphosphorylated form of the rb protein. Thus, inactivation of p53/rb can occur by means of mutation, phosphorylation, or their sequestration either by viral or cellular proteins such as the 18A2/mts1 leading to transition of cells from G_1 to S phase of the cell cycle (Figure 11). It is imperative therefore that we take serious cognisance of the contribution of genes involved in cell cycle control and how the so-called metastasis-associated genes such as the 18A2/mts1 of the S-100 protein family impinge upon their functions before we finally pronounce upon their potential in relation to the diverse processes of cancer invasion and metastasis.

In the light of their importance in cell cycle regulation, the cyclins may be expected to be prominently associated with neoplastic transformation and progression. G_1 cyclins have been regarded as oncoproteins. Cyclin D1, isolated from parathyroid adenomas, has been reported to be over-expressed in many tumour types (Arnold et al., 1989; Lammie et al., 1991; Motokura et al., 1991; Rosenberg et al., 1991a,b; Withers et al., 1991). In B-cell malignancies, reciprocal chromosomal translocation t(11;14)(q13;q32) occurs at break points around the Bcl1 locus of 11q13 and this is thought to activate cyclin D1 gene (Rosenberg et al., 1991a). Several genes which might be relevant to malignant transformation have been assigned to this locus and complex amplification events take place here, with several core amplicons covering the whole locus (see below).

Buckley et al. (1993) found higher expression of one or more of cyclins A, B1, D1 or E in seven out of 20 breast cancer cell lines; cyclin D1 was over-expressed in five out of 20 cell lines. Of 124 breast cancer biopsies investigated, 56 specimens showed higher cyclin D gene expression compared with normal breast tissue. Amplification of chromosome 11q13 which contains the bcl1/PRAD1 (cyclin D1) together with EMS1, (and hst1 and int2 only rarely

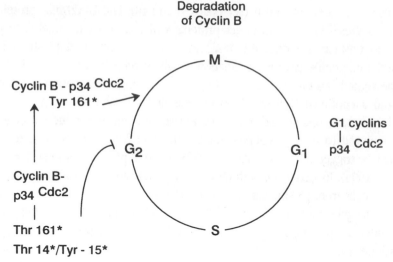

Figure 11. Interaction of cyclins and cdks during the cell cycle. The cyclin D/CDK-4 complexes are activated by CAKs and this activated complex can now phosphorylate rb and release transcription factors required for the activation of genes whose expression is required for transition of the cells into the S-phase (see Figures 9 and 10). Cyclin B is synthesised during the S-phase and, in the G_2 phase, it forms a complex with p34^{cdc2}. Phosphorylation of tyrosine-161 is believed to activate p34 and this enables the cells to make the G_2-M transition. A proposed control mechanism of this transition is the phosphorylation of threonine-14/tyrosine-15 which are believed to inactivate p34.

expressed in breast cancer) genes has been reported (Faust and Meeker, 1992; Schuuring *et al.*, 1992). Schuuring *et al.* (1992) observed that 11q13 amplification showed a positive association with lymph node involvement and significantly shorter relapse-free interval and on this basis have suggested that this may be a predictor of diminished survival in operable breast cancer. Elevated cyclin D1 expression has also been reported in a B-cell non-Hodgkin's lymphoma called mantle cell lymphomas (Bosch *et al.*, 1994; Yang *et al.*, 1994), squamous cell carcinomas of the head and neck (Callender *et al.*, 1994; Lucas *et al.*, 1994), hepatocellular carcinomas (Nishida *et al.*, 1994) and colorectal carcinomas (Bartkova *et al.*, 1994a). In breast cancer an over-expression of the gene has been reported in half of a batch of 170 primary carcinomas studied by Bartkova *et al.* (1994b); this occurred as an early event and was maintained through the progression of the tumours to the metastatic stage. In human laryngeal carcinomas cyclin D1 gene amplification and also elevated levels of its messenger RNA were associated with advanced local invasion and metastasis of the tumour to the lymph nodes (Jares *et al.*, 1994). Cyclin D1 gene amplification was found in advanced stages of hepatocellular carcinomas exhibiting high growth rates, suggesting its association with aggressiveness of the disease (Nishida *et al.*, 1994). However, in tumours of the head and neck cyclin D1 amplification did not correlate with tumour grade, stage, or degree of aneuploidy (Callender *et al.*, 1994). It should be pointed out that amplification is not always accompanied by increased cyclin D1 gene expression (Buckley *et al.*, 1993). Furthermore, murine tumour cell lines, produced by the use of benzo(a)pyrene, show high invasive potential *in vitro* and do possess other features such as p53 mutations, without attendant amplification or rearrangement of cyclin D1 gene (Ruggeri *et al.*, 1994). Besides, *int-2 (FGF3)* and *hst (FGF4)*, which encode growth factors of the fibroblast growth factor family, have been assigned to the same chromosomal locus as cyclin D1, namely 11q13. The *int-2* gene has been reported to be co-amplified with cyclin D1 gene in hepatocellular carcinomas. Several of these genes may be amplified in breast cancer and amplicons at the 11q13 locus encompasses a large tract of DNA containing several cores of amplification (Karlseder *et al.*, 1994). Jaakkola *et al.* (1993), however, found no amplification of any of these genes of the 11q13 locus. Nonetheless, the possibility that cyclin D1 may be only one of the genes in the amplicon relevant in the process of tumorigenesis is worth further investigation.

Induction of cyclin D1 expression does release cells from G_1-arrest (Musgrove *et al.*, 1994) and there is the suggestion that over-expression of cyclin D1 may correlate with *rb* expression (Schauer *et al.*, 1994) and is presumably therefore mediated by E2F activation of cell cycle related genes. In this context, it is of some interest that Lovec *et al.* (1994a) have recently reported that over-expression of cyclin D1 by means of transfection induces transformation of primary rat embryo fibroblast lines, with the cooperation of the activated H-*ras* oncogene. Cyclin D1 appears to cooperate also with *myc* gene homologues (Lovec *et al.*, 1994b), but there are no reports of possible involvement of B-*myb* and other cell cycle associated genes. Nevertheless, there is a general perception that a deregulation of cyclins might be involved with cellular transformation and tumour progression.

Cyclin-dependent kinase (cdk) inhibitors as tumour suppressors

In recent years, a number of genes which encode proteins capable of functioning as inhibitors of cyclin-dependent kinases have been identified and cloned. Cyclin-dependent kinases (cdks) regulate cell cycle progression. The cdks phosphorylate the rb protein which then allows the progression of cells from G_1 into the S-phase. The cdks are activated by phosphorylation by cdk-activating kinases (CAK). The cdk inhibitors block this activation of cdks by CAK. The inhibition of cdk activation results in the inhibition of rb phosphorylation and consequently in cell cycle arrest in G_1 phase. Therefore, consistent with the recognition of *p53* and *rb* genes as tumour suppressor genes, the cdk inhibitor genes have also been regarded as putative tumour suppressors. The cdk inhibitors can be considered as two distinct groups of enzymes. Group 1 includes waf1/cip1/[p21][CDKN1], kip1/[p27][CDKN4] and kip2/[p57] and Group 2 includes the cdk inhibitors which are known as ink4B [p15][MTS2], ink4A/[p16][CDKN2] and p18. There are major differences in the physiological properties of group 1 and group 2 cdk inhibitors; waf1/cip1, kip1 and kip2 are known to bind cyclins D1, D2, D3, cyclins-E and A and cyclin B to a lesser extent. The group 1 inhibitors do not bind or associate with the kinase subunit unless the cyclins are present. In contrast, the ink4B or ink4A members do bind to cdk4 and cdk6 even in the absence of cyclins, suggesting differences in their specificity (Hall *et al.*, 1995). There are also some differences in their structural features, e.g. the presence of ankyrin repeat motifs in group 2 cdk inhibitors (Kawamata *et al.*, 1995).

Structural and functional features of group 1 cdk inhibitors

The cdk inhibitors of group 1 share several features relating to their genomic structure and functional elements (Table 3). The mouse kip2 protein has four major functional domains: the *N*-terminal with cdk inhibitory function, a proline-rich domain, a domain containing tandem repeat motifs consisting of four acidic amino acid residues and a *C*-terminal domain. This last domain contains nuclear targeting and possible cdk phosphorylation regions. The kip2 protein has sequence similarity to kip1 but not to waf1/cip1 (Lee *et al.*, 1995; Matsuoka *et al.*, 1995). The *N*-terminal domain of waf1/cip1 and kip1, as in kip2, possesses cdk inhibitory activity. Proliferating cell nuclear antigen (PCNA) binding ability resides in the *C*-terminal domain, but neither kip1 or kip2 have PCNA-binding ability (Luo *et al.*, 1995). Waf1/cip1 and kip1 have a common DNA-inhibitory motif, which corresponds to residues 49–61 in waf1/cip1 and residues 60–76 in kip1 (Nakanishi *et al.*, 1995a). A most important criterion by which a distinction can be made between the members of the group 1 cdk inhibitors is their response to DNA damage and cell–cell contact and antiproliferative signals. As discussed in the following sections, *waf1/cip1* proves to be a downstream target of p53, regulated by *p53* and induced by DNA damage, whereas kip1 and kip2 tend to respond to growth inhibitory signals from inhibitory growth factors and cell–cell contact phenomena (Reed *et al.*, 1994; Datto *et al.*, 1995a,b). Finally, there are also notable differences in their tissue distribution. Whereas kip2 has been reported to show tissue-specific distribution, e.g. in the placenta, heart, skeletal muscle, the distribution of waf1/cip1 and kip1 appears to be more widespread (Polyak *et al.*, 1994a,b; Lee *et al.*, 1995; Matsuoka *et al.*, 1995).

Regulation of *waf1/cip1* gene expression by p53

Several genes have been identified whose expression the *p53* gene is able to modulate and, conversely, others have been identified that may affect p53 supressor function. However, the mechanism by which *p53* exerts control over cell proliferation and growth is poorly under-stood. The *waf1/cip1* is another target gene whose expression has been recently found to be regulated by *p53*. El-Deiry *et al.* (1993) identified this target gene *waf1* (*w*ild-type p53 *a*ctivated *f*ragment 1) which suppresses tumour cell proliferation in culture. Concurrently, Harper *et al.*

Table 3. Structural and functional features of cyclin dependent kinase inhibitors waf1/cip1, p27 (kip1), and p57 (kip2)

Waf1/cip1	Kip1	Kip2
Loc: 6p21.2[1]	12p12.3[2]	11p15.5[3]
p53 regulated		Not regulated by p53[3]
DNA damaged-induced[9]		Induced by cell–cell contact, antiproliferative signals[4,10]
May be up-regulated by TGF-β		Up-regulated by TGF-β[4,9]
Cyclin D1, D2, D3, E, A, B?[8]		Cyclin E-cdk2; D2-cdk4; A-cdk2[5]
2 exons similar intron-exon organisation		
		Four domains[3,5]
N-terminal cdk inhibition[3,5,11]	N-terminal cdk inhibition[3,5]	1. N-terminal CDK inhibition
		2. Proline-rich
		3. acidic repeats
	C-terminal conserved	4. C-terminal nuclear targeting; cdk phosphorylation
PCNA inhibition C-terminal[6]		No PCNA inhibition[6]
DNA inhibition motif[7] residues 49-61	Residues 60-76[7]	
	Widespread tissue distribution[4]	Tissue-specific placenta, heart, skeletal muscle, terminally diff. cells[3,5]

[1] El-Deiry et al. (1993); Demetrick et al. (1995).
[2] Martin E et al. (1995); Pietenpol et al. (1995); Poncecastaneda et al. (1995).
[3] Matsuoka et al. (1995).
[4] Polyak et al. (1994a,b).
[5] Lee MH et al. (1995).
[6] Luo et al. (1995).
[7] Nakanishi et al. (1995a).
[8] Hall et al. (1995).
[9] Datto et al. (1995b).
[10] Reed et al. (1994).
[11] Goubin and Ducommun (1995).

(1993) described the gene as *cip1* (*cdk interacting protein 1*) and Xiong *et al.* (1993a) as gene *p21*, and Noda *et al.* (1994) as *sdi1*. The product of *waf1/cip1* has been found to associate with and inhibit cyclin-cdk complexes and suppress the transition of cell from G_1 into the S-phase of the cell cycle (Harper *et al.*, 1993; Xiong *et al.*, 1993b). The gene has been mapped to chromosome 6p21.2 (El-Deiry *et al.*, 1993).

There is now considerable evidence that *waf1/cip1* is regulated by the wild-type, but not mutant, *p53* gene, as originally reported by El-Deiry *et al.* (1993). Expression of *waf1/cip1* is low in LN-Z308 cells where *p53* is not expressed. Transfection of wild-type, but not mutant, *p53* into these cells, inhibits cell growth with accompanying *waf1/cip1* expression (Jung *et al.*, 1995a). Katayose *et al.* (1995) constructed two adenovirus vectors, one expressing *waf1/cip1* cDNA (AdWaf1) and a second one expressing wild type *p53* (Adwtp53). When cells were infected with AdWaf1 high levels of *waf1/cip1* gene expression were found and these were comparable to levels found in cells infected with the vector carrying wild-type *p53*.

The waf1/cip1 protein is known to form a quaternary complex with cyclin/cdk and proliferating cell nuclear antigen (PCNA) (Xiong *et al.*, 1992, 1993a,b). The *C*-terminal region of waf1/cip1 protein is involved in binding to PCNA, but the importance of PCNA binding to its ability to inhibit DNA synthesis is unclear, since deletion mutants which are unable to bind to PCNA and/or cdk2 still retain their ability to inhibit DNA synthesis (Nakanishi *et al.*, 1995b). A cdk inhibitor from 3T3 cells described by Gu *et al.* (1993) may be a homologue of the human waf1/cip1 protein.

The *waf1/cip1* promoter contains a p53-binding site and p53 has been found to induce *waf1* expression (El-Deiry *et al.*, 1993, 1994). p53 binding sites occur upstream of the transcription site in the *waf1/cip1* promoter (El-Deiry *et al.*, 1995). The *C*-terminal basic domain of p53 is not essential for the regulation of *waf1/cip1* transcription. The expression of this gene is induced by DNA damage in cells carrying wild-type, but not mutant, *p53* (El-Deiry *et al.*, 1994). The induction of waf1/cip1 would then be expected to inactivate the cyclin–CDK complex and restrain the cells from entering the S-phase. However, it is worthwhile acknowledging that there may be pathways other than waf1/cip1 mediation by which *p53* may control cell proliferation (Hu *et al.*, 1995).

The *waf1/cip1* gene could be regulated by a *p53*-independent mechanism. Human breast carcinoma cells show increased *waf1/cip1* gene expression upon DNA damage, regardless of whether they carried wild-type or mutant *p53*. In these cells serum starvation caused enhanced gene expression, although the expression of *p53* was unaffected (Sheikh *et al.*, 1994). Serum stimulation and EGF can induce waf1/cip1 in quiescent embryonic fibroblasts derived from *p53* knock-out mice (Michieli *et al.*, 1994). TGF-α-responsive MCF7 breast carcinoma cells, show an increase in waf1/cip1 expression, whereas in the TGF-α-resistant MCF7 variant no such changes in waf1/cip1 expression have been encountered (Mazars *et al.*, 1995). TGF-β, which produces G_1 arrest, enhances waf1/cip1 protein in colorectal cancer cell lines, but this induction does not occur if the cells are not TGF-β responsive (Li CY *et al.*, 1995). In fact, TGF-β activates the transcription of *waf1/cip1* and a 10 bp sequence has been identified in the *waf1/cip1* promoter which is required for TGF-β mediated activation (Datto *et al.*, 1995a). Indeed, TGF and p53, activate transcription through two distinct elements in the *waf1/cip1* promoter (Datto *et al.*, 1995b). The suppression of proliferation by TGF-β is believed to be a result of reduced cyclin E kinase activity which, in turn, leads to suppression of phosphorylation of the *rb* gene product. When cells are treated with TGF-β, waf1/cip1 protein and other cyclin-dependent kinase inhibitors, such as kip1 and ink4B, bind to and inhibit the activity of cyclin–cdk complexes (Li CY *et al.*, 1995).

There is an old adage that cell proliferation and differentiation are mutually exclusive phenomena - or to put more accurately, cells withdraw from the cell division cycle when they are committed to the path of differentiation. The *waf1/cip1* gene can be induced during the differentiation of human promyelocytic leukaemia cells with a *p53*-null phenotype into macrophage/monocyte pathway by TPA, 1,25-dihydroxyvitamin D3, retinoic acid and dimethyl-sulphoxide (Jiang *et al.*, 1994). Similar results have been obtained by Zhang W *et al.* (1995), but only using TPA, okadaic acid and inteferon-γ (IFN-γ). In *p53*-deficient MG-63 osteosarcoma cells, waf1/cip1 is induced in early G_1 phase in the absence of any detectable p53 protein (Wu LT *et al.*, 1995). Induction of *waf1/cip1* expression in leukaemic and hepatoma cells in response to exposure to differentiation-inducing agents has also been demonstrated by Steinman *et al.* (1994).

The members of the MyoD family of basic helix–loop–helix transcription factors play an esssential role in myogenic cell differentiation and in the transcription of muscle-specific genes. The muscle differentiation model has been used to investigate the role of *waf1/cip1* in cell differentiation and the withdrawal of cells, committed to the path of differentiation, from the cell cycle. Terminal differentiation of a variety of cell types, e.g. skeletal muscle, skin, cartilage, etc., correlates with *waf1/cip1* gene expression (Parker *et al.*, 1995). Induction of waf1/cip1 protein and mRNA was seen during skeletal muscle differentiation, but in 10T1/2 fibroblasts this occurred only in those cells that had been transfected with MyoD, a skeletal muscle-specific transcription regulator. MyoD mediated induction of waf1/cip1 occurred independently of *p53*. Furthermore, transient transfection of cells with MyoD and induction of waf1/cip1 correlated with cell cycle arrest (Halevy *et al.*, 1995).

Is the *waf1/cip1* gene altered in cancer?

The *waf1/cip1* gene functions as a downstream target for the *p53* gene in its function of G_1-S transition control. As we have seen before, *waf1/cip* can function independently of *p53* to produce G_1 arrest and therefore can be regarded as a suppressor gene itself. Using this reasoning some attempts have been made to seek possible aberrations in *waf1/cip1* in human cancers. Marchetti *et al.* (1995c) investigated a large number of breast carcinomas, non-small cell lung tumours and ovarian adenocarcinomas for mutations in the gene. A polymorphism at codon 31 was seen in a small proportion (16 out of 183) of cancers and no mutations were encountered in the *waf1/cip1* open reading frame. Polymorphism of codon 31 has also been reported in colorectal cancer and somatic mutations have not been found in codons 9 through 139 that were screened (Li YJ *et al.*, 1995). Multiple polymorphisms were seen in human brain tumours, most frequently of codon 31 – again there were no somatic mutations (Koopmann *et al.*, 1995). Codon 31 polymorphism occurs also in normal individuals (Li YJ *et al.*, 1995; Marchetti *et al.*, 1995c) and, in the brain tumour study, the polymorphisms did not relate to histological type (Koopmann *et al.*, 1995). Jung *et al.* (1995b) also investigated gliomas for *waf1/cip1* abnormalities. Surprisingly, waf1/cip1 protein levels were low in normal brain tissue and in reactive gliosis, but were highly elevated in gliomas irrespective of grade. Glioblastoma multiforme showed elevated protein levels, in tumour samples carrying either wild-type or mutated *p53*. No elevation of protein occurred in anaplastic astrocytomas carrying mutant *p53*. Jung *et al.* (1995b) also stated that *waf1/cip1* gene is not deleted in gliomas. The observations of enhanced gene expression in gliomas irrespective of grade is somewhat incongruous since glioma grading closely reflects the enhanced degrees of proliferative capacity and loss of differentiation. In support of this apparent incongruity one should cite the observations of Barboule *et al.* (1995), who found no correlation between proliferation index and levels of *waf1/cip1* expression in ovarian carcinomas. Jung *et al.* (1995b) have argued, however, that in their study over-expression of waf1/cip1 did not completely inhibit cdk activity. It would appear that cdk inhibition is stoichiometrically regulated, only when waf1/cip1 occurs in molar excess. In other words, when its levels are below stoichiometric parity, there is no inhibition (Zhang *et al.*, 1994; Harper *et al.*, 1995). There may be interference on account of growth factors, such as PDGF, which are present in gliomas. Conceptually, why a putative suppressor gene might be upregulated in these tumours in response to mitogenic growth factors is a conundrum, but mitogen-activated protein kinases have been evoked in the transcriptional activation of the *waf1/cip1* gene (Liu *et al.*, 1996). Somatic mutations have been reported in three (out of 18) primary prostate cancers, whereas none was found in matched normal tissues (Gao *et al.*, 1995a). Nonetheless, the overall assessment at this point is that aberrations of this gene may not be associated with the neoplastic changes.

Response of *kip1/kip2* genes to antiproliferative signals

Extraneous signals such as cell-cell contact and those imparted to the cell by antiproliferative growth factors, such as TGF-β, arrest cells in the G_1 phase, and it follows therefore that the transduction of these signals might affect the expression of cdk inhibitors which appear to exert a regulatory effect on cell proliferation.

TGF-β represents a family of peptides which regulate growth and differentiation. It is composed of two identical 25 kDa dimers containing 112 amino acid residues. Several isoforms of TGF-β have been described (Massague, 1987, 1990; Sporn *et al.*, 1987; Roberts and Sporn, 1990). TGF peptides are multifunctional. They inhibit growth in a variety of cell types, such as epithelial, endothelial and haemopoietic cells and also in keratinocytes, lymphocytes and hepatocytes (Sporn and Roberts, 1987, 1988; Roberts and Sporn, 1990). The mechanism by which TGF-β brings about growth inhibition involves cdk inhibitors. Accumulation of kip1 occurs in mammalian cells as a result of exposure to antiproliferative agents such as TGF-β. It was recognised some time ago that the inhibitory effects of TGF-β were related to the inhibition of phosphorylation and the accumulation of unphosphorylated rb protein (Ewen et al. 1993b; Koff et al., 1993). This has led to the suggestion that cyclin dependent kinases might be involved in bringing about the inhibition of cell proliferation. The antiproliferative effect of this growth factor is not restricted to kip1, and indeed, it has been shown that TGF-β also enhances waf1/cip1 and p15/ink4B protein levels (Hannon and Beach, 1994; Datto et al., 1995b; Reynisdottir et al., 1995). Contact inhibition of cell proliferation also seems to involve cdks, as shown by Polyak et al., 1994a,b); they found that a 27 kDa protein (kip1) which binds to and inhibits cyclin E-cdk complexes can be isolated from contact-inhibited and TGF-β-arrested cells but not from proliferating cells.

Macrophages exposed to mitogenic stimulation by colony stimulating factor 1, show G_1 arrest upon cyclic-AMP treatment, and this block of proliferation is associated with an increase in kip1 (Kato et al., 1994). Another instance is that of TPA which inhibits the growth of malignant melanoma cells and blocks G_1-S and G_2-M transitions. In this tumour model, Coppock et al. (1995) found high levels of wap1/cip1 and kip1 in G_1 cells and these levels dropped as the cells entered the S-phase. This drop in the level of the cdk inhibitors could be prevented by treating the cells with TPA. Similarly, an increase in the levels of kip1 and waf1/cip1 has been observed in the inhibition of proliferation of MCF-7 breast carcinoma cells (Watts et al., 1995). Interferon, which is a powerful antiproliferative agent causes G_1 arrest of Daudi–Burkitt lymphoma cells, increases kip1 expression, but does not appear to affect waf1/cip1 (Yamada H et al., 1995a). Conversely, cdk inhibitors are inactivated by mitogenic signals. Proliferation of human T-lymphocytes depends upon two mitogenic signals. The first signal, provided by the T-cell antigen receptor stimulation, causes the induction of the appropriate cyclins and cdks, but activation of the kinases does not occur owing to the presence of kip1. Interleukin-2 provides the second signal which facilitates G_1-S transition by inactivating kip1 (Firpo et al., 1994; Nourse et al., 1994). kip2 shows tissue-specific expression and is found predominantly in differentiated cell types and kip2 mRNA patterns may be related to embryonic development (Lee et al., 1995; Matsuoka et al., 1995). Therefore kip2 and, indeed also waf1/cip1, may serve as a signal to differentiating cells to exit from the cell cycle.

kip1 gene expression in neoplasia

The kip1 and kip2 proteins have been regarded as potential suppressors of tumorigenicity, by virtue of their ability to regulate the entry of cell into the S-phase through the inhibition of cdk phosphorylation and consequent inhibition of phosphorylation of rb protein. Inevitably therefore there have been some attempts to see if any abnormalities occur in the kip genes in human cancers. These early studies do not suggest the involvement of these genes in the pathogenesis of cancers. Poncecastaneda *et al.* (1995) investigated a large number of human primary solid tumours and detected no mutations in the *kip1* gene. Kawamata *et al.* (1995) also examined a large number of human cancers (432 cases) and cancer cell lines but failed to find any aberrations associated with the *kip1* gene.

There are a few studies in haemopoietic malignancies which have suggested some alterations in *kip1*. A non-sense mutation that can result in the production of truncated kip1 protein has been reported in codon 76 in one out of 42 cases of adult T-cell leukaemia/ lymphoma (ATL), but is not in matched normal tissue. Some polymorphisms have also been identified in non-Hodgkin's lymphoma. One non-Hodgkin's lymphoma and one ATL showed homozygous deletion of *kip1* (Morosetti *et al.*, 1995). Loss of heterozygosity has been detected in acute lymphoblastic leukaemia (ALL) but in none of these cases had inactivation of the second allele occurred (Cave *et al.*, 1995). Pietenpol *et al.* (1995) have also not found any mutations of *kip1*. It must be recognised, however, that deletions of this region (chromosome 12p12-13) do occur in leukaemias in a small proportion of childhood ALL and possibly other genes occurring at this location may be involved. The *tel* gene (an *ets* family gene coding for transcription factors) is located approximately 1-2 Mbp telomeric from *kip1* (Sato *et al.*, 1995). Stegmaier *et al.* (1995) found loss of heterozygosity at the *tel* gene locus in 15% of informative cases. Allelic loss on chromosome 12, not involving *kip1*, has been reported also by Takeuchi S *et al.* (1995).

Polymorphisms relating to *kip1* G → A transition at codon 109 in one case and T → G transversion in 26% of breast cancer DNA samples and 31 out of 80 normal individuals were detected by Ferrando *et al.* (1996), but they found no somatic mutations of the gene. These initial studies, albeit a few in number, suggest that *kip1* alterations may be rare events in the pathogenesis of cancer. There are no studies on the involvement of *kip2*. But Matsuoka *et al.* (1995) point out that *kip2* region of the human chromosome may be involved in sporadic and with the familial cancer syndrome - the Beckwith-Wiedemann syndrome.

p16/ink4 putative multiple tumour suppressor gene in tumour development and progression

We have seen above how the p21/*waf1*, a powerful inhibitor of cyclin-dependent kinases induced by p53, is involved in cell cycle progression. Recently, the *p16/ink4* and the closely related *p15/ink4b* genes which code for an inhibitor of cyclin-dependent kinases, have been cloned. The product of this gene negatively regulates cell cycle traverse and has been reported to function as a tumour suppressor gene. A suggested mechanism of action of p16/ink4 is by repression of E2F transcription factor. The latter regulates the E2F promoter of adenovirus 5 (Kovesdi *et al.*, 1986) and E2F protein-binding sites have been found in several genes, such as the B-*myb* (Lam and Watson, 1993) and the dihydrofolate reductase gene (Means *et al.*, 1992), which are known to be associated with cell cycle progression. It is also known that the underphosphorylated form of rb protein binds to E2F transcription factor and represses its function (Hiebert et al., 1992; Zamanian and La Thangue, 1992) leading to suppression of growth. Phosphorylation of rb protein by cyclin D1-dependent kinase will activate E2F and its target genes and remove the block on cell proliferation; inhibition of this kinase by p16/ink4 will re-impose rb-mediated control of cell cycle progression (see Figure 10, page 54).

This putative suppressor gene (p16/ink4) is located on chromosome 9p21 (Kamb et al., 1994; Marx, 1994a,b; Nobori et al., 1994) and both homo and heterozygous deletions involving this region as well as point mutations have been reported in a variety of human cancers, providing evidence for its function as a classical tumour suppressor gene.

Kamb et al. (1994) reported that homozygous deletions of p16/ink4 occurred at high frequencies in cell lines derived from a wide variety of human tumours. Somatic mutations and homozygous deletions were reported to occur at a high frequency in solid tumours, e.g. pancreatic adenocarcinomas (85%) (Caldas et al., 1994), human non-small cell lung carcinomas (30%) (Hayashi et al., 1994), oesophageal carcinomas (52%) (Mori et al., 1994). Deletion of the gene was reported in 80% of human astrocytoma cell lines and deletion mapping demonstrated allelic loss of chromosome 9p in 15 out of 30 astrocytomas. However, direct analysis of p16/ink4 itself revealed only a single missense mutation in a high-grade tumour that had lost the second allele (Ueki et al., 1994). In primary breast cancers also, no mutations of the gene have been found, although one in five tumour cell lines has shown homozygous deletion (Xu et al., 1994). In haematological malignancies also the initial reports of its deletions at high frequency have not been borne out by subsequent studies. Thus initially, Hebert et al. (1994) found homozygous deletions of p16/ink4 in 20 out of 24 and of p15/ink4b in 16 out of 24 T-cell acute lymphoblastic leukaemia (ALL) but only one out of 31 ALL of B-cell lineage. Duro et al. (1994) also reported similar results for T-ALL; they found that such deletions were far less frequent in lymphomas. In acute paediatric lymphoblastic leukaemia homozygous deletions of both ink4 and ink4b have been found (Okuda et al., 1994). A study by Guidat et al. (1994) of a series of 60 consecutive childhood primary ALL has suggested that the frequency of p16/ink4 alterations may be far lower than originally believed.

There are two important points which need to be taken into account while considering the significance of chromosome 9p deletions. One is the possibility that deletions may involve not only chromosome 9p p16/ink4 genes but also flanking genes (Miller et al., 1994; Silly et al., 1994; Ueki et al., 1994). It is unclear from these early studies whether there have been mutations of other cell cycle controlling genes such as p53 and rb. Inactivation of these genes has been reported, together with molecular abnormalities of p16/ink4 (Caldas et al., 1994; Miller et al., 1994). This putative suppressor gene does not appear to be deleted in cellular transformation produced by viruses. At present it may be premature to attempt to assess how critical the changes in this gene are in tumour development and progression.

Heat shock proteins in development, differentiation and tumorigenesis

Heat shock proteins (HSPs) constitute a family of proteins which are induced in the cell in response to exposure to environmental stress such as increase in temperature, and exposure to heavy metals, toxins, bacterial and viral infections (Table 4). These proteins are generally known as heat shock proteins because they were first discovered in *Drosophila* cells exposed to heat shock (Tissieres *et al.*, 1974). The ubiquitous nature of the response across the species barrier (Fink and Zeuther, 1978; Kelly and Schlesinger, 1978; Lemaux *et al.*, 1978; Yamamori *et al.*, 1978) has suggested a common mechanism by which cells cope with environmental stress. Viral and certain environmental factors have been regarded as the aetiological agents in carcinogenesis, therefore the study of heat shock proteins has assumed some significance in the context of tumorigenesis and cell proliferation. HSPs are known to associate with microtubules and participate in their assembly (Gupta, 1990). Furthermore, there is much evidence that exposure of cells to heat shock disrupts cytoskeletal organisation and affects cytoskeletal components such as actin filaments, intermediate filaments and microtubules (Coss *et al.*, 1982; Lin *et al.*, 1982; Welch and Suhan, 1985). The disruptive effects of heat shock on these cytoskeletal elements may be seen as alterations in cellular morphology (Wiegant *et al.*, 1987). Such a disruption of cytoskeletal integrity may also bring in its wake changes in the proliferative and invasive behaviour of cells.

The HSP family is made up of several members which are known by the molecular weights of their component subunits, e.g. as HSP15-30, HSP70, HSP90, and ubiquitin which, in

Table 4.   Heat shock proteins in normal and aberrant cell physiology

Environmental signals	*Physiological functions*
Heat shock	Protein transport
Viral agents	Protein folding/assembly
Heavy metals	Protein stabilisation
Toxins	Protein ubiquitination
Oxidants	Embryonic development
	Cell differentiation
	Modulation of cell morphology
Cell cycle related target genes	Cell mobility?
p53	Polymerisation of tubulin
rb	DNA repair
18A2/mts1	Hormone receptor transformation

(Based on literature cited in the text)

comparison with other members of this family, is a small protein of 8 kDa. The high molecular weight isoforms are highly conserved (Ingolia *et al.*, 1982; Voellmy *et al.*, 1982; Hacket and Lis, 1983; Hunt and Morimoto, 1985; Rochester *et al.*, 1986). The low molecular weight HSPs are less highly conserved but much homology is seen between members from different species, although ubiquitin itself is a highly conserved protein (Bond and Schlesinger, 1985, 1986; Finley and Varshavsky, 1985; Finley *et al.*, 1987; Ozkaynak *et al.*, 1987).

Functions of HSPs

HSPs have been referred to as molecular chaperones in the light of the role they play in the regulation of protein synthesis, and in the folding, assembly and transport of proteins (reviewed by Pechan, 1991; Craig, 1993; Hendrick and Hartl, 1993). HSPs may also subserve the function of stabilising cellular proteins and thereby preventing their degradation (Munro and Pelham, 1984; Pechan, 1991). Conversely, the proteolysis of polypeptides is mediated by ubiquitin, which has been identified as a heat shock protein (Bond and Schlesinger, 1985). Ubiquitin is activated by ATP at the *C*-terminal glycine and this activation results in the process described as ubiquitination which involves the attachment of ubiquitin to the ε-lysine groups of proteins and these then become targets for proteolysis. The importance of these proteins in the control of cell proliferation has been greatly enhanced by their ability to function as molecular chaperones, and their role in stabilising and or ubiquitinating certain cell cycle related nuclear proteins such as p53, c-myc, E1A, c-fos, etc. These proteins appear to be specific targets for ubiquitin-mediated proteolysis *in vitro* (Ciechanover *et al.*, 1991) and possibly also their intracellular degradation. Conversely, p53 may be stabilised and its half-life substantially increased by HSPs.

HSPs in embryonic development and differentiation

HSPs are a group of developmentally regulated proteins. Changes in the pattern of HSP gene expression has been reported during yeast sporulation (Kurtz and Linquist, 1984). They show a defined spatial and temporal expression pattern in *Drosophila* development (Mason *et al.*, 1984; Glaser *et al.*, 1986; Kurtz *et al.*, 1986; Palter *et al.*, 1986). Response to thermal stress appears to be dependent upon developmental stage in early embryonic development of *Xenopus*. The induction of HSPs in response to heat shock is seen in *Xenopus* oocytes but this ceases upon fertilisation (Browder *et al.*, 1987), although HSP induction occurs again in the neurula stage embryos (Nickells and Browder, 1985; Heikkila *et al.*, 1987). The HSP isoforms also appear to be differentially regulated with development (Bienz, 1984; Krone and Heikkila, 1988). This raises the question whether the regulation of these isoforms might be cell type specific. This has been shown to be the case in *Xenopus* oocytes. Bienz (1984) showed that HSP30 gene injected into oocytes was strongly heat-inducible. In contrast, HSP70 gene was found to be expressed at the normal temperature, i.e. constitutively expressed. This could not be increased by heat shock. Mouse embryos at the two-cell cleavage stage constitutively express HSP70 subtype proteins (Bensaude *et al.*, 1983) and some of these may continue to be synthesised up to the eight-cell stage (Bensaude and Morange, 1983; Hahnel *et al.*, 1986). There are also indications of possible presumptive tissue- or lineage-specific synthesis of HSPs (Kothary *et al.*, 1987). A differential expression of HSPs also occurs in erythroid differentiation (Banerji *et al.*, 1984; Morimoto and Fodor, 1984).

HSPs are cell cycle regulated proteins

The past few years have seen an accumulation of evidence that HSPs are closely associated with the growth phase of cells. Serum, mitogen or growth factor-mediated stimulation of growth results in the synthesis of HSPs and it has been suggested that HSP70 expression may be linked with DNA synthesis (Wu and Morimoto, 1985; Ferris *et al.*, 1988). Milarski and Morimoto (1986) found that HSP70 expression may be regulated at the G_1-S transition of cells. Pechan (1991) has further pointed out the occurrence of sequence homologies between HSPs and cyclin dependent kinase promoters. The yeast cyclin-dependent kinase cdc25 shares 76% sequence homology over a 42 base region with HSP22 of *Drosophila* and 79% homology over a 19 base sequence with HSP70 of *Xenopus* (Southgate *et al.*, 1983; Camonis *et al.*, 1986) in the promoter regions. The DnaK gene of *Escherichia coli*, which is required for lambda DNA replication, codes for a protein which shows 50% amino acid sequence homology with human HSP70 (Zylicz *et al.*, 1983, 1984; Liberek *et al.*, 1988; Sakakibara, 1988).

Interaction of p53 with HSPs

The phosphoprotein p53, as we have discussed previously, is able to regulate the G_1-S transition in the cell cycle. It would appear that p53 is involved, together with HSPs, in a regulatory loop with several genes whose expression is required for cell proliferation. Thus, p53 protein down-regulates the activity of the promoters of several genes, prominent among these are promoters of c-*fos* and c-*jun*, the immediate early response genes, and also the β-actin gene and the HSP70 gene (Ginsberg *et al.*, 1991). The oncoproteins c-myc and E1A also stimulate the HSP70 promoter (Wu *et al.*, 1986; Kaddurah-Daouk *et al.*, 1987) and E1A is also known to enhance transcription of *p53* (Braithwaite *et al.*, 1990). Wild-type p53 can down-regulate the HSP70 promoter (Agoff *et al.*, 1993), but mutant p53 causes transactivation of HSP promoter (Tsutsumiishii *et al.*, 1995). The transcriptional regulation of HSP genes is mediated by *cis*-acting element, known as the heat shock element (HSE). HSE occurs upstream of the

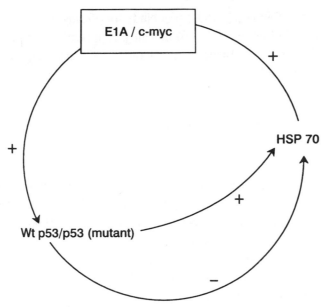

Figure 12. The possible involvement of heat shock proteins in the control of cell cycle progression by p53 is presented here, albeit based on circumstantial evidence. Wild-type p53 down-regulates and mutant p53 up-regulates HSP70 expression. The oncoprotein E1A is also known to be able to stimulate HSP70 promoter as well as enhance p53 transcription. Based on sources cited in the text.

transcription start site and has a defined nucleotide sequence consisting of two or three modules composed of alternately arranged GAA or TTC blocks at 2-nucleotide intervals (Amin *et al.*, 1988). Tsutsumiishii *et al.* (1995) showed that the HSE responds to mutant p53 protein. Further support for the view that wild-type p53 negatively regulates HSP70 comes from studies of He *et al.* (1995) using embryonic fibroblasts derived from p53-deficient transgenic mice. These authors found that cells with p53−/− phenotype contained 1000-fold more HSP70 than cells with p53+/+ phenotype, and the p53 null cells grew three- to fourfold faster than the p53+/+ cells. Thus, HSPs appear to be integrated with wild-type 53 or mutant p53 and oncogenic proteins such as c-myc and E1A in the machinery that controls cell cycle progression (Figure 12).

    The implication of HSPs in cell proliferation has been strengthened by several reports of the binding of HSPs or cognate proteins often referred to as heat shock cognate (HSCs) proteins with p53. We have discussed previously the significance of the formation of complexes between p53 and cellular proteins in the inactivation or sequestration of p53 that leads to a suppression of its negative control over cell cycle progression. The mutant inactivated form of p53 exerts no such suppressor control. It has been found to bind HSP70 subtype proteins (Pinhasi-Kimhi *et al.*, 1986; Sturzbecher *et al.*, 1987; Clarke *et al.*, 1988; Finlay *et al.*, 1988). Matsumoto *et al.* (1994) have recently reported the co-precipitation of wild-type p53 with

HSP72/73. According to Nihei *et al.* (1993) p53 binds specifically to HSP73, but in the rodent system studied by Pinhasi-Kimhi *et al.* (1986) mutant p53 appeared to bind to HSP70 (HSC68) and to another 90 kDa protein. Hainaut and Milner (1992) also suggest specific complex formation of mutant p53 protein with HSP70.

rb protein and HSPs in cell proliferation

Interaction between the retinoblastoma-susceptibility gene (*rb*) encoded protein, which is another negative regulator of cell cycle progression, and HSP70 has also been demonstrated. The HSP-binding site on the rb protein has been determined to be residues 373–579 (Inoue *et al.*, 1995). Of further interest is the observation by these investigators that the binding of HSP to rb protein is inhibited by phosphorylation. Binding of HSPs to the underphosphorylated form of rb would allow the cells to enter the S-phase of the cell cycle. Once again, this demonstrates the involvement of HSPs in cell cycle progression.

18A2/mts1 protein and HSPs in cell proliferation

Another cellular protein which appears to be associated concomitantly with both cell cycle progression and HSPs, is the 18A2/mts1 protein, a Ca^{2+}-binding protein which is associated with the invasive and metastatic behaviour of cancer cells (see page 191). The cell cycle related expression of the 18A2/mts1 protein is now well documented. A high level of expression of *18A2/mts1* is invariably associated with large S-phase fractions in murine and in human carcinoma cells (Parker *et al.*, 1994a; Sherbet *et al.*, 1995). Parker *et al.* (1994b) have further demonstrated, by means of gene transfer technology, that switching on the exogenous *18A2/ mts1* in B16 murine melanoma cells induces them to undergo G_1-S transition, and it also appears to control the cell cycle traverse. In parallel, these studies have revealed an increase in the detectability of p53 protein (Parker *et al.*, 1994a,b), suggesting that G_1-S transition may be induced by the sequestration of p53. The concomitant involvement of HSPs in this putative p53/ 18A2/mts1-mediated mechanism has emerged from the studies of Cajone *et al.* (1994) who have demonstrated that exposure of B16-BL6 melanoma cells to heat shock down-regulates the *18A2/mts* gene and, further, that in the heat-resistant derivative cell line HTG of the B16-BL6 melanoma, the gene is constitutively down-regulated. In both heat-shocked cells and the heat-resistant cells significant changes occur in the pattern of expression of the high molecular weight proteins (Cajone *et al.*, 1994). The heat-resistant HTG variant cells show a three- to four-fold enhancement in the expression of HSP28 and a marked reduction in the S-phase fraction (Sherbet *et al.*, 1996). These experiments suggest that HSP28 may be associated with inhibition of cell proliferation. This proliferation inhibitory property of HSP28 has been recorded before.

For instance, HSP28 is highly expressed in quiescent keratinocytes compared with their proliferating counterparts (Honore *et al.*, 1994). In mitogen-stimulated human B lymphocytes HSP28 induction coincides with peak proliferation and the onset of arrest of growth (Spector *et al.*, 1992). HSP28 appears to be regulated in human leukaemic HL-60 cells when they are induced to differentiate by retinoic acid, since a transient increase of HSP28 levels occurs upon exposure to retinoic acid with concomitant G_1 arrest (Spector *et al.*, 1994). The expression of HSP27 is related to the state of differentiation in cervical cancer and its expression in breast cancer is considered to be an indicator of good prognosis (see Ciocca *et al.*, 1993). Thus, a spectrum of studies supports the view that HSP28 is associated with inhibition of cell proliferation.

Alterations in HSP28 are not simply restricted to changes in their levels, but also involve the state of its phosphorylation; it appears to be phosphorylated prior to growth inhibition. When HL-60 cells are induced to differentiate by the phorbol 12-myristate 13-acetate (PMA), HSP28 becomes rapidly phosphorylated and this precedes the increase in its levels (Spector *et al.*, 1993). PMA is an activator of protein kinase C. TGF-β1, which is a growth inhibitor, increases HSP28 phosphorylation in the G_1 phase of the cell cycle when the cells are susceptible to growth inhibition by this factor. TNF also induces a rapid increase in HSP28 phosphorylation (Vietor and Vilcek, 1994). Growth stimulatory agents such as the epidermal growth factor TPA etc., do not affect HSP28 phosphorylation status (Shibanuma *et al.*, 1992). This suggests that phosphorylation might activate the growth inhibitory function of HSP28, just as protein ubiquitination requires the phosphorylation of ubiquitin.

The studies discussed above suggest the possibility that the 18A2/mts1 protein, p53 and HSPs may all be involved in a coordinated fashion in the control of the transition of the cells from G_1 to the S phase. The implication that HSPs may be targeting the products of cell cycle control genes should not detract from its involvement with the regulation of growth response of cells to glucocorticoid and steroid hormones. HSPs are known to modify the activity of the receptors for both these classes of hormones. The high molecular weight HSPs form complexes with these receptors (Sanchez *et al.*, 1990; Wilhelmsson *et al.*, 1990). The receptors dissociate from HSPs before binding to DNA. Thus, HSPs could be transforming these receptors for binding to DNA. The precise nature of this transformation is unclear but these receptors are in the phosphoryl-ated form and the transformation and binding to DNA seems to require their dephosphorylation (Sanchez *et al.*, 1990).

HSPs in cancer and their possible relevance to prognosis

Heat shock proteins have been reported to exert a marked suppressive effect on cellular transformation. The suppressive effect could be a consequence of the formation of complexes between HSP and the transforming agents. For instance, transfection of HSP70 into cells transformed by mutant p53 and ras/myc oncogenes suppresses the process of transformation

(Yehiely and Oren, 1992). Complex formation between p53 and HSPs has also been shown to occur in several human tumours. Davidoff *et al.* (1992) demonstrated p53/HSP70 complexes in breast cancer. The tumours investigated in this series have been described as primary invasive breast carcinomas. Unfortunately, no information is available from this study by Davidoff *et al.* (1992) about the relationship between the detection of these complexes and the invasive nature of the carcinomas. Perhaps the value of this approach may be diminished because Iwaya *et al.* (1995) state that only a part of the p53 pool may enter into complex formation with HSPs. Nevertheless, it is noteworthy that the expression of HSP correlated positively with oestrogen receptor expression and inversely with epidermal growth factor receptor expression (Takahashi *et al.*, 1994). This suggests that changes in HSP expression could be one of the events associated with the progression of breast cancer. Elledge *et al.* (1994) did not note any correlation between HSP detection and accumulation of p53. But patients with p53−/HSP+ tumours showed better overall survival than those with p53−/HSP− tumours.

HSP expression has also been examined in other forms of human cancer. The expression of high molelcular weight (60-90 kDa) HSP levels are said to be significantly higher in circulating cells of patients with acute myeloid leukaemia than in cells from patients with chronic myeloid leukaemia, and in both these cases HSP levels were higher than in mononuclear cells of normal peripheral blood (Chant *et al.*, 1995). The occurrence of high molecular weight HSPs has also been described in lung cancers (Bonay *et al.*, 1994). Prostate cancers have been reported to show positive cytoplasmic staining for both p53 and HSP72/73 (van Veldhuizen *et al.*, 1993). The median intensity of immunochemical staining for HSP70 did not differ markedly between oral squamous cell carcinoma, epithelial dysplasia and benign oral mucosal lesions (Sugerman *et al.*, 1995). In summation, it may be premature to judge the value of HSP expression as a marker of cancer progression and as a tool for predicting prognosis.

Postulated functions of HSP complexes

Several functions have been attributed to protein complexes involving heat shock proteins. The function of translocating proteins has been of particular interest with the implication that HSPs might ferry proteins across intracellular membranes and enable efficient antigen presentation for eliciting immunological responses (Chirico *et al.*, 1988; Deshaies *et al.*, 1988; van Buskirk *et al.*, 1991). This view is supported by the observation that wherever immune response to p53 was encountered in breast cancer patients p53 protein was found to be complexed with HSP70. In contrast, patients who had no detectable anti-p53 antibodies contained no p53/HSP70 complexes (Davidoff *et al.*, 1992). p53 protein is known to form complexes with SV40 large T antigen and tubulin and this may be an event associated with the intracellular translocation of these proteins (Maxwell *et al.*, 1991). Although p53/HSP complexes have not been proven to involve the translocation of p53 to the plasma membrane, this seems to be a possible explanation for the detection of higher anti-p53 antibody titres in patients where p53 occurs in a complex with HSP70.

HSPs may be involved in the translocation of cellular protein, which may be crucial in maintaining the integrity of cell shape, and in cell mobility and intercellular adhesion. HSP70, for instance, has been reported to bind to actin microfilaments (Tsang, 1993). It is also involved in the folding and dimerisation of tubulin (Paciucci, 1994). It has been suggested that proteins such as the 18A2/mts1 which appear to possess the property of promoting cytoskeletal depolymerisation may be recruited to the sites of microtubule assembly by HSPs (Sherbet and Lakshmi, 1997). This is supported by much circumstantial evidence. For example, S-100β, a Ca^{2+}-binding protein closely related to the 18A2/mts1 protein, also shows association with tubulin (Donato, 1991). HSP70 has a calmodulin-binding site and is known to form a complex with calmodulin (Stevenson and Calderwood, 1990). By anology with these proteins, it is conceivable that HSPs form complexes with 18A2/mts1 protein.

Weinberg (1991) has suggested a further function for the formation of p53–HSP complexes, that they may provide the machinery by which the aberrant p53 is trapped and rendered ineffective. HSP70 (HSC70) has, in fact, been reported to suppress transformation of rat embryo fibroblasts by mutant p53. However, HSP does not form complexes exclusively with mutant p53, although early studies may have suggested a selective, or even a preferential process (Hainaut and Milner, 1992). The C-terminal domain of p53 is essential for p53 oligomerisation (Milner et al., 1991) and it is also required for its interaction and binding with HSP which is dependent upon the tertiary structure of p53 (Hainaut and Milner, 1992).

6

Apoptosis in tumour growth and metastasis

Apoptosis or programmed cell death is a natural physiological phenomenon occurring in embryonic development, differentiation and morphogenesis. It represents a pathway of control of growth by a selective elimination of cells as distinct from the regulatory pathway of growth control. Apoptosis is also induced by exposure of cells to various agents and aberrant physiological conditions. Thus, apoptosis of thymocytes is induced by exposure to glucocorticoids (Caron-Leslie et al., 1991; Compton and Cidlowski, 1992), cytotoxic agents such as the topoisomerase-reactive drugs etoposide and teniposide (Walker et al., 1991; Onishi et al., 1993), gamma irradiation (Sellins and Cohen, 1987; Clarke et al., 1993, 1994) and hyperthermia (Sellins and Cohen, 1991a). Differentiation-inducing agents such as retinoids and sodium butyrate are known to induce apoptosis (Sadaie and Hager, 1994; Delia et al., 1995). Apoptotic changes are induced in target cells by cytotoxic T cells (Sellins and Cohen, 1991b; Cohen et al., 1992). The DNA fragmentation associated with apoptosis is a Ca^{2+}-dependent process (McConkey et al., 1989), and initial studies have claimed that calcium ionophores induce apoptosis and calcium chelators suppress it. However, this does not appear to be the case. For instance, in neutrophils, calcium ionophores suppress apoptosis but apoptosis is promoted by calcium chelators and the calmodulin-inhibitor W7 (Whyte et al., 1993). Kluck et al. (1994) also believe that enhanced intracellular Ca^{2+} levels are not involved in the induction of apoptosis.

The nature of apoptotic changes

Cells undergoing apoptosis display distinctive morphological changes involving the condensation of nuclear chromatin and shrinkage of the cytoplasm. The cells break up into apoptotic bodies comprising membrane-bound cell fragments. The apoptotic bodies are phagocytosed but not accompanied by an inflammatory response. This sharply distinguishes apoptosis from necrosis, which is characterised by cell swelling and rupture leading to a marked inflammatory response. The major biochemical feature of the apoptotic process is the fragmentation of nuclear DNA by Ca^{2+}-Mg^{2+}-dependent endonucleases which cleaves the DNA at internucleosomal sites. The fragmentation of the DNA is visualised in agarose gel electrophoresis by the ladder pattern of 180–200 bp oligomers (Wyllie, 1980, 1987, 1993; Cohen and Duke, 1984; Caron-Leslie et al., 1991). It has been recognised that nascent RNA and protein synthesis are often an important requirement of apoptosis and this has led to the suggestion that apoptosis is mediated by the activation of a genetic programme designed for a natural process of cell destruction (Montpetit et al., 1986; Ovens et al., 1991).

Genetic regulation of apoptosis

Several genes that are closely associated with cell proliferation and neoplastic development are also associated with the apoptotic pathway and this suggests that the regulation of these processes may be interlinked. It follows from this that deregulation of apoptosis may be expected to lead to tumorigenesis and further that deregulation of cell cycle control would sway the cells into apoptotic pathway. An appraisal of this complex scenario is attempted here by analysing the genetic regulation of apoptosis and assessing the interaction of the cell cycle control genes in these regulatory mechanisms.

bcl-2 *and related genes in the regulation of apoptosis*

The *bcl-2* gene was identified as an oncogene in follicular lymphoma associated with the chromosomal translocation occurring between chromosomes 18 and 14. The *bcl-2* gene occurs on chromosome 18q21 (Bakhshi et al., 1985; Cleary and Sklar, 1985; Tsujimoto et al., 1985a,b, 1987). Upon translocation this appears juxtaposed with the immunoglobulin heavy chain gene located on chromosome 14q32. Because the break point in chromosome 18 occurs in the 3'-untranslated region of the *bcl-2* gene, this translocation produces a *bcl-2/Ig* fusion gene. The t(14;18) translocation occurs in a vast majority of follicular lymphomas and, as a consequence of this translocation, there is an over-expression of *bcl-2* RNA and protein, even though the coding regions of the gene are unaltered (Cleary et al., 1986a,b; Graninger et al., 1987; Seto et al.,

1988). This is supposed to be the result of deregulation of the *bcl-2/Ig* fusion gene. But T-cell lymphomas which do not show this translocation do express bcl-2 protein (Pezzella *et al.*, 1990; Kondo *et al.*, 1992), albeit at a lower level than B-cell lymphomas (Zutter *et al.*, 1991). Therefore, there might be other mechanisms by which *bcl-2* expression is deregulated. Two bcl-2 proteins, bcl-2α and bcl-2β, produced by mRNA splicing have been identified (Seto *et al.*, 1988). The bcl-2 protein is associated with the inner and outer mitochondrial membranes (Hockenbery *et al.*, 1990; Monaghan *et al.*, 1992; Nakai *et al.*, 1993; Nguyen *et al.*, 1993a; Lithgow *et al.*, 1994). However, apoptosis can occur in human mutant cell lines that lack mitochondrial DNA and can be protected from apoptosis by an over-expression of bcl-2 protein. Apoptosis also occurs in anucleated cytoplasts and is prevented by bcl-2 over-expression (Jacobson *et al.*, 1993, 1994). This suggests that the bcl-2 protein may occur at several intracellular sites. It has since been found to be present in the nuclear membrane and the endoplasmic reticulum (Chen-Levy *et al.*, 1989; Alnemri *et al.*, 1992a; Monaghan *et al.*, 1992; Jacobson *et al.*, 1993; Lithgow *et al.*, 1994). The bcl-2 protein suppresses lipid peroxidation and its location may be related to its function as a suppressor of the generation of free radicals (Hockenbery *et al.*, 1993) and in this way it suppresses apoptotic cell death. The opposite view that bcl-2 acts as a pro-oxidant has been expressed by Steinman (1995). It is known that bcl-2-mediated apoptosis can occur under anaerobic conditions suggesting that reactive oxygen species are not required for apoptosis (Jacobson and Raff, 1995).

The bcl-2 appears to extend cell survival and inhibit apoptosis (Liu *et al.*, 1991; Strasser *et al.*, 1991; Borzillo *et al.*, 1992; Jacobson *et al.*, 1993). This appears to require the full-length bcl-2. The truncated form of the protein does not appear to be able to prolong cell survival (Alnemri *et al.*, 1992b). Expression of *bcl-2* extends the life span of memory B-lymphocytes and maintains long-term immune responsiveness (Nunez *et al.*, 1991). This gene is also expressed in cell types with characteristically long life spans. For example, neurones and haemopoietic stem cells and also stem cells of differentiating epithelia of skin and intestine show *bcl-2* expression. The gene is also involved in glandular epithelia where hyperplasia and involution are controlled by hormones. In most instances, gene expression is associated with zones of tissues containing cells with long life spans or proliferating cells (Hockenbery *et al.*, 1991). This suggests that its expression exerts a homeostatic effect on cell numbers. In contrast, apoptosis occurring during the involution and remodelling of the mammary gland is regulated by the induction of *bax* (bar) and bcl-x(S) proteins (Heermeier *et al.*, 1996). The induction of differentiation of leukaemic cells by interleukin-6 and dexamethasone differentially modulates the expression of several bcl-2 family genes (Lotem and Sachs, 1995).

A family of genes related to *bcl-2* have now been identified (Table 5). The protein products of these genes show high sequence homology within two high conserved domains called BH1 and BH2 (Yin *et al.*, 1994). The bax protein identified by Oltvai *et al.* (1993) is a 21 kDa protein possessing a high sequence homology to the bcl-2 protein. This protein forms homodimers and also heterodimers with bcl-2. Over-expression of this protein appears to promote apoptotic cell death and to counteract bcl-2 mediated inhibition of apoptosis. Substitution of an amino acid residue in the BH1 domain can interfere with heterodimer formation between the bax and bcl-2

Table 5.   The bcl-2 family of apoptosis related proteins

Protein nomenclature	References
Inhibitors of apoptosis (promoters of cell survival)	
bcl-2	Cleary *et al.* (1986a,b)
bcl-x(L)	Boise *et al.* (1993)
bcl-x(β)	Gonzalez-Garcia *et al.* (1995)
A1 (mouse)	Lin *et al.* (1993)
Promoters of apoptosis	
bcl-x(S)	Boise *et al.* (1993)
bad	Yang *et al.* (1995)
bak	Farrow *et al.* (1995)
bax	Oltvai *et al.* (1993), Craig (1995)

proteins and negates the normal bcl-2 function of inhibition of apoptosis (Yin *et al.*, 1994). It has been postulated that the relative levels of bax and bcl-2 proteins might define the pathway of survival or apoptosis and that the dimerisation between the different components is an essential event in the differential regulation of *bcl-2* function. The bax protein has been found to undergo selective dimerisation with other bcl-2 family proteins (Thomas *et al.*, 1995). Bcl-x(L) and Bcl-x(S) (see below) can themselves regulate cell survival and bcl-x(S) can counteract the apoptosis-inhibitory effect of bcl-x(L). However, *in vitro*, the binding of bcl-x(S) and bcl-x(L) is far weaker than to the bax protein (bar) (Minn *et al.*, 1996). On similar lines, selective dimerisation has been shown to occur between bcl-x(L) and another member of the bcl-2 family, namely the bad protein (Yang *et al.*, 1995). Thus, the bcl-2 family proteins show a wide spectrum of activity ranging from inhibition of cell apoptosis to promotion of the process of cell death. The formation of dimeric complex may provide a mechanism by which cell population homeostasis is finely controlled (see Craig, 1993; Thomas *et al.*, 1995). In other words, the nature of the competing proteins, the strength and the selectivity of their binding can produce a hierarchy of complexes with apoptotic function. These genes also may be differentially regulated, so that the relative levels of the proteins available for dimerisation will vary and thereby control and determine the degree of apoptosis. Among alternative mechanisms suggested is the loss of apoptosis suppressor function of bcl-2 due to enhanced phosphorylation. Agents which affect microtubule dynamics are believed to act in this way (Croce, 1997).

Boise *et al.* (1993) isolated another *bcl-2*-related gene, *bcl-x*, which also appears to be involved in the regulation of apoptosis. The bcl-x protein occurs in two forms, bcl-x(L) and bcl-x(S), by the alternative splicing of bcl-x mRNA. A third form of bcl-x protein, the bcl-x(β), has been described, which is produced from the unspliced bcl-x mRNA (Gonzalez-Garcia *et al.*, 1994). The bcl-x(L) protein can inhibit apoptosis and promote cell survival, whereas bcl-x(S) promotes apoptosis and counteracts bcl-2-mediated inhibition of apoptosis. This is compatible with the high bcl-x(L) mRNA levels found predominantly in cells which have a long life span, e.g. in neurones and adult CNS. In contrast, bcl-x(S) mRNA levels found in cell types which show a high turnover (Boise *et al.*, 1993; Gonzalez-Garcia *et al.*, 1995). Microinjection of bcl-x(L) and bcl-x(β) mRNA prevents the apoptosis of primary sympathetic neurones induced by the withdrawal of nerve growth factor (Gonzalez-Garcia *et al.*, 1995). Furthermore, transfection of *bcl-x(L)* gene into the interleukin-2-dependent CTTL-2 cells promotes their survival even in the absence of the cytokine (Boise *et al.*, 1996). Cells that over-express bcl-x(L) have been found to be resistant to apoptosis following DNA damage inflicted by chemotherapeutic agents (Minn *et al.*, 1995), but no differences in the expression of bcl-2, bcl-x or bar proteins have been encountered between drug-resistant and sensitive cell lines isolated from small cell and non-small cell lung cancers (Reeve *et al.*, 1996). The *ced-9* gene of *Caenorhabditis elegans* is an inhibitor of apoptosis (Hengartner *et al.*, 1992) and it codes for a protein which shows sequence similarities to the bcl-2 protein (Hengartner and Horvitz, 1994). Certain other members of the *bcl-2* family have also been found to function antagonistically to *bcl-2*, such as the *bak* (Farrow *et al.*, 1995) and *bad* (Yang *et al.*, 1995). The *bad* protein bears sequence homology to the BH1 and BH2 domains of bcl-2 protein and dimerise selectively with bcl-2 and bcl-x(L) proteins. It is obviously involved in the regulation of the apoptosis inhibitory function of the bcl-x(L)/bax protein complex. It can displace the bax protein and restore apoptosis (Yang *et al.*, 1995).

Regulation of bcl-2 *gene expression by* p53

The wide spectrum of biological processes that encompass cell differentiation, morphogenesis and growth show an absolute dependence on reaching a homeostasis in the kinetics of cell population expansion. This can be accomplished either by regulation of cell growth, or by the regulation of apoptotic loss of cells, or by a combination of both. The deregulation of these mechanisms leads to the population expansion which characterises tumour growth and the development of overt metastasis. The size of the primary tumour is an important parameter which relates to its biological behaviour. If the cell growth within a metastatic deposit were to remain under impeccable control, that secondary deposit would remain dormant. The appearance of these deposits as overt distant neoplasms may depend upon stimulation of cell proliferation by growth factor signals. Equally, overt metastasis can appear if population kinetics were perturbed by deregulation of apoptotic loss of cells. The demonstration that genes controlling the cell cycle are involved in the pathogenesis of a vast majority of cancers and the association of *bcl-2* family genes with a wide variety of human tumours has suggested that the operation of a mechanism which co-ordinates their function may be inherent in biological systems. Therefore, the cell cycle control genes have been a natural target of attention and, fittingly, investigation of whether they regulate the expression of the apoptosis genes.

The suppressor gene *p53* not only controls the transition of cells from the G_1 to the S-phase of the cell cycle, but it is also capable of inducing apoptosis. Yonish-Rouach *et al.* (1991) demonstrated some years ago that introduction of wild-type *p53* into a murine myeloid cell line lacking normal p53 function induced their apoptosis. Shaw *et al.* (1992) transfected wild-type *p53* gene under the control of the metallothionein MT-1 promoter. Switching on the transfected gene using zinc chloride produced DNA fragmentation and laddering characteristic of apoptosis. The *p53*-induced apoptosis was inhibited by interleukin-6 (Yonish-Rouach *et al.*, 1993), which suggests that the induction of apoptosis was a function of *p53* quite distinct from its ability to regulate the cell cycle. It is possible that the function of p53 as a sequence-specific transcription factor can be modulated causing a reduction or inhibition of p53-mediated apoptosis without affecting the ability to control the cell cycle progression. The presence of *p53* is essential for radiation-induced apoptosis of mouse thymocytes. Immature thymocytes lacking *p53* are resistant to ionising radiation (Clarke *et al.*, 1993; Lowe *et al.*, 1993). The adenovirus E1A protein stabilises and induces high levels of p53 and causes a loss of cell viability by a process akin to apoptosis (Lowe and Ruley, 1993). The E1B protein, on the other hand, blocks E1A-induced apoptosis bringing p53 protein to normal levels (Rao *et al.*, 1992; Lowe and Ruley, 1993). Human cervical cancer cell lines with low *p53* expression have been experiment-ally infected with adenovirus carrying the wild-type *p53* gene. These infected cells were found to undergo apoptosis and greatly reduced cell growth compared with cells not infected with the adenoviral vector (Hamada *et al.*, 1996). In nasopharyngeal carcinoma *p53* expression inversely correlates with *bcl-2* expression (Harn *et al.*, 1996). Therefore, the expression of *p53* does seem to be able to influence that of *bcl-2* family genes. However, apoptosis can also occur independently of *p53*. Mouse thymocytes that are p53-deficient are susceptible to apoptosis upon exposure to glucocorticoids (Clarke *et al.*, 1993; Lowe *et al.*, 1993). The apoptotic process set in motion in prostatic glandular cells by the ablation of androgen does not require *p53* (Berges *et al.*, 1993). The topoisomerase II inhibitor etoposide and Ca^{2+} ionophores also induce apoptosis in the absence of *p53* (Clarke *et al.*, 1993). These experiments suggest the possibility that the *p53*-mediated pathway to apoptosis is adopted only where DNA damage in the form of strand breaks might have occurred (Clarke *et al.*, 1994). The induction of *p53* expression is a response to DNA damage so that the cell does not traverse in the cycle into the S-phase before it can repair the DNA damage and at this juncture the cells which have sustained extensive and irreparable DNA damage can be selectively destroyed by apopotosis. Consistent with this is the observation that mutant p53 is unable to induce apoptosis (Lotem and Sachs, 1993). Furthermore, Wang *et al.* (1996) have shown that human papilloma virus (HPV)-16 E7 protein is able to prevent G_1 arrest induced by wild-type *p53* but did not affect the degree of *p53*-induced apoptosis.

It is becoming increasingly evident that p53 may be functioning as a transcription factor in the mediation of apoptosis. Impairment of this function does affect *p53*-mediated apoptosis (Roemer and Mueller-Lantzsch, 1996). There has also been elegant demonstration of this by using temperature-sensitive *p53* mutants. M1 myeloid leukaemia cells that do not express endogenous p53 have been transfected with a temperature-sensitive *p53* mutant (Selvakumaran *et al.*, 1994a).

They found that apoptosis is induced when wild-type *p53* expression is induced at the permissive temperature of 32.5°C and the kinetics of induction of apoptosis by *p53* expression is far more rapid than that induced by transforming growth factor (TGF)-β. Both wild-type *p53* expression and TGF-β down-regulated the expression of bcl-2 protein, and *p53* alone up-regulated bax protein expression in the cells. Miyashita *et al.* (1994) have also demonstrated the down-regulation of *bcl-2* and up-regulation of *bax* expression at the mRNA and at the protein level by wild-type *p53*. This suggests that *p53* and TGF-β induce apoptosis by two distinct pathways, although TGF-β mediated apoptosis may still operate through genes such as *GADD45* and *Myd118*, which may be seen as downstream effectors of p53 function. Selvakumaran *et al.* (1994b) have, in fact, demonstrated that *Myd118* does influence TGF-β induced apoptosis. Transcription of the *bax* gene may be directly activated by p53, but over-expression of bax protein alone is insufficient to drive the cells to the apoptotic pathway (Brady *et al.*, 1996).

The involvement of p53 as a transcription factor in mediating apoptosis is supported by the observation that mdm2 protein can counteract p53-mediated apoptosis (Chen *et al.*, 1996; Haupt *et al.*, 1996). The protective effect of mdm2 is seen only when mdm2/p53 complexes are formed, which suggests that abrogation of apoptosis is usually a consequence of the abolition of the transcription factor function of p53.

Induction of apoptosis by myc and ras oncogenes

The proliferative response produced by cells to growth factor stimuli is a normal physiological event. However, deregulation of cell proliferation in the absence of such stimuli may induce apoptosis under certain conditions (Green *et al.*, 1996). The withdrawal of cytokines from cells dependent upon them for normal proliferation initiates an apoptotic cell loss which is prevented by the over-expression of *bcl-2* (Hockenbery *et al.*, 1990; Nunez *et al.*, 1990). The *myc* and *ras* oncogenes promote cell proliferation in the presence of growth factors, but in their absence the cells undergo apoptosis (Evan *et al.*, 1992; Wyllie, 1993; Tanaka *et al.*, 1994). Wyllie (1993) has argued that the *myc* oncogene has a dual function and it leads to cell proliferation when growth factors are present, but that cells apoptose when growth stimuli are withdrawn or blocked by the use of some other agent. Furthermore, the cells may be rescued from apoptosis by the expression of *ras* or *bcl-2* gene. Thus, the mutated form of the *ras* oncogene enables the cells to proliferate without undergoing apoptosis (Wyllie *et al.*, 1987).

The retinoblastoma susceptibility gene rb and apoptosis

The tumour suppressor *rb* gene which also participates in regulating G_1-S transition of cells in the cell cycle (see page 52), is associated with apoptosis together with other cell proliferation related genes such as the myc protein, the transcription factor E2F-1, cdc2, and cyclin A. The phosphorylation of the rb protein is the key to its function as a regulator of cell proliferation. The underphosphorylated form of the rb protein inhibits cell proliferation by binding to E2F-1 and preventing it from activating cell cycle genes. However, upon being phosphorylated by specific cyclin–cdk complexes E2F is released from its complex with rb and this leads to the derepression of cell cycle genes with E2F-1 responsive promoters (Figure 10). We have seen in the preceding section, the myc protein can induce apoptosis. Other rb-binding proteins such as the adenovirus protein E1A and HPV E7 proteins (Debbas and White, 1993; Lowe and Ruley, 1993; White *et al.*, 1994); E2F-1 (Qin *et al.*, 1994; Kowalik *et al.*, 1995) induce apoptosis apparently by interfering with the negative regulatory function of rb. Apoptosis induced by serum-deprivation causes the up-regulation of a number of genes including c-*myc*, c-*jun*, c-*fos* and *cdc2* together with the phosphorylation of the rb protein (Pandey and Wang, 1995). Conversely, mutant rb protein which cannot bind to its regular partners, is unable to protect cells from apoptosis (Haas-Kogan *et al.*, 1995). In the absence of rb protein, the p53-mediated pathway to apoptosis may be opened up. In the developing lens of the mouse, the loss of *rb* function leads to uncontrolled proliferation and also to the disappearance of differentiation markers and to the apoptosis of lens fibres. This form of deregulation of cell proliferation can activate p53-dependent apoptosis (Morgenbesser *et al.*, 1994). The exposure of *rb* − / − mouse embryo fibroblasts to the anticancer drug methotrexate has been found to induce *p53* expression, activation of E2F-1 responsive genes and apoptosis (Almasan *et al.*, 1995). It thus seems possible that E2F-1 may interact with p53 as well as with rb. Wu and Levine (1994) transfected a murine cell line carrying a temperature-sensitive *p53* mutant with a human E2F-1 expression vector. When the wild-type *p53* was expressed by these cells at 32°C, the transfectants showed enhanced apoptosis. This suggests a close link-up between the rb- and p53-mediated pathways to apoptosis.

Deregulated expression of bcl-2 family genes in cancer

The *bcl-2* genes have been regarded as potential oncogenes in view of their function in apoptotic cell death and consequent perturbation of the delicate homeostasis of cell population growth. Transcriptionally deregulated *bcl-2* genes would obviously alter tumour growth kinetics and may profoundly influence clinical outcome. Indeed, over-expression of this gene has been reported in a variety of human tumours, e.g. adenocarcinoma of the prostate, squamous carcinoma of the lung, nasopharyngeal carcinoma and haemopoietic malignancies (McDonnell *et al.*, 1992; Lu *et al.*, 1993; Pezzella *et al.*, 1993b; Akagi *et al.*, 1994). Despite this widespread association, the significance of deregulated *bcl-2* expression, in terms of its relevance to the expansion of the primary tumour and to the growth of metastatic tumours, is uncertain. This is partly attributable to the present state of comparative knowledge of the operation of apoptosis in primary and secondary tumours. A major source of error resides in the assumption that both primary tumours and their distant metastases follow similar or comparable kinetics of apoptosis. This may not be the case as shown by Matsuda *et al.* (1996). Primary and secondary tumours differ markedly in respect of the degree apoptosis. As expected, primary tumours show an inverse relationship between tumour growth and apoptosis but, in contrast, there is an increase of apoptosis in metastatic tumours. This should be taken as a note of caution in order to avoid over-interpretation of the state of expression of *bcl-2* genes in tumours as independent predictors of their biological behaviour. Equally, high metastasis variants of the B16 murine melanoma have been reported to be more resistant to apoptosis than variants with low metastatic potential (Glinsky and Glinsky, 1996), and apoptosis index *per se* may also directly relate to patient survival (Aihara *et al.*, 1995).

There are preliminary indications that the deregulation of *bcl-2* expression may be an event in neoplastic development. The *bcl-2* gene is frequently expressed in colorectal carcinomas and cell lines. A majority (19 out 22) of adenocarcinomas and 12 out of 13 adenomas have been reported to be *bcl-2* positive. Expression was also found in metastastic tumour in the lymph nodes and in cell lines established from nodal metastases (Hague *et al.*, 1994), on the basis of which these authors suggested that the deregulation of its expression may be an early event in the progression of colorectal carcinoma. The bcl-2 protein has been reported to increase from cervical intraepithelial neoplasia (CIN) 1/II to CIN III which is consistent with their degree of dysplasia (mild to severe dysplasia from CIN 1/II to III). Surprisingly, there was also a marked decrease of expression in the progression to invasive carcinoma (Saegusa *et al.*, 1995).

bcl-2 expression has been studied in a large number of human breast carcinomas, but this has revealed an ambivalent correlation between gene expression and the accepted clinical criteria such as nodal involvement, tumour size or differentiation (Leek *et al.*, 1994). Sierra *et al.* (1995) have reported that lymph node metastases were more likely to occur in patients with *bcl-2* positive tumours than those with *bcl-2* negative tumours. Both these studies show that *bcl-2* gene expression correlates positively with oestrogen receptor (ER) status, with 80% of *bcl-2* positive tumours being ER positive. Breast tumours that are ER positive tend to be epidermal growth factor receptor (EGFr)-negative. Compatible with this, *bcl-2* positivity correlated inversely with (EGFr) status (Leek *et al.*, 1994). They make a further interesting observation that there is a strong association of *bcl-2* expression with invasive breast carcinomas. Since low ER and high EGFr are regarded as strong indicators of poor prognosis in breast cancer (see page 153) and it has been suggested that *bcl-2* may be hormonally regulated (Leek *et al.*, 1994). Although these studies indicate that *bcl-2* might serve as an independent prognostic indicator in breast cancer, the work of Lipponen *et al.* (1995a) does not appear to support this view; they believe that it has no independent prognostic value in node-negative breast cancer, but do state that it might be a weak prognostic factor in node-positive breast cancer. However, in head and neck cancer, *bcl-2*-positive status appears to correlate with significantly superior disease-free survival as compared with *bcl-2*-negative status (Gasparini *et al.*, 1995). Here, one should consider the possibility that the patients may have been sensitised to radio- and chemotherapy by concurrent up-regulation of apoptosis promoting genes, which do not appear to have been studied.

These reports should be balanced by the findings in other forms of cancer of a lack of relationship between *bcl-2* and prognosis. In a short series of 70 patients with laryngeal squamous cell carcinoma, bcl-2 protein was found to have no prognostic value (Spafford *et al.*, 1996). There was no correlation between *bcl-2* expression and overall survival in high-grade B-cell lymphoma, but when coupled with p53 protein expression there was a significant correlation with survival. Expression of both p53 and bcl-2 proteins correlated with poorer prognosis than p53 protein expression alone (Piris *et al.*, 1994). Similar additive effects or complementation of *bcl-2* expression may occur with the expression of other oncogenes, such as c-*myc*, as demonstrated in an experimental lymphoma model. Double transgenic c-*myc/bcl-2* mice showed a rapid development of lymphomas (Marin *et al.*, 1995). Lipponen *et al.* (1995b) examined the expression of *bcl-2* together with *rb* and c-*myc* genes and noted no correlation between their expression and prognosis of renal carcinomas.

The apoptosis-promoting genes can be viewed as suppressors of tumorigenesis. Among these, the *bax* gene has received some attention. Bargou *et al.* (1995) found that *bax-α*, a splice variant of *bax*, is highly expressed in normal breast tissue but it is considerably down-regulated in breast tumour tissues. Following upon this, Wagener *et al.* (1996) transfected this gene into breast cancer cell lines R30C and MCF-7 and found that the transfectant cells became sensitive to the chemotherapeutic agent epirubicin. They further demonstrated that this sensitivity was due to the promotion of apoptosis. Over-expression of *bax* also sensitises MCF-7 cells to radiation-induced apoptosis (Sakakura *et al.*, 1996). However, Chou *et al.* (1996) found no alterations in the *bax* in human gliomas and believe that it may not be involved in their pathogenesis. The importance of focusing on both apoptosis-promoting and apoptosis inhibitory genes is illustrated by the observations made by Aguilar-Santelises *et al.* (1996) on cells derived from progressive chronic lymphocytic leukaemia. In these cells bcl-2 and bax proteins did not individually relate to progressive disease but the ratio of bcl-2/bax-α mRNA expression was higher in the group with progressive disease.

Perhaps, it would be appropriate also to conduct more incisive studies than mere measurements of the expression of *bcl-2* genes may be required. For example, point mutations have been found in the translocated *bcl-2* alleles in human lymphomas and leukaemia, and there is therefore the implicit potential of these mutated genes to provide tumour cells with a growth and survival advantage, leading to tumour progression (Reed and Tanaka, 1993). Meijerink *et al.* (1995) have reported the presence of mutations in the highly conserved BH1 and BH2 domains of *bax* gene of cell lines derived from haematological malignancies. Such changes may affect the process of homo- or hetero-dimerisation of the proteins and in this way affect their function. Thus, point mutations can be activating or gain of function mutations or loss of function mutations as, for example, the point mutation occurring in *ced-9* and *bcl-2* (Hengartner and Horvitz, 1994; Yin *et al.*, 1994). One should be also be mindful of the fact that the array of apoptosis-related genes discovered to date exhibit a range of properties and the formation of dimers between various members of the family provides exquisite control over apoptosis and cell survival. Inevitably, therefore, a range of these genes need to be evaluated in order to obtain a complete picture of the homeostasis of cell growth in tumours.

7

Angiogenesis in cancer

Angiogenesis or neovascularisation is an important requirement for several biological processes such as embryonic development, wound healing and chronic inflammation. Angiogenesis is also a key prerequisite for the successful establishment, growth and dissemination of tumours. It was demonstrated many years ago that the growth of tumour is dependent upon adequate vascularisation (Folkman et al., 1971; Folkman, 1972). Two distinct phases of tumour growth can be identified: the avascular and vascular phases (Folkman, 1975). The avascular phase constitutes a self-limiting phase of growth because of constraints on the diffusion of nutrients and catabolic products imposed by the tumour surface area in relation to its volume. In contrast, the vascular phase of growth constitutes a phase of rapid exponential expansion. Gimbrone et al. (1972) demonstrated that tumours implanted into the avascular environment of the anterior eye chamber show limited growth, but when they attach to the vascular bed of the iris they become vascularised and grow rapidly. Recent work has shown that tumour growth is adversely affected by agents which block angiogenesis (Hori et al., 1991; Kim et al., 1993), but it is stimulated by factors that enhance angiogenesis (Ueki et al., 1992). The inhibition of angiogenesis has therefore provided a potentially valuable target for a new therapeutic strategy (Harris et al., 1996).

Induction of neovascularisation by tumours

There has been a clear perception of the association of neovascularisation with tumours for several decades, but the idea that a humoral factor may mediate the induction of angiogenesis was mooted by Greenblatt and Shubik (1968). Subsequently, Folkman (1974, 1975) demonstrated that tumours possessed the ability to induce the proliferation of proximal capillaries. New capillaries arise mainly from small venules in response to the angiogenic stimulus imparted by the tumour. Initially, local dissolution of the basement membrane occurs, possibly caused by proteinases whose synthesis in endothelial cells has been found to be induced by the angiogenic factor, basic fibroblast growth factor (bFGF) (Moscatelli *et al.*, 1986). This is followed by migration of endothelial cells towards the source of the angiogenic factor. The endothelial cells then align themselves end to end and form a 'sprout' which subsequently develops a lumen (Ausprunk and Folkman, 1977). Angiogenic growth factors such as the bFGF (see below) are also known to be able to stimulate endothelial cell motility and the *ras* oncogene might be involved in this process. The injection of Ha-*ras* proteins into bovine endothelial cells appears to stimulate their motility; antibodies to the ras protein can inhibit bFGF-stimulated motility and indeed inhibit even the initiation of the process. These experiments demonstrate that presence of the ras protein is required in the transduction of the motility signal (Fox PL *et al.*, 1994).

Several factors with angiogenic ability have now been identified and some of them are known to be secreted by the tumour (Table 6). Prominent among these are certain growth factors. An important group embraces growth factors which are described as heparin binding growth factors, namely the vascular endothelial growth factor (VEGF), fibroblast growth factors (FGFs), transforming growth factor-β (TGF-β) and the hepatocyte growth factor (HGF). The binding of these growth factors to heparan sulphate proteoglycans (HSPG) has been seen as a mechanism for localising the growth factors on the cell surface and presenting them to their appropriate receptors in the most favourable conformation, in order to facilitate the interaction of the growth factors with the receptors. The isoform of FGF known as the basic fibroblast growth factor (bFGF) has been shown to bind reversibly to a secreted protein which protects it from degradation (Wu *et al.*, 1991; Czubayko *et al.*, 1994).

The vascular endothelial growth factor (VEGF)

The vascular endothelial growth factor (VEGF) was originally isolated as the vascular permeability factor (Senger *et al.*, 1983) and subsequently by Ferrara and Henzel (1989) as a growth factor which induced proliferation of endothelial cells but not mitogenic to fibroblasts or epithelial cells. Four isoforms of VEGF have been identified and these are designated as $VEGF_{121}$, $VEGF_{165}$, $VEGF_{180}$ and $VEGF_{206}$, distinguished by subscript numbers which refer to the numbers of amino acid residues in the mature protein in each case. The major subtype, $VEGF_{121}$, may be described as providing the primary pattern consisting of exons 1-5 encoding 141 amino acids of the N-terminal region and six C-terminal amino acids encoded by exon 8. The other isoforms represent addition of exon 7 in $VEGF_{165}$, exons 6 and 7 in $VEGF_{189}$. $VEGF_{206}$ carries, in addition to exons 6 and 7, an extra short exon 6'. Exon 6 encodes a stretch of highly basic amino acids and exon 7 encoded region of VEGF shows a mild heparin-binding ability (Ferrara *et al.*, 1991;

Table 6.   Inducers and inhibitors of angiogenesis

Inducers of angiogenesis
Growth factors
  Basic fibroblast growth factor (bFGF)
  Vascular endothelial growth factor (VEGF)
  Hepatocyte growth factor (Bussolino *et al.*, 1992)
  Transforming growth factor β (TGF-β) (Roberts *et al.*, 1986)
  Tumour necrosis factor (TNF) (Leibovich *et al.*, 1987; Frater-Schroder *et al.*, 1987)
  Interleukins: IL-8 (Koch *et al.*, 1992); IL-1,4,6
  Angiogenin (King and Vallee, 1991)
Prostaglandins E_1, E_2
Plasminogen activators (Hildenbrand *et al.*, 1995a,b)
Oestrogen
Angiotensin (Fett *et al.*, 1985)
Substance P
Lipopolysaccharide (Mattsbybaltzer *et al.*, 1994)
Thymidine phosphorylase (Platelet-derived endothelial growth factor) (Moghaddam *et al.*, 1995)
E- and P- selectin (Koch *et al.*, 1995; Fox *et al.*, 1995c)
Ganglioside GD3 (Koochekpour and Pilkington, 1996)
Polyamines (spermine and spermidine) (Takigawa *et al.*, 1990a)
Cathepsin B (Mikkelsen *et al.*, 1995)
Cell adhesion molecules (CAMs, selectins)
Integrin receptors (Drake *et al.*, 1991; Bauer *et al.*, 1992; Brooks *et al.*, 1994)

Inhibitors of angiogenesis
Wild-type p53 (van Meir *et al.*, 1994b)
Interleukin-1 (?)
Interferons (Sidky and Border, 1987; White *et al.*, 1990)
Thrombospondin-1
Tissue inhibitors of metalloproteinases (TIMPs) (Takigawa *et al.*, 1990a; Johnson *et al.*, 1994)
Polysulphonated naphthylureas (Suramin and analogues)
Multimeric YIGSR laminin motif (Iwamoto *et al.*, 1996)
Isosorbide mono- and di-nitrates via nitric oxide generation (Pipili-Synetos *et al.*, 1995)

References in text or as cited in the Table; and partly based on Diaz-Flores *et al.* (1994); Fidler and Ellis (1994).

Houck *et al.*, 1991, 1992). The *N*-terminal region accommodates eight cysteine residues which might be enabling the molecules to dimerise. A 32 kDa fragment generated by the use of plasmin has been found to possess both VEGF activity and the ability to regulate vascular permeability (Houck *et al.*, 1992). Subsequently, Keyt *et al.* (1996) have shown that residues

111-165 from the C-terminal portion of this region are essential for the mitogenic activity of VEGF. $VEGF_{121}$ is a soluble form of VEGF and possesses no heparin-binding ability: $VEGF_{189}$ and $VEGF_{165}$ do bind to heparin but $VEGF_{189}$ binds more strongly than does $VEGF_{165}$. Therefore, the different isoforms may have distinct biological activity, and the differences in their ability to regulate vascular permeability or their mitogenic activity may involve splicing out of these important domains of the molecule. Two VEGF-related placental growth factors, PIGF1 and PIGF2, have been described which may be produced by alternative splicing of pre-mRNA transcribed from the VEGF gene (Hauser and Weich, 1993; Maglione et al., 1993).

The promoter of the VEGF gene does not possess a TATA box, but has six GC boxes for transcription factor SP-1 binding and also sites for AP-1 and AP-2 binding (Tischer et al., 1991). The expression of the gene is modulated by several growth factors such as EGF (Goldman et al., 1993), TGF (Harada et al., 1994; Pertovaara et al., 1994), and, significantly, by hypoxia (Ladoux and Frelin, 1993). In some cell types VEGF expression appears to be regulated by other growth factors such as interleukin-1 (Kvanta, 1995), and bFGF, epidermal growth factor and platelet-derived growth factors (Koochekpour et al., 1995). A commonality of mediation of protein kinase C in the regulation of VEGF by these growth factors is suggested by the experiments of Kvanta (1995) where enhanced VEGF expression was induced by phorbol esters which activate the kinase. Ikeda et al. (1995) showed that hypoxia induces VEGF in C6 glioma cells. The VEGF gene appears to be activated by hypoxia, the effect being mediated by the presence of hypoxia responsive elements in the 5′-flanking region of the VEGF gene. The oncogene c-src has been implicated in the pathway of hypoxia-mediated induction of VEGF. Mukhopadhyay et al. (1995) showed that an inhibition of protein kinases inhibits the induction of VEGF. Hypoxia increases the kinase activity of $pp60^{src}$. In addition to this circumstantial evidence, Mukhopadhyay et al. (1995) have gone on to show that the induction of VEGF by hypoxia is impaired in c-src negative cells. Therefore, they have suggested that VEGF gene might be a downstream target for c-src function. Among other oncogenes implicated in angiogenesis is ras, which is frequently mutated in cancers. The expression of mutant ras has been found to be associated with an up-regulation of VEGF mRNA and with the secreted protein in human and rodent cell lines. VEGF expression can be down-regulated by treatment of cells with agents that disrupt the function of the ras protein (Rak et al., 1995).

VEGF is specific for vascular endothelium, because it binds to receptors which are found only on endothelial cells. The membrane receptors belong to the tyrosine kinase family of growth factor receptors. The VEGF receptors constitute a family of which the recognised members are flt-1 (fms-like-tyrosine kinase) (Shibuya et al., 1990; Finnerty et al., 1993; Yamane et al., 1994), flt-4 (Finnerty et al., 1993; Galland et al., 1993; Pajusola et al., 1994), and flk-1 (also known as KDR) (Matthews et al., 1991; Terman et al., 1991, 1992; Sarzani et al., 1992). These receptors share several features with other tyrosine kinase receptors. They are transmembrane proteins, with an extracellular, a transmembrane and an intracellular tyrosine kinase domains. The extracellular domain resembles fms, kit and PDGFr proteins with regard to the distribution of cysteine residues. The extracellular sections of both flt-1 and flk-1 have been shown to possess seven immunoglobulin-like domains. The second of these domains may be involved in the binding of VEGF. The introduction of the second immunoglobulin-like domain into flt-4, which does not normally bind VEGF, enables the chimeric flt-4 to bind the ligand (Davis-Smyth *et al.*, 1996). The VEGF receptor molecule also shares some features of the cytoplasmic tyrosine kinase domain.

The angiogenic effect of VEGF has been elegantly demonstrated by Zhang HT *et al.* (1995) who transfected a cDNA clone of an isoform of VEGF into MCF7 cells. They showed that the transfectant clone (called V12) stimulated a directional outgrowth of capillaries upon implantation into rabbit cornea. V12 tumours grew faster as xenografts than untransfected cells; V12 tumours were also more vascular. VEGF expression has been closely correlated with the degree of angiogenesis in human epidermoid lung carcinoma. It is also a potent mitogen: for instance, VEGF levels correlate with high proliferation as indicated by the expression of PCNA, the proliferation related nuclear antigen (Mattern *et al.*, 1996).

VEGF functions as a major angiogenic factor in normal and in pathological conditions. Its role in the development of rheumatoid arthritis is well known (Koch *et al.*, 1994). VEGF has a prominent function in embryogenesis. It is found in developing organs. Three isoforms of VEGF occur in the developing human kidney together with two VEGF-specific receptors of the tyrosine kinase type, flt-1 and KDR (flk-1) (Simon *et al.*, 1995). Both VEGF and its receptors are required for angiogenesis, and regulation of the process of angiogenesis may relate to the regulation of the individual components of the ligand–receptor system. Both VEGF and VEGF-receptor expression is modulated by several agents. As mentioned earlier, VEGF gene expression is up-regulated by EGF, TGF-β and hypoxia. TGF-β and hypoxic conditions also affect the expression of the receptor. TGF-β down-regulates expression of flk-1 (Mandriota *et al.*, 1996), but hypoxia produces a 13-fold up-regulation of flk-1 expression (Brogi *et al.*, 1996). Tumour necrosis factor α (TNF-α) is known to inhibit VEGF-mediated proliferation of human endothelial cell. This appears to occur by the down-regulation of flk-1 expression (Patterson *et al.*, 1996). There also may be some affinity of interaction between the VEGF isoforms and the various receptors. Isoform PlGF has been found to bind to flt-1 but not to flk-1 (Sawano *et al.*, 1996). Whether this has a functional significance is yet unclear. Flt-4, on the other hand, does not bind VEGF at all.

Mutations in the ligand lead to its inactivation and this has serious consequences for their function. Mutation even in one allele of the VEGF gene is lethal for mouse embryos, with attendant aberrations in angiogenesis. Interestingly, VEGF null embryonic stem cells failed to form tumours when implanted into nude mice (Ferrara *et al.*, 1996).

Very little information is available regarding the activation of expression of VEGF in tumours. The expression of VEGF, but not flt-1, is reported to be greatly increased in carcinomas of the breast (Yoshiji *et al.*, 1996). In endometrial carcinomas, the expression of VEGF was very strong, as detected by *in situ* hybridisation; the endothelial cells of the microvessels associated with these tumours showed a marked expression of flt-1 and flk-1 mRNAs (Guidi *et al.*, 1996). The expression of both VEGF and receptor have also been found to be up-regulated in human germ cell tumours and this correlates with the degree of vascularisation of the tumours (Viglietto *et al.*, 1996). VEGF is abundant in gliomas. Both flt-1 and KDR mRNA are expressed in endotheial cells of high-grade gliomas, but not in low-grade gliomas. VEGF receptors are not expressed in the normal brain endothelium. It is therefore suggested that the neovascularisation associated with high-grade tumours may be a paracrine response initiated by a coordinated up-regulation of the receptor genes (Plate et al., 1994). Similarly, in haemangioblastoma associated with von Hippel–Lindau syndrome, isoforms of VEGF are secreted by stromal cells. VEGF then interacts with the flt-1 and flk-1 receptors situated on the tumour endothelium (Wizigmannvoos et al., 1995). The flk-1 receptor is now known to be involved in the growth of a variety of human tumours (Millauer et al., 1996).

Fibroblast growth factors in angiogenesis

Fibroblast growth factors (FGFs) constitute a large family of growth factors which are structurally related to each other and participate in several biological processes such as cell differentiation, motility, proliferation, wound healing and also in angiogenesis and in the pathogenesis of cancer. The best characterised members of the family are the acidic and basic fibroblast growth factors. The following discussion is restricted to bFGF and the growth factor FGF-3 encoded by the int-2 oncogene.

bFGF, an 18 kDa polypeptide belonging to the fibrobast growth factor family, is a potent angiogenic factor (Shing et al., 1985). It is strongly implicated in cell proliferation, cell motility, embryonic development, differentiation, wound healing and also in angiogenesis (Shing et al., 1984; Gospodarowicz et al., 1986; Thomas and Gimenez-Gallego, 1986; Rifkin and Moscatelli, 1989). It would appear that bFGF is not secreted by cells in the conventional manner since it does not contain the signal sequence for secretion (Abraham et al., 1986) but it may be released by damaged or dying cells. Furthermore, it is sensitive to degradation by proteolytic enzymes. Moscatelli et al. (1991) have shown that bFGF might become localised at the site of its biological function and indeed retain its activity by virtue of its ability to form complexes with heparan sulphate proteoglycans. FGF is released with greater ease from complexes with heparan sulphate than with FGF receptors. The release of FGFs from these complexes occurs by the action of heparinase (Vlodavsky et al., 1988, 1991; Bashkin et al., 1989; Moscatelli, 1992). The function of FGF (both the basic and the acidic isoforms) involves its binding to receptors which possess features characteristic of tyrosine kinase receptors of other growth factors such as the epidermal and platelet-derived growth factors. There are several forms of the FGF receptor, which may arise from alternative splicing of a single pre-mRNA product. Since both isoforms of FGF can bind with equal affinity to these receptor isoforms, there must exist a complex system of regulation of FGF signalling (Dionne et al., 1991). Inhibition of bFGF by LAM5, a polysulphate derivative of glucan laminarin, inhibits angiogenesis (Hoffman et al., 1996). Conversely, enhancement of bFGF promotes angiogenesis; for example, the angiogenic ability of TNF-α is attributed to its ability to enhance the production and secretion of bFGF (Okamura et al., 1991).

int-2 *protein (FGF-3)*

The *int-2* oncogene encodes a growth factor which bears high sequence homology with bFGF. This is known as FGF-3. The *int-2* oncogene is located on chromosome 11q13. The *hst-1, EMS1, PRAD1* and *bcl-1* genes also occur at the *int-2* locus. The *int-2* oncogene is known to be involved in embryonic development (Jakobovits *et al.*, 1986; Wilkinson *et al.*, 1988, 1989; Represa *et al.*, 1991) and in mouse mammary tumour virus (MMTV)-induced tumorigenesis. MMTV induces transcriptional activation of this gene (Gordon *et al.*, 1983; Peters *et al.*, 1983; Dickson *et al.*, 1984). Recent work shows that MMTV integration results in the mutation of several other genes, e.g. *wnt-1,3, 10b, FGF-4*, and *FGF-8* among others (Callahan, 1996), all of them with considerable potential for influencing the path of tumour progression. Nonetheless, *int-2* gene expression and amplification, in particular, has been studied in several human tumours. It is over-expressed in carcinoma of the breast (Fanti *et al.*, 1989), oesophagus (Kitagawa *et al.*, 1991), ovary (Rosen *et al.*, 1993) and in Kaposi's sarcoma (Huang *et al.*, 1993). Amplification of *int-2* correlates strongly with the presence of lymph node metastases in breast cancer and is significantly associated with a greater risk of recurrence (Nagayama and Watatani, 1993; Champeme *et al.*, 1995; Pauley *et al.*, 1996). Oral squamous cell carcinomas contain homogeneously staining regions (HSRs) at 11q13, which indicate that gene amplification may be occurring there. In fact, *int-2* and *hst-1* appear to be co-amplified in these tumours (Lese *et al.*, 1995). No amplification of *int-2* gene has been found in breast and ovarian cancers (Jaakkola *et al.*, 1993) and in carcinomas of the prostate (Latil *et al.*, 1994).

Amplification of the 11q13 amplicon can affect several genes occurring within the amplicon, and therefore weighting of individual genes in terms of their relevance to progression is liable to be a complex exercise. The *hst-1* gene is another member of the FGF family which occurs in the 11q13 amplicon, 35 kbp downstream of *int-2* in the same transcriptional orientation at 11q13.3 (Wada *et al.*, 1988; Yoshida *et al.*, 1988). *hst-1* is often co-amplified with *int-2* (Yoshida *et al.*, 1988; Adnane *et al.*, 1989; Tsuda H *et al.*, 1989; Tsuda T *et al.*, 1989; Lese *et al.*, 1995). The *hst-1* encoded protein is a potent mitogen, but it has not been tested for angiogenic ability. The association of *int-2* with the aggressive behaviour of tumours may be due to the ability of its product (FGF-3) to induce angiogenesis (Costa *et al.*, 1994).

The hepatocyte growth factor (HGF)

The hepatocyte growth factor (HGF) described by Rubin *et al.* (1991) was discovered as the scatter factor (Gherardi *et al.*, 1989; Gherardi and Stoker, 1990) and the cytotoxic factor (Higashio *et al.*, 1990). HGF is secreted by fibroblasts and is mitogenic for epithelial and endothelial cells as well as melanocytes, but does not affect fibroblasts (Rubin *et al.*, 1991). For example, the addition of HGF to pancreatic cell lines greatly promotes their motility and proliferation (Direnzo *et al.*, 1995a) (see also page 127). The paracrine effect of HGF is mediated by its binding to the tyrosine kinase type receptor protein encoded by the c-*met* oncogene.

The expression of the c-*met* protein has been studied in several human tumours. In colorectal tumours the expression of the protein increased from five- to 50-fold with progression in approximately 50% of 123 primary carcinomas and in 70% of 25 liver metastases examined. Amplification of the c-*met* gene was also detected in only 10% of the primary tumours but at a far greater frequency (eight out of nine) in liver metastases (Direnzo *et al.*, 1995b). A high proportion (45% of 128) of prostatic carcinoma show the presence of the c-*met* protein. In metastatic tumour the frequency has been found to increase to 75% (Humphrey *et al.*, 1995). Furthermore, c-*met* protein staining has been found to be related to tumour grade in another study of prostatic tumours (Pisters *et al.*, 1995). Expression of the protein in gastric carcinomas has also been found to correlate with lymph node involvement, serosal invasion and the dissemination into the peritoneal cavity (Yonemura *et al.*, 1996). Yonemura *et al.* (1996) also state that c-*met* positive tumours were liable to show distant metastases; however, such a clear relationship with tumour progression has not emerged from studies on breast (Nagy *et al.*, 1995) or head and neck carcinomas (Muller *et al.*, 1995). Nagy *et al.* (1995) found a loss of heterozygosity at the c-*met* locus (7q31) in only 4% of the tumours, but c-*met* protein expression was significantly greater in carcinomas than in tissues derived from benign breast disease. In contrast, in head and neck tumours loss of heterozygosity occurred in 23% of the tumours but this was not associated with lymph node involvement (Muller *et al.*, 1995).

HGF induces angiogenesis and its levels have recently been measured in primary breast cancer by Nagy *et al.* (1996). They found tumour vascular volume, determined by immunostaining using anti-CD34 antibody, correlated with HGF levels in the tumour and with tumour proliferation as measured by Ki-67 index. This accords with the elevation of expression of its receptor protein to correspond with tumour progression. The involvement of HGF-mediated angiogenesis in progression is also implied in the observations by Hiscox and Jiang (1996). They found that c-*met* transcripts and also the protein are up-regulated by bFGF and TGF-β, which are powerful inducers of angiogenesis. In contrast, IFN-γ, which inhibits angiogenesis, also down-regulated them. These studies emphasise in a substantial way the paracrine mechanism by which HGF and c-*met* protein confer upon tumour cells selective advantages of growth, invasive and metastatic properties.

Other angiogenic mediators

The platelet-derived endothelial growth factor, now known to be thymidine phosphorylase (TP) has been found to be angiogenic and to stimulate tumour growth. The induction of angiogenesis by TP in *in vitro* models can be inhibited by neutralising anti-TP antibodies (Fox *et al.*, 1995a; Moghaddam *et al.*, 1995). Fox *et al.* (1995b) raised a monoclonal antibody against recombinant TP and tested for the state of TP expression in a variety of human tissues. They found TP expression in endothelial cells, but the expression did not correlate with sites of new vessel growth. The expression of TP was found to be up-regulated in both tumour epithelium (in 53% of 240 primary breast cancers) and tumour endothelial cells, prominently with peripheral endothelial cells (Fox *et al.*, 1996).

There are also other angiogenic mediators, such as plasminogen activators, which may function indirectly by promoting the dissolution of the basement membrane to enable exposure of endothelial cells to angiogenic agents. Hildenbrand *et al.* (1995a,b) compared urokinase (plasminogen activator uPA) levels of 42 primary invasive breast carcinomas and tumour angiogenesis, as determined by microvessel density. They found that uPA levels correlated with microvessel density, rate of proliferation and vascular invasion. Conversely, angiogenic factors might themselves induce the production of proteinases.

Cell adhesion molecules such as the vascular endothelial cell adhesion molecule-1 (VCAM-1), E-selectin, sialyl Lewis-X/A glycoconjugates, etc. (Nguyen *et al.*, 1993b; Koch *et al.*, 1995) also take part in angiogenesis. The cell adhesion molecules, E- and P-selectins, for instance, may be expressed more intensely in invasive breast cancer than in corresponding normal tissues and such expression is prominent at the tumour periphery (Fox *et al.*, 1995c). Antibodies raised against E-selectin and VCAM inhibit the angiogenic property and the chemotactic effect towards endothelial cells exerted by rheumatoid synovial fluid. This is compatible with the observation that TNF is able to up-regulate the expression of ICAM-1 and also induce angiogenesis. These molecules are involved in the adhesive interactions between tumour and endothelial cells (see page 113), but whether they are associated with tumours is uncertain.

In sharp contrast, the active site of laminin which also participates in cell adhesion and migration (page 102) has an inhibitory effect on angiogenesis. The $\beta 1$ chain of laminin has an active site composed of the sequence tyrosine-isoleucine-glycine-serine-arginine (YIGSR) residues 929–933 (Graf *et al.*, 1987). Synthetic peptides containing this amino acid sequence promote cell adhesion and migration (Iwamoto *et al.*, 1988). The YIGSR sequence is also able to inhibit experimental metastasis (Iwamoto *et al.*, 1987). The inhibitory effect on metastasis and angiogenesis appears to be related to the number of YIGSR motifs in the polypeptide. Thus, synthetic molecules containing 16 motifs were far more inhibitory than the monomeric YIGSR motif (Iwamoto *et al.*, 1996). The ability of the pentapeptide to inhibit metastasis has been attributed to its ability to inhibit angiogenesis (Sakamoto *et al.*, 1991; Iwamoto *et al.*, 1996). Although this is an attractive hypothesis, it is possible that the multimeric YIGSR peptide may saturate laminin-binding sites and inhibit the adhesion of tumour cells to the basement membrane. Kim WH *et al.* (1994) found that the multimeric YIGSR peptide can induce apoptosis of human fibrosarcoma cells.

Inhibitors of neovascularisation

Several factors that inhibit angiogenesis occur naturally. Sidky and Borden (1987, 1989) reported the inhibition of angiogenesis as well as tumour growth by interferons α and β. IFN-α has also been used successfully in the treatment of pulmonary haemangiomatosis and angiosarcomas (White *et al.*, 1990). The role of interleukin-1 in angiogenesis is still uncertain. It has been shown to inhibit angiogenesis in some *in vivo* models but not in others. It has been described as a mitogen for vascular smooth muscle cells and fibroblasts (Sunderkotter *et al.*, 1991).

Angiogenesis has provided a valuable target for developing anti-tumour agents. Earlier, we alluded to the binding of bFGF to heparan sulphate proteoglycans (HSPG) as a mechanism by which bFGF may be localised at the site of its action and protected from degradation. This has inevitably led to the use of heparinoids and related compounds to inhibit the heparin-binding growth factors. The polysulphonated naphthylurea suramin is a moderate inhibitor of these growth factors (Myers *et al.*, 1991; Zugmaier *et al.*, 1992). It appears to inhibit the binding of bFGF to endothelial cells (Takano *et al.*, 1994). Suramin also inhibits VEGF and VEGF-induced chemotaxis of endothelial cells. The inhibition seems to result from inhibition of VEGF-mediated phosphorylation of the VEGF receptors (Waltenberger *et al.*, 1996); possibly a mechanism by which suramin exerts its anti-angiogenic effect could be by interfering with the binding of angiogenic growth factors with their receptors. Braddock *et al.* (1994) synthesised several polysulphonated naphthylureas resembling suramin in their structure and showed that these could inhibit bFGF-mediated angiogenesis *in vitro*. Sulphonated derivatives of distamycin A have been found to be capable of complexing with bFGF and inhibiting angiogenesis (Ciomei *et al.*, 1994). Firsching *et al.* (1995) believe that the anti-angiogenic potential of these compounds is related to structural features other than merely their polyanionic nature. Nevertheless, the polyamines putrescine and spermidine are inducers of angiogenesis. Firsching *et al.* (1995) showed that polyamine-induced angiogenesis can be inhibited by the ornithine carboxylase inhibitor α-difluoromethylornithine (DFMO). DFMO can also inhibit B16 melanoma-induced angiogenesis in the chorioallantoic membrane (Takigawa *et al.*, 1990a,b).

Nitric oxide, which is regarded as a regulator of many physiological systems, may have anti-angiogenic properties. Pipili-Synetos *et al.* (1995) found that isosorbide mono- and di-nitrates inhibited angiogenesis in chick chorio-allantoic membrane (CAM) assays. These compounds also effectively inhibited growth and metastasis of Lewis lung carcinomas implanted into compatible mice. Both isosorbide nitrates function through the release of nitric oxide and, furthermore, the nitric oxide synthase inhibitor L-NAME enhanced pulmonary metastatic spread of animal tumours.

The suppressor gene *p53* which controls the progression of the cell cycle has been shown to be able to inhibit bFGF-mediated angiogenesis (van Meir *et al.*, 1994b). These authors transfected wild-type p53 into glioma with $p53-/-$ null phenotype. The induction of expression of the wild-type, but not the mutant, gene appeared to produce a factor that inhibited angiogenesis. Another pathway by which *p53* might inhibit angiogenesis is by modulating the production of thrombospondin-1 (TSP-1). TSP-1 is an extracellular matrix glycoprotein containing RGD (arginine-glycine-aspartic acid) recognition sequences and binds to $\alpha_v\beta_3$ integrin receptors. TSP-1 regulates cell adhesion, motility and has often been found to inhibit tumour growth and metastasis. The latter effects have been attributed to its ability to inhibit angiogenesis. However, in a recent review Roberts (1996) pointed out that TSP-1 can interact with several cell surface receptors and that under certain conditions may enhance metastatic spread and has, therefore, suggested that the modulation of cell behaviour by TSP-1 could be cell-type specific. Nevertheless, that TSP-1 can negatively regulate tumour growth is demonstrated by the observation that the cell cycle controlling genes *p53* and *rb* (see pages 28 and 50), both up-regulate TSP-1 gene transcription. Thus, the transfection of wild-type *p53* gene into fibroblasts from patients with Li–Fraumeni syndrome who carry germ line mutations in the *p53* gene up-regulates the expression of TSP-1 gene (Dameron *et al.*, 1994). In a similar vein, Chinese hamster embryo cells transformed by nickel show reduced TSP-1 expression while in the normal cells it is abundantly expressed in the cytoplasm; however, co-transfection with the retinoblastoma-susceptibility gene *rb* causes an increase in the transcription of the gene encoding TSP-1 (Salnikow *et al.*, 1994). Thrombospondin-1 inhibits angiogenesis by suppressing bFGF function. A loss of wild-type *p53* or its mutation may therefore be expected to allow the normal angiogenic function of bFGF together with the removal of growth restraint. This link-up of the loss of control of tumour growth with a switch to the vascular phase of development may prove to be an important event in tumour progression.

Angiogenesis as a predictor of prognosis of cancer

The process of neovascularisation of the tumour is a critical step in the progression of the disease. Adequate vascularisation is not only essential for continued tumour growth, but also in dissemination of the tumour to distant metastatic sites on account of the fact that the vascular and lymphatic systems are the major vehicles of transport of cancer cells released from the primary tumour. At the metastatic site also, the growth of the secondary deposits is dependent upon angiogenesis. This was demonstrated by Holmgren *et al.* (1995) by using dormant lung metastases produced under conditions where angiogenesis had been experimentally suppressed. They found that a rapid growth of the metastases ensued upon removal of inhibition of angiogenesis. An intriguing observation was that the dormant metastases exhibited the same rate of proliferation. This contradiction was explained by the greater than threefold increase in apoptosis in the dormant metastases compared with actively growing secondary deposits. It appears, therefore, that in the absence of adequate angiogenesis, metastatic deposits remain dormant on account of a steady state being reached between the rates of proliferation and apoptosis of cells. In the light of the enormous significance of angiogenesis to the total process of metastatic spread, a logical advance would be to explore if the state of angiogenesis can be employed in predicting prognosis of the disease.

The transformation of cells to the neoplastic state is associated with the acquisition of angiogenic property (Gimbrone and Gullino, 1976; Brem *et al.*, 1977, 1978; Maiorana and Gullino, 1978). According to Ziche and Gullino (1982), this precedes the transformation of cells to the tumorigenic state. Maiorana and Gullino (1978) implanted tissues of rat mammary gland from virgin, pregnant and lactating animals and noted that only a small proportion (5%) of implants elicited angiogenesis. Hyperplastic tissue also produced a low angiogenic response but far more frequently than normal tissues. At the other extreme, 75–100% of implants of rat mammary carcinomas induced an angiogenic response. Similar observations were then made in respect of human breast tissues. Benign tissues, such as those derived from fibroadenomas or fibrocystic disease, failed to elicit an angiogenic response upon implantation into rabbit iris. Roughly one-quarter of hyperplastic tissue fragments induced angiogenesis. In contrast, out of 63 tissue fragments tested from 10 carcinomas, 41 fragments induced strong angiogenic response – apparently a clear intensification of the angiogenic response with neoplastic progression. Recently, the exploration of this relationship and the assessment of the clinical value of the degree of tumour-associated angiogenesis has taken two forms: microvessel counting and the assessment of the expression of angiogenic factors in tumours (Craft and Harris, 1994).

Clinical significance of microvessel density

The density of microvessels associated with tumours is usually measured by immunohistochemical staining, e.g. using antibodies against von Willebrand factor (factor VIII)-related antigen, endothelial specific antigens such as platelet/endothelial cell adhesion molecule (PE-CAM) (CD31), or CD34.

The possible correlation of tumour microvessel density with clinicopathological features and clinical outcome of breast cancer have been investigated by several laboratories. Horak *et al.* (1992) used antibodies against E-CAM and counted microvessels associated with 103 primary breast cancers. They found significantly greater vascularisation of tumour tissue compared with normal breast tissue and, furthermore, the higher microvessel density correlated with lymph node metastasis. Thus, only two out of 50 tumours with microvessel density of 99 or less per mm^2 showed lymph node metastasis as compared with 31 out of 39 tumours which had microvessel density >140 mm^{-2}. They also found that neovascularisation related to tumour size, grade and differentiation. In another series of 165 early stage breast cancers with median follow-up of 5 years, tumour angiogenesis was found to be a significant and independent prognostic indicator (Gasparini *et al.*, 1994). This is supported also by Nagy *et al.* (1996) who found tumour vascularisation to correlate with relapse of the disease. In contradistinction, however, Miliaras *et al.* (1995) found no correlation between microvessel counts and tumour size and grade. Tumours with lymph node metastases and those with no nodal involvement showed similar microvessel density. A study which included 155 invasive breast cancers showed no correlation between microvessel density and tumour size, histological grade or lymph node status. However, high microvessel counts were found to correlate strongly with shorter disease-free and overall survival in these patients (Ogawa *et al.*, 1995).

Among other forms of human cancer studied are gastric carcinomas. Maeda *et al.* (1995) investigated 108 gastric carcinomas for microvessel density and determined the expression of PCNA to measure cell proliferation. Both features were associated with poor prognosis. High microvessel density was also significantly associated with high risk for hepatic metastasis. Similarly, high microvessel count correlated with poor survival of patients with non-small cell lung carcinoma (Fontanini et al., 1995). These authors have also found, upon follow-up of 94 patients, that high microvessel count correlated positively with development of metastases. Microvessel density appears to be a good prognostic indicator for transitional cell carcinoma of the bladder, although stage and grade of tumours was not related to microvessel count (Dickinson et al., 1994). But, Philip et al. (1996) reported a highly significant correlation between microvessel density and tumour stage, and both TNM stage and also that microvessel density were significant predictors of survival.

Some of the ambiguities in the data may have resulted from the number of areas of vascularisation counted. Miliaras et al. (1995) state that they counted three most active areas of neovascularisation. Whether such a selection produces a bias in the results should be considered. Furthermore, ability to induce angiogenesis may be another feature of heterogeneity. In addition, it should be borne in mind that the vascular endothelium is itself antigenically heterogeneous (Kazu et al., 1992). Furthermore, PE-CAM (CD31), believed to be a more sensitive marker, may be more appropriate than factor VIII for the quantification of microvessel density (Vermeulen PB et al., 1995). Ideally, more than one marker should be employed for assessing angiogenesis.

The expression of angiogenic factors in tumours

The second approach advocated by Craft and Harris (1994) for assessing the significance of neovascularisation associated with tumours as a prognostic marker is the assessment of the expression of angiogenic factors and their receptors in tumours. They postulate that angiogenic factors produced by tumours may bind to appropriate receptors occurring on tumour-associated endothelia in a paracrine fashion, and further that the expression of both may be coordinately regulated in producing the angiogenic response so essential for tumour dissemination. This postulate has attracted considerable support. Furthermore, as discussed earlier, the expression of angiogenic growth factors in tumours correlates with the degree of neovascularisation. This has inevitably led several investigators to focus on the production of these factors in human tumours. Several angiogenic growth factors, e.g. VEGF, acidic and bFGF and TP, among others, are expressed in breast cancer (Moghaddam et al., 1995; Harris et al., 1996). The hepatocyte growth factor is also known to be produced by breast cancers and its expression correlates with disease relapse and overall survival (Nagy et al., 1996). Basic FGF and FGF receptor (FGFr) mRNAs have been found to be expressed in a majority of advanced gastric carcinomas - mostly undifferentiated tumours and invasive adenocarcinomas. In addition, the expression of bFGF and FGFr correlated with higher incidence of nodal metastasis and poorer survival (Ueki et al., 1995). The ganglioside, GD3, has been implicated in the release of VEGF by human glioma cell lines. Koochekpour and Pilkington (1996) found that GD3 was invariably detected in glioblastoma multiforme and in a majority of anaplastic astrocytomas, but it was not detectable in low-grade gliomas. A potential source of incorrect attribution will be the ability of host cell infiltrates, e.g. macrophages, to produce angiogenic factors (Sunderkotter *et al.*, 1991). Macrophages do produce angiogenic factors (Koch *et al.*, 1992). This is also suggested, for example, by the low levels of bFGF found in human colon cell cultures compared with higher levels of the growth factor found in cells derived directly from tumours grown as xenografts (McCarty *et al.*, 1995). Furthermore, microvessel density has been found, at least in one study of invasive breast cancer, to correlate with macrophage count (Hildenbrand *et al.*, 1995a,b). This is an important issue to resolve because the degree of host cell infiltration is directly related to differentiation of the tumour and therefore inversely related with the degree of malignancy. It is essential that the expression of these factors resides demonstrably with tumour cells themselves.

The expression of the endothelial adhesion factor VCAM-1 shows a close asssociation with tumour progression. It occurs in 62% of primary melanomas less than 1.5 mm thick and in only 6% of primaries of greater thickness. VCAM is also present on 14% of lymph nodes metastases. When compared with the presence of this adhesion molecule in 79% of benign naevi, the conclusion is inescapable that a loss of VCAM may be important in metastasis (Denton *et al.*, 1992). Presumably, this could be a reflection of its ability to promote angiogenesis. Thus, a consensus view may be emerging that the expression of angiogenic agents could provide a practical prognostic tool.

The cardinal query to which most of these studies have addressed themselves was whether angiogenesis is related to tumour progression, but the answer may be deemed self-evident. Metastatic disease is the major cause of cancer deaths and the vascular and lymphatic systems are the carriers of the tumour cells to the metastatic sites. Admittedly, the identification of angiogenic factors has provided important targets for designing new drugs that can effectively inhibit angiogenesis and metastatic spread. However, it is of crucial importance that attention is focused sharply upon the coordinated regulation of genes encoding the angiogenic factors, and their receptors, and its integration with the complex system of control of cell proliferation. The ability to elicit angiogenic response apparently seems to precede the state when transformed cells become tumorigenic. However, tumorigenicity itself does not imply malignancy. The latter subsumes the notion that tumours have also acquired the invasive ability and the ability to induce neovascularisation as a means to accomplish metastatic dissemination. Therefore, it would be legitimate to inquire into how and when the appropriate genes are switched on in this process of transition to the tumorigenic state and from there to malignant disease. Some of the angiogenic factors also enhance endothelial permeability, and this may assist the entry of tumour cells into the vascular system and their extravasation at the metastatic site.

8

Cell surface glycoproteins and their receptors

Several families of adhesion molecules have been identified over the past several years and their synthesis and expression on the cell membrane studied in relation to the invasive and metastatic behaviour of cancers. These adhesion molecules may be deleted selectively or exhibit specific patterns of expression. They may also be differentially expressed as a metastasis-associated phenomenon (Nicolson *et al.*, 1986). Intercellular interactions and also interactions of cell surface macromolecules with the extracellular matrix are obviously of great significance in many biological processes of growth, apoptosis, differentiation, cell migration and pattern formation. Intercellular and cell-matrix (substratum) interactions are also a major element of cancer cell invasion and dissemination. These functions are mediated by many cell adhesion molecules and cell surface receptors, of which the integrin receptor family has been studied extensively.

Integrin receptors and their function

Integrins belong to a well-characterised family of receptors. These receptors recognise signals from the extracellular matrix and these are transduced via the cytoskeletal structures (Arregui *et al.*, 1994). A new paradigm is emerging in which integrin receptors are regarded as true receptors capable of tyrosine kinase-mediated transduction of extracellular signals (Juliano and

Haskill, 1993). The integrins, heterodimeric glycoproteins which form the receptors for the adhesion-mediating glycoproteins, have also been the focus of much research. They are composed of two subunits, the α and β subunits. A large number of the α and β subunits have been identified and these combine to form a variety of heterodimers and these serve as receptors for a large variety of ligands such as fibronectin, laminin, vitronectin, thrombospondin, tenascin, osteopontin, and cell adhesion molecules such as VCAM, ICAMs 1 and 2, among others (see Dedhar, 1990).

The possible role of integrins in tumour progression and use as prognostic markers have been studied and reviewed extensively (Dedhar, 1990; Chammas and Brentani, 1991; Natali et al., 1991; Seftor et al., 1992). The integrins appear to be involved with the transduction of extracellular biochemical signals and their expression is regulated during development and differentiation. Thus, Kornberg et al. (1991) have recently shown that antibody-mediated clustering of integrin receptors results in the phosphorylation of tyrosine residues of a complex of substrate proteins. Recently, in the search for a mechanism by which the src oncogene produces malignant transformation, an intracellular substrate protein now known as the $p125^{FAK}$ was discovered (Schaller et al., 1992), which is itself a protein kinase. The $p125^{FAK}$ is phosphorylated not only by the $pp60^{src}$ protein kinase but integrins also trigger its phosphorylation consequent upon occupancy of the receptor by the appropriate ligand (Guan et al., 1991; Guan and Shalloway, 1992). Zachary et al. (1992) have found that bombesin, vasopressin, endothelin and mitogenic neuropeptides also stimulate phosphorylation of $p125^{FAK}$. This is a most significant development, as Zachary and Rozengurt (1992) point out, because the process of transduction of this variety of biological signals focuses upon the phosphorylation of a single substrate protein. Some recent work by Vuori and Ruoslahti (1994) suggests that these processes might be related to growth factor stimulation of cells. Thus, a co-ordinated function of growth factors, integrins, and cytoskeletal elements, may be recognised as an essential ingredient of signal transduction.

Vitronectin receptors

The expression of vitronectin, another adhesion-mediating glycoprotein, appears to be associated with glioblastomas but it was not detectable in normal glial cells or low-grade gliomas (Gladson and Cheresh, 1991). The progression of cutaneous melanoma appears to be associated with the emergence of the vitronectin receptor, $\alpha_v\beta_3$ integrin. In MeWo human melanoma cells, retinoic acid has been shown to inhibit cell differentiation, increase melanogenesis and induce morphological changes, together with higher levels of vitronectin receptors (Santos et al., 1994). The emergence of the $\alpha_v\beta_3$ vitronectin receptor in melanoma progression has also been described by Danen et al. (1994). These authors investigated a spectrum of cutaneous tissues including common naevocellular naevi, dysplastic naevi, primary cutaneous melanomas and metastatic melanoma. The vitronectin receptor was found to be associated only with primary melanoma and metastasis, but little is known to date regarding the significance of the association or patterns of emergence of vitronectin receptors with tumour progression. The expression of $\alpha_v\beta_3$ integrin has been reported to increase by 50- to 100-fold during the progression of human melanomas to a more metastatic stage (Gehlsen *et al.*, 1992). Glioblastomas not only express vitronectin but also one of its integrin receptors, the $\alpha_v\beta_3$ integrin. The latter was not found in low-grade gliomas or normal glial cells (Gladson and Cheresh, 1991). The integrins α_7, α_v, and β_3 have been implicated in the invasion of the basement membrane by glioma cells on the basis of the observation that antibodies against these integrins inhibit the invasion by glioma cells of reconstituted basement membrane (Matrigel) *in vitro* (Paulus and Tonn, 1994).

Laminin receptors

Laminin is a major adhesion-mediating glycoprotein occurring in the basement membrane. Laminin derived from tumour cells is a cruciform trimer of α-1(A), β-1 (B1) and γ-2 (B2) subunits of 400, 210 and 200 kDa size, respectively. The long arm of the cruciform structure is composed of three strands in a coiled-coil conformation (see Timpl, 1989; Burgeson *et al.*, 1994). Laminin interacts with other macromolecules of the basement membrane, such as type IV collagen, heparan sulphate proteoglycans and with itself to provide stability and preserve the stability of the basement membrane. The integrins $\alpha_6\beta_1$ (Sonnenberg *et al.*, 1988) and probably also $\alpha_6\beta_4$ (Hemler *et al.*, 1989; Kajiji *et al.*, 1989) are involved in the binding of laminin molecules to the cell surface.

There have been several attempts recently to examine the possible correlation between laminin receptor expression and tumour invasion and metastasis. Initial work by Dedhar and Saulnier (1990) on chemically transformed human cells demonstrated that, upon transformation, these cells show a greater than 10-fold enhancement of expression of laminin and collagen receptor integrins $\alpha_6\beta_1$, $\alpha_2\beta_1$ and $\alpha_1\beta_1$, but fibronectin receptor levels remain unchanged. Some studies with human tumours have reported a direct correlation between laminin receptor positivity and lymph node involvement and the presence of distant metastases in gastric and colorectal cancers (Grigioni *et al.*, 1986; Cioce *et al.*, 1991). In human small cell lung carcinoma the expression of the 67 kDa receptor for laminin was related to tumour cell proliferation (Satoh *et al.*, 1992). In contrast, Marques *et al.* (1990) found an inverse relationship between laminin receptor levels and relapse-free survival in breast cancer. In node negative breast cancer, a 6-year follow-up study revealed that laminin receptor status does not possess the potential to predict prognosis (Daidone *et al.*, 1991). High expression of $\alpha_6\beta_1$ integrin has been found in the highly metastatic B16/129 melanoma and in KLN-205 carcinoma. An antibody, EA-1, which recognises the α_6 chain inhibits lung colonisation by B16/129 cells when injected into the tail vein (Ruiz *et al.*, 1993), suggesting that inhibition of integrin-mediated adhesion to laminin may inhibit lung colonisation.

Cadherins

Cadherins are transmembrane glycoproteins which mediate calcium-dependent cell-cell adhesion (Takeichi, 1990, 1991). The extracellular domain of cadherins contain several Ca^{2+}-binding domains and these self-associate and cause intercellular adhesion. Several intracellular proteins, α- and β-catenins and plakoglobin, have been postulated to participate in the linking of the cytoplasmic domains of cadherins to cytoskeletal elements (Ozawa et al., 1989; McCrea and Gumbiner, 1991; Nagafuchi et al., 1991; Knudsen and Wheelock, 1992). The participation of catenins is essential for the process of cadherin-mediated adhesion and cell aggregation to take place (Hirano et al., 1992). The cadherin–catenin complex binds to the cytoskeletal elements and phosphorylation of catenins appears to regulate the adhesive function of the complex (Ponta et al., 1994).

Several cadherins and cadherin-like molecules have been identified (Takeichi, 1988; Magee and Buxton, 1991). Of these E-cadherin has been studied extensively in relation to its role in cancer invasion. The E-cadherin gene has been mapped to chromosome 16q22.1. The gene encompasses approximately 100 kb and has 16 exons. Intron 1 contains a 5'-CpG island which may be involved in the regulation of its transcription (Berx et al., 1995a). In association with this process of regulation, changes have been found to occur in chromatin structure in the regulator region of the E-cadherin promoter and in the methylation status of the CpG sites. The chromatin structure is loosened in cells expressing E-cadherin, but condensed during the state of repression of transcription of the gene (Hennig et al., 1995). E-cadherin has been regarded as a suppressor of invasion in vitro (Vleminckx et al., 1991a,b). There has been notable progress in our understanding of the mechanisms associated with the loss of function of this gene as a suppressor of invasive potential. Three distinct modes can be identified. It has been consistently demonstrated that down-regulation of E-cadherin expression occurs concomitantly with acquisition of invasive capacity. The down-regulation results from a repression of transcription of the gene (Frixen et al., 1991; Vlemnickx et al., 1991a,b; Brabant et al., 1993). A mutation of the E-cadherin gene would result in a non-functional product. Biochemical modification such as the state of phosphorylation of the intermediate components, catenins and plakoglobin, which link E-cadherin to the cytoskeleton, or a loss of one of these elements also may be expected effectively to render the cadherin non-functional (Figure 13).

The loss of E-cadherin is a characteristic feature of invasive cell types and this invasive ability can be inhibited by transfecting the invasive cells with the E-cadherin gene. The transformation by H-ras of Madin–Darby canine kidney (MDCK) cells has been found to reduce E-cadherin levels in association with changes in cellular morphology and with increased malignancy. However, when the cadherin levels were restored by gene transfer the cells were found to regain normal morphology and revert to a benign condition (Behrens et al., 1989; Mareel et al., 1991). Behrens et al. (1989) demonstrated that MDCK cells acquired invasive ability upon treatment with antibodies against E-cadherin. MDCK cells transformed with Harvey or Moloney

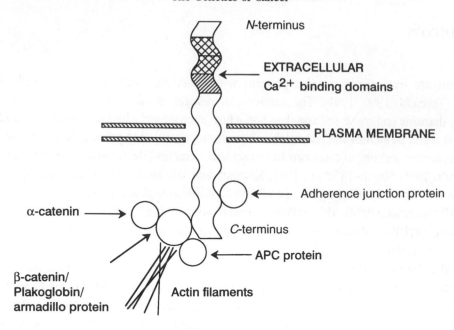

Figure 13.   A schematic diagram of the transmembrane protein E-cadherin and its interaction with cytoskeletal elements and APC protein. Based on van Roy *et al.* (1992).

virus were able to invade collagen gels and embryonal heart tissue and showed no E-cadherin expression at the cell surface.

The apparent close relationship between the invasive ability of tumours and the state of expression of E-cadherin has been upheld by several later studies. Pizaro *et al.* (1994) found that cadherin levels were reduced in 10 out of 15 infiltrating basal cell carcinomas as compared with superficial and nodular basal cell carcinomas. Vleminckx *et al.* (1991b) found that E-cadherin was not present in invasive MMTV-transformed mouse mammary tumour cells, whereas non-invasive cells contained high amounts of this glycoprotein. Again, the invasive ability could be abrogated by transfecting the cells with the E-cadherin gene. Frixen *et al.* (1991) also showed that invasion could be prevented by transfecting E-cadherin cDNA into cell lines derived from a variety of human carcinomas, e.g. from bladder, breast, lung and pancreas. Using a three-dimensional collagen gel matrix Chen and Obrink (1991) demonstrated that cells not expressing E-cadherin invaded the gels but those that expressed it were less invasive. Infiltrating lobular carcinomas appear to exhibit E-cadherin loss (Palacios *et al.*, 1995a), and this loss may often be associated with the infiltrating cells (Gamallo *et al.*, 1993). According to Siitonen *et al.* (1996), the frequency with which E-cadherin loss or reduction in its expression occurs, increases from 20% in intraductal carcinomas (four out of 20) to 52% (124 out of 239) of invasive ductal carcinomas and 64% (18 out of 28) of recurrent carcinomas. It has been reported that E-cadherin loss may be accompanied by the loss of α-catenin (Rimm *et al.*, 1995). A majority of breast cancer lines investigated by Pierceall *et al.* (1995) have revealed a loss of E-cadherin as well as its

RNA transcripts. The relationship between E-cadherin loss and invasive nature is apparent also from studies on bladder cancer. E-cadherin expression is high in normal bladder epithelium and in cystitis; reduced expression is seen in only 20% of superficial bladder cancers compared with 75-90% of invasive cancers (Bringuier et al., 1993; Syrigos et al., 1995).

There have been reports that cadherin expression is related to tumour differentiation. Retinoic acid, which is known to induce differentiation and inhibit the invasive ability of cancer cells, up-regulates the E-cadherin–catenin functional complex (Vermeulen SJ et al., 1995). In vivo, E-cadherins are highly expressed in well-differentiated hepatocellular carcinomas, whereas in poorly differentiated tumours only low levels of the cadherin can be found (Shimoyama and Hirohashi, 1991a); in a subsequent report of an investigation of gastric adenocarcinomas, however, Shimoyama and Hirohashi (1991b) failed to find such a clear-cut association between cadherin expression and differentiation. Schipper et al. (1991) studied E-cadherin expression in 32 squamous cell carcinomas of the head and neck and reported that expression was inversely related to both degree of differentiation and lymph node metastasis. Reduced expression of E-cadherin has also been reported in poorly differentiated squamous cell and small cell lung carcinomas. Most metastases also showed reduced levels of E-cadherin (Bohm et al., 1994).

These studies suggest that E-cadherin might participate in contact and adhesion processes and could function as an anti-invasive gene. It may be reasonable to suggest, therefore, that E-cadherin might act to suppress invasion and metastasis. Katayama et al. (1994) found that sera of cancer patients contained higher than normal levels of E-cadherin fragments. The possibility should therefore be considered that a deletion of E-cadherin may enable tumour cells to invade. It is essential, therefore, to examine E-cadherin gene expression as well as the protein in order that a coherent picture may be drawn of the involvement of this protein in cancer invasion and metastasis.

Consistent with the potential anti-invasive and metastasis-supressing properties of E-cadherin, a loss of this adhesion protein has been associated with poor prognosis in patients with several forms of cancer, e.g. squamous and small cell lung carcinoma (Bohm et al., 1994) and bladder carcinomas (Otto et al., 1994). Reduced levels of E-cadherin in bladder cancer was found to be related not only to invasive ability but also to shorter recurrence-free survival (Lipponen and Eskelinin, 1995). In breast cancer, E-cadherin expression was related to tumour grade, with grade 1 tumours being more immunoreactive than grade 2 (Gamallo et al., 1993). Lipponen et al. (1994) found that its expression was not related to nodal status of patients, the presence of distant metastases at presentation, or to the size of the S-phase fraction and mitotic index. The findings of Palacios et al. (1995b) generally support this view. However, it should be noted that these authors found E-cadherin expression in myoepithelial cells and luminal epithelium of normal breast tissue and in benign breast lesions, but infiltrating ductal carcinomas showed no E-cadherin expression.

Most of these studies have been prompted by the putative invasion suppressor function of E-cadherin and have concentrated upon establishing a link between loss of its expression with acquisition of invasive potential. However, recent studies show that this might be a simplistic interpretation of the invasion suppressor postulate. For instance, there is a tacit assumption that surface cadherin normally occurs in a functional state: such an assumption is erroneous because Bracke *et al.* (1994) found that the E-cadherin occurring on the surface of MCP-7/6 breast cancer cell lines is non-functional but that it can be activated by treating the cells with tamoxifen, which leads to the restoration of E-cadherin activity as assessed by cell aggregation and inhibition of the invasive potential of the cells. In addition, the invasion-suppressor function of E-cadherin depends upon its ability to form successful attachment to the actin cytoskeleton. For this, other linking elements of the cadherin complex not only need to be present but they have to be functionally sound. For instance, a reduced expression or loss of the linking α-catenin has been reported in breast cancers (Takayama *et al.*, 1994). However, one can also envisage a situation where E-cadherin may be non-functional on account of the loss of α- or β-catenin, where the cadherin expression will be seen as not conforming to the accepted view of tumour suppression. Sommers *et al.* (1994) tranfected the E-cadherin gene into the E-cadherin-negative invasive breast cancer lines, BT549 and HS578t and found that the morphology and the invasive behaviour of the cells was not suppressed even though E-cadherin was expressed, as indicated by the Ca^{2+}-dependent aggregation exhibited by the transfected cells. The reason for this has been suggested to be a defective linkage of the transfected E-cadherin to the actin cytoskeleton because they found that the transfected E-cadherin occurred mainly in a soluble (in Triton X-100) form, whereas the normally functioning E-cadherin of another breast cancer cell line MCF7 was found at the cell–cell interphase. Furthermore, Sommers *et al.* (1994) found that the level of tyrosine phosporylation of β-catenin of the E-cadherin-transfected BT549 and HS578t cells was higher than that of MCF7 cells, which may have resulted in a defective interaction with E-cadherin. These experiments demonstrate that the suppression of invasive potential of cells requires all the components of the E-cadherin complex to be in place and fully functional.

Other molecular mechanisms may be involved in the regulation of the invasive behaviour by cadherins. Mutations affecting the exons 8 and 9 coding for the putative Ca^{2+}-binding domains have been found in 50% of diffuse-type gastric carcinomas (Becker *et al.*, 1994). Other types of mutation have been reported in endometrial carcinomas (Risinger *et al.*, 1994). Mutations of the gene and allelic loss at its locus (chromosome 16q22.1) may result in the production of inactive E-cadherin or loss of its expression (Berx *et al.*, 1995b). Truncation of the extracellular domain of *N*-cadherin, for instance, leads to an impairment of intercellular contact and adhesion (Hertig *et al.*, 1996). To date, no mutations have been detected in the α- or β-catenin genes (Candidus *et al.*, 1996).

It would be worthwhile pointing out that although investigations have been focused on one or two major cadherins, the cadherin family has several other members. Suzuki *et al.* (1991) have reported eight new molecules with overall structure similar to the well-known cadherins. The diversity of this family and the function of several putative members is largely unknown.

Tenascin

The extracellular matrix glycoprotein called tenascin has been regarded as a regulator of cell migration and organogenesis, e.g. the migration of neural crest cells (Crossin *et al.*, 1986; Bronner-Fraser, 1988). This glycoprotein is reportedly found in higher levels in breast carcinomas than in fibrocystic disease or normal breast tissue. Tenascin is found more strongly associated with infiltrating ductal carcinomas than with *in situ* ductal and lobular carcinomas of the breast (Gould *et al.*, 1990). Compatible with this is the report that in human astrocytomas, tenascin expression strongly correlated with the degree of dedifferentiation (Higuchi *et al.*, 1993). Contradictory results have been reported by Sakakura and Kusakabe (1994) who found high levels of tenascin expression associated with favourable prognosis in breast and colon cancers. Moch *et al.* (1993) also reported no recognisable pattern in tenascin expression with reference to other prognostic factors such as nodal involvement, invasion of blood vessels, the S-phase fraction or ploidy, in breast cancer. Tenascin is found in non-neoplastic lung parenchyma and benign lung tumours, and also in lung carcinomas (Sakakura and Kusakabe, 1994; Soini *et al.*, 1993).

It would be premature to attempt any rationalisation of these conflicting reports, but tumour cells appear to be capable of synthesising tenascin in response to extracellular stimuli (Sakakura and Kusakabe, 1994). One should recall that Chiquetehrisman *et al.* (1994) have presented evidence for the existence of more than one member in this family of tenascins. However, the observation that mice lacking a functional tenascin gene do develop normally, argues quite strongly against a premature attribution of a role to these glycoproteins in tumour progression.

CD44 and its isoforms

A recent development is the identification of a transmembrane glycoprotein, CD44. CD44 is expressed as one or more isoforms derived from alternative splicing of the RNA and differences in the patterns of glycosylation. The splice variants or isoforms have been reported to be expressed differentially between non-metastatic and metastatic tumours of the pancreas (Gunthert *et al.*, 1991). The CD44 glycoprotein (also referred to as the *Hermes-1* antigen, Pgp-1 protein, extracellular matrix receptor, lymphocyte homing receptor, etc.) are found on the surface of diverse cell types such as lymphocytes, bone marrow prothymocytes, fibroblasts, astrocytes and epithelial cells. CD44 appears to participate in cellular adhesion and binding to extracellular matrix components, which may be mediated by cytoskeletal elements (see Haynes *et al.*, 1989). CD44 promotes adhesion to a variety of substrates, e.g. collagen types I and IV, endothelial cells, etc., and it is the major receptor for the extracellular matrix component glycosaminoglycan hyaluronate (Aruffo *et al.*, 1990; Miyake *et al.*, 1990), but it may also bind other ligands such as fibronectin. The CD44 cDNA does not appear to be related to other families of adhesion receptors such as the integrins or to cadherins (Berg *et al.*, 1989). By virtue of these properties, CD44 could participate in normal physiological functions such as T-cell maturation and activation (Haynes *et al.*, 1989; Huet *et al.*, 1989; Denning *et al.*, 1990) and its expression may be developmentally regulated (Patel *et al.*, 1995).

Gunthert *et al.* (1991) demonstrated that one of the splice variation of CD44 conferred metastatic properties on a non-metastatic variant of a rat pancreatic carcinoma cell line. Sy *et al.* (1991) stably transfected B cell lymphoma cells with either CD44-H (haemopoietic) or E (epithelial) isoforms. Cells transfected with the H form produced tumours in four out of five nude mice upon subcutaneous implantation, while no tumours were formed by the CD44-E transfectant. In experimental metastasis assays, the CD44-H transfectants produced tumours in 90% of animals injected. In comparison, CD44-E transfected cells showed a greatly reduced (20%) metastatic localisation.

In gliomas CD44 has been reported to be highly expressed in high-grade tumours compared with low-grade gliomas and meningiomas (Kuppner *et al.*, 1992). Radotra *et al.* (1994) found no correlation between glioma grade and tumour-associated CD44 and Li H *et al.* (1993) reported that they could not detect any CD44 in human glioblastomas or glioma cell lines. The isoform CD44H (the haemopoietic form) is believed to figure prominently in normal brain tissue and brain tumours and they do not express the larger molecular weight variants such as the v6 (Nagasaka *et al.*, 1995), the isoform which has been associated with metastatic spread. This may be significant in the light of the general observation that brain tumours do not normally metastasise to extracranial sites, but do show local invasion and will spread to other sites within the CNS (Sherbet, 1987). Radotra *et al.* (1994) found that the adhesion of glioma cells to a variety of extracellular matrix components could be blocked by CD44 antibodies. CD44 may be associated with the invasive behaviour of these tumours, as indicated by the inhibition by anti-CD44 antibodies of *in vitro* invasion by glioma cell lines. Invasion was completely inhibited by an antisense oligonucleotide for CD44, which, in parallel, also inhibited CD44 expression (Merzak *et al.*, 1994c). This also appears to be the case in breast cancer cell lines where invasion *in vitro* has been found to correlate with the amounts of associated CD44 (Culty *et al.*, 1994).

In neuroblastomas the CD44 story is entirely different; virtually all early stage tumours expressed CD44 whereas only 50% of advanced tumours were CD44 positive (Combaret *et al.*, 1995; Gross *et al.*, 1995). As these authors have themselves pointed out, this is the first tumour model where the absence of CD44, rather than its over-expression, correlated with tumour aggressiveness and proved to be highly predictive of clinical outcome. It ought to be pointed out, however, that Combaret *et al.* (1995) used an antibody which was generated against an epitope common to all CD44 isoforms. Since we know that the isoforms tend to be expressed differentially in different tumour models, it would be more meaningful to know whether any specific isoforms might show this correlation between loss of expression with clinical aggressiveness of the tumour. Nevertheless, an inverse relationship between CD44 and the state of progression has also been noted by Gross *et al.* (1995). CD44 expression was lower in later stages of the disease where n-*myc* oncogene expression was found at an enhanced level. Gross *et al.* (1995) show, however, that CD44 expression and n-*myc* amplification are not directly related, but the former is related to the state of differentiation, as indicated by the fact that retinoic acid up-regulates CD44 expression in parallel with induction of differentiation. This ties in with the loss of CD44 with associated n-*myc* over-expression, since this gene is known to down-regulate class I HLA antigen expression. This may exemplify cooperative function of genes.

Tanabe *et al.* (1993) have reported that 12 out of 14 primary colonic tumours and all metastatic tumours that they examined expressed the epithelial variant CD44R1 compared with two out of 13 normal mucosal specimens. However, the haemopoietic variant CD44H was found to be expressed in all the specimens studied, suggesting enhanced CD44R1 expression relative to CD44H in colonic carcinomas. Mulder *et al.* (1994) have found that CD44v6 variant expression relates to progression of colorectal tumour in man, with expression associated closely with tumour-related death and have suggested that CD44v6 expression may reflect a propensity of the tumours to metastasise. In another study, the expression of CD44 isoforms v8–v10 has been reported to be significantly greater in carcinomas associated with liver metastasis; the metastatic tumours themselves showed far greater CD44 v8-10 expression than the primary tumours (Takeuchi K *et al.*, 1995). The recent report of Ichikawa's (1994) claims that CD44-H expression showed no correlation with tumour size, grade, Duke's stage, or growth patterns of colorectal carcinomas, but CD44-H positivity correlated significantly with liver metastases and patient survival. In contrast, however, Heider *et al.* (1993) found that CD44 variants were expressed even in early stages of colorectal carcinogenesis, e.g. in adenomatous polyps. Indeed, CD44 variants v2-v10 may be commonly expressed in normal colonic crypt epithelium, and the v6 variant, which is often claimed to be important for metastatic spread, is found in benign colonic tumours and also occurs in normal basal crypt epithelium as well as in colon carcinoma cells (Gotley *et al.*, 1996).

There have also been investigations into possible correlation of CD44 expression with other markers, such as p53 expression, which are closely associated with the progression of colonic carcinomas. Consistent with their previous study, Mulder *et al.* (1995) reported statistically significant increases in both CD44 and p53 expression in the late stages of progression. Furthermore, a significant correlation was also noted between CD44 and p53. Ichikawa (1994) also studied p53 and nm23 expression in this tumour model but found that only CD44 expression correlated with the incidence of hepatic metastasis and recurrence. Unfortunately, unlike Mulder *et al.* (1995), Ichikawa does not appear to have examined possible correlations between CD44 and other markers.

In gastric cancers, invasive carcinomas have been reported to stain more strongly for CD44 than dysplasia or intramucosal carcinomas and there is also a correlation between degree of CD44 staining and patient survival (Washington *et al.*, 1994). Serum CD44 levels have also been suggested as indicators of tumour burden and metastatic spread, with 20-fold greater amounts of CD44 being detected in serum from gastric and colonic carcinoma patients compared with normal subjects (Guo *et al.*, 1994). In general support are the findings of Harn *et al.* (1995) who found no CD44 expression in normal gastric mucosa, but high expression in intestinal metaplasias and in adenocarcinomas. The metaplasias expressed both v5 and v6 variants, but tubular and signet-ring cell types of adenocarcinoma were significantly v5 positive, although v6 was also expressed in 30% of the tubular type. Most significantly, only v5 was the most frequently expressed variant (18 out of 20) in adenocarcinomas which had metastasised to lymph nodes, compared with v6 expression (seen only in four out of 20). In breast cancer the v6 isoform appears to correlate with clinical aggressiveness of the disease. CD44 is not expressed in normal epithelium or hyperplasias, but v3, v5 and v6 are found in most tumour tissues. The v6 isoform is expressed in 84% of primary tumours and 100% of tumours metastatic to the lymph node, and v6 negativity has been found to be a good prognostic factor (Kaufmann *et al.*, 1995).

Of gynaecological tumours, cervical and ovarian cancers have been studied for CD44 expression. In cervical cancer, tumours expressing v6 metastasised frequently to pelvic lymph nodes and vascular invasion, and patients with CD44v6-positive tumours showed poor overall survival (Kainz *et al.*, 1995). However, in ovarian epithelial cancers where CD44 expression was common, there was no association of CD44 expression with standard prognostic factors, such as stage and grade of disease or survival (Cannistra *et al.*, 1995). In typical contrast that has characterised most CD44 studies, patients with CD44v-positive ovarian carcinoma had a significantly shorter disease-free survival than patients with CD44v-negative tumours (Uhlsteidl *et al.*, 1995).

The v6 isoform was not detectable in melanocytic lesions, but v5 and v10 were differentially expressed. In two cell lines generated from metastatic melanomas, the v5 isoform was strongly expressed (Mantenhorst *et al.*, 1995). Contrary to this, Guttinger *et al.* (1995) found strong expression of v4, v6 and v9 isoforms in hyperproliferative skin disorders, but expression appeared to be down-regulated in primary skin tumours and their metastases.

In a recent report Fox SB *et al.* (1994) described a study of CD44 protein expression in a variety of human tumours and normal tissues using a comprehensive panel of CD44 exon-specific monoclonal antibodies generated against recombinant CD44 (v3–v10). They found that CD44v expression varied greatly. Some tumours were found to express low levels of CD44v or none at all. CD44 variants carrying v3, v4/5 and v8/9 were also expressed in human tumours. Furthermore, normal epithelial cells expressed high levels of the glycoprotein. Normal urothelium has been reported to express the v6 isoform and its expression may be down-regulated in urothelial carcinogenesis (Hong *et al.*, 1995). CD44 expression has been studied in lung carcinomas by using an antibody which detects all the isoforms (Clarke *et al.*, 1995). They found CD44 in moderately to poorly differentiated adenocarcinomas, but this did not correlate with pleural invasion or angio-lymphatic invasion. Consistent with the strain of contradiction which seems to run virtually through most CD44 studies, Jackson *et al.* (1994) had previously found no CD44v6 in any form of lung cancer; not even metastatic deposits expressed CD44v6. These observations quite clearly argue against the relevance of CD44v6 in metastatic dissemination. Even if CD44 may have appeared on occasion to dominate the metastatic process, we are unsure as to the relative significance to metastatic spread of the CD44v6 variants. Conversely, in the B16 melanoma model, Sherbet and Lakshmi (1995) found no changes in the overall expression of CD44v6 in association with increased metastatic spread induced by the expression of the metastasis-related *18A2/mts1* gene, but they noted that upon up-regulation of this gene, the distribution of CD44v6 changed from a uniform to a focal or capping pattern. The *18A2/mts1* gene promotes depolymerisation of cytoskeletal structures and therefore these authours have attributed the changes in the topographical distribution of CD44v6 to changes in the lateral mobility of the CD44 receptors consequent upon up-regulation of the gene. The phenomenon of CD44 redistribution and capping has also been reported in lymphocyte-endothelial adhesion interactions; it is an energy-dependent process and is cytoskeletally driven (Rosenman *et al.*, 1993). Hyaluronic acid, which is the ligand for CD44 receptor, has been shown to induce CD44 capping and adhesion of mouse T-lymphoma cells to hyaluronic acid-coated substratum and together with this a preferential accumulation of and binding to the membrane cytoskeletal protein ankyrin occurs underneath these CD44 caps (Bourguignon *et al.*, 1993; Welsh *et al.*, 1995). The highly conserved intracellular domain is of CD44 essential for cytoskeletal interaction. Lokeshwar and Bourguignon (1992) found that GTP binding significantly increases CD44 interaction with ankyrin. There are indications that phosphorylation of CD44 *in vivo* requires the presence of serine-323 and serine-325 residues, although phosphorylation of these residues does not control membrane localisation or cytoskeletal interaction (Neame and Isacke, 1992); binding of CD44 to hyaluronic acid may also be independent of phosphorylation (Uff *et al.*, 1995). Hyaluronic acid binding has been described in the absence of the cytoplasmic domain, but dimerisation of the extracellular domain is essential in this case (Pershl *et al.*, 1995a). But Pure *et al.* (1995), while confirming that serine-325 and serine-327 are required for the phosphorylation of CD44, also found that substitution of these residues, e.g. serine-325 to glycine or serine-327 to alanine resulted in defective hyaluronate binding. These substitutions also affected CD44-mediated adhesion of T cells to smooth muscle cells and ligand-induced modulation of CD44 receptor. This suggests that phosphorylation of serine-325/327 may be required for the interaction of the cytoplasmic domain with the cytoskeletal components.

It is obvious, therefore, that CD44 capping indicates membrane activity related to cell adhesion and change of cell shape. The redistribution of CD44v6 demonstrated by Sherbet and Lakshmi (1995) may be interpreted as indicating a change in such membrane activity in the B16 melanoma system in association with increased metastatic potential brought about by enhanced expression of *18A2/mts1* gene. Although these studies show the importance of the extracellular domain of CD44 in adhesion-dependent phenomena, there have been suggestions that the transmembrane portion of the molecule may play an important part in the redistribution of CD44 (Perschl *et al.*, 1995b).

Many of these studies have concentrated upon the total CD44 expression or have focused on one or two splice variants in relation to progression. The pattern of relative expression of the various splice variants has recently received attention and Yokozaki *et al.* (1994) have pointed out that the expression of aberrant patterns can show some relationship to gastric carcinoma progression. According to these authors, all the primary and metastatic tumours that they studied over-expressed CD44 variants larger than 1.0 kb compared with corresponding normal gastric mucosa. Whereas six out of nine well-differentiated cancers over-expressed more than three aberrant transcripts, 10 out of 11 poorly differentiated tumours over-expressed only one or two aberrant transcripts. Although it is too early to determine the value of this approach, it would appear that such a qualitative assessment of the abnormal expression and the generation of splice-variants may be potentially more valuable than assessing the expression of generic CD44 or a selected splice-variant.

It would be reasonable to conclude, that although different CD44 glycoprotein isoforms could be associated with different tumour or cell types, there is no incontrovertible evidence of any pattern in the expression of the CD44 splice variants in relation to tumour type, tumour progression or cell lineage. It is certainly premature in the light of the above review of recent work to consider CD44 expression as a non-invasive method for assessing the progression of tumours, however desirable maybe the availability of such techniques for determining progression and prognosis.

Implicit in some studies is the suggestion that the CD44 gene is a candidate metastasis gene. At present there is only limited evidence to support such a concept. Possibly, CD44 is just another adhesion mediating protein which is controlled distally by gene(s) that may confer invasive properties upon cells by linking extracellular matrix proteins to cytoskeletal elements. Hoffmann et al. (1993) have reported that induction of ras expression brings about changes in levels of CD44s, a variant said to be associated with lung colonisation, and produces a transient increase in the CD44v6 variant, believed to be a marker for the metastatic phenotype. The induction of CD44 over-expression by activated ras and src genes has been demonstrated also by Jamal et al. (1994). This suggests that CD44 may be only a target gene which might come into its own at a specific stage of metastatic progression. Further work is needed to establish whether any other transforming gene or metastasis-associated gene might alter CD44 expression in parallel with changes in biological behaviour.

Miyake et al. (1990) have shown that hyaluronate is a ligand for CD44 in adhesive interactions. A number of studies have reported that tumour cells produce far greater amounts of hyaluronates than corresponding normal cells and large differences have also been reported between metastasising and non-metastasising tumours (Kimata et al., 1983; Turley and Tretiak, 1985). Kimata et al. (1983) found 27- to 54-fold greater incorporation of labelled precursors into hyaluronic acid in carcinoma cells with high metastatic potential than in those with low metastatic potential. This mechanism, however, may not be a general one since hyaluronate is not synthesised by some cells, e.g. B16 melanomas (Edward and MacKie, 1989). But B16 melanomas do show adhesion to hyaluronate substratum (East et al., 1992). Furthermore, Edward et al. (1992) have shown that normal fibroblasts can synthesise hyaluronate if they are grown in melanoma-conditioned medium. It is possible that the different isoforms of CD44 may differ functionally. Alternatively, CD44 may be bound by other ligands such as fibronectin which has been regarded as an alternative ligand for CD44.

In summary, it would appear that some glycoprotein mediators of cell adhesion and invasion, together with their appropriate receptors, may be associated with greater malignancy. These observations are consistent with the important part that adhesive interactions play in tumour cell invasion and metastasis.

Cell adhesion molecules (CAMs) in cancer invasion

The interaction of tumour cells with the microvasculature is an essential prerequisite in cancer invasion and metastasis. The adhesion of tumour cells to endothelial cells involves recognition mechanisms that operate also in leukocyte adhesion to endothelial cells. Hence, the expression of certain leukocyte adhesion factors and their regulation by growth factors have been studied in cancer cells, in relation to their function in cancer invasion and metastasis.

Leukocyte adhesion factors can be classified into three families: (a) the leukocyte integrins CD11/CD18; (b) the intercellular adhesion molecules (ICAMs) comprising ICAMs-1, 2 and 3 and the vascular cell adhesion molecule (VCAM-1); and (c) the carbohydrate-binding molecules called the selectins, comprising L-selectin, E-selectin (also known as the endothelial leukocyte adhesion molecule or ELAM-1) and P-selectin. The cell adhesion molecules function as ligands for the leukocyte integrins CD11 and CD18. These integrins are normally non-adhesive, but they are activated by binding to ICAMs. Li R et al. (1993, 1995) showed that a peptide derived from ICAM-2 can bind to leukocyte integrins and activate leukocyte adhesion. This peptide specifically binds to CD11a,b/CD18 and stimulates aggregation of monocytic cell lines. It also induces integrin-mediated binding of the monocytic cells to the substratum. Evidence has been presented recently that the binding of ICAM-2 occurs with the immunoglobulin-like domain of the integrin and, further, that certain threonine and aspartic acid residues occurring in the immunoglobulin-like domains of the integrins are essential for the binding of ICAM-1 and C3Bi molecules (Kamata et al., 1995; Xie et al., 1995). A conserved amino acid motif has been identified in ICAM-3 which functions as its binding site for the integrin receptor LFA-1. This may be a common integrin-binding motif, since it has been found to operate also in ICAM-1 and VCAM-1 (Sadhu et al., 1994). Similarly, E-selectin binds to the sialyl Lewis (x) carbohydrate epitope of the leukocyte integrins (Kotovuori et al., 1993).

Among other adhesion molecules that have been studied in the context of human cancer invasion is the neural cell adhesion molecule (NCAM) and the neuroglial cell adhesion molecule (NG-CAM). Telencephalin (TLN) is a 130 kDa transmembrane glycoprotein found exclusively in neurones of the telencephanon and localised in the dendritic membrane of the soma, but not in the membrane of the axons. TLN shows homology with the immunoglobulin-like domains of the ICAMs (Yoshihara et al., 1994) (Table 7).

The cell adhesion molecules (CAMs) are constitutively expressed in leukocytes and also induced to express on vascular endothelial cells. Prominent among CAMs that participate in the interaction between leukocytes and endothelial cells are ICAM-1, E-selectin and VCAM-1. ICAM-1 is a glycosylated protein, of approximately 90 kDa size, belonging to the immunoglo-bulin family of adhesion factors and it is expressed in haemopoietic cells as well as in vascular endothelial cells, mucosal epithelial cells and T-lymphocytes. ICAM-1 has five extracellular immunoglobulin-like domains. ICAM-1 may be shed from the cell surface in a soluble form

Table 7.   Cell adhesion molecules (CAM) and their integrin/ECM counter receptors

CAM ligand	Integrin/ECM counter-receptor
ICAM-1 (CD54)	CD11a (LFA-1),b/CD18
	LFA-3 (CD58)
ICAM-2 (CD102)	
ICAM-2 (CD50)	LFA-1
VCAM-1	$\alpha_4 \beta_1$ (VLA-4)
E-selectin (ELAM-1, endothelial leukocyte adhesion molecule)	Carbohydrate epitopes of sialyl Lewis (x)/ Lewis (a) antigens
	sPan-1 (Yamada N *et al.*, 1995)
L-selectin	
P-selectin	
NCAM (CD-56)	
NGCAM (Grumet *et al.*, 1993)	Laminin
Telencephalin	

Based on references cited in the Table and those in text; LFA: lymphocyte function associated antigen.

which contains these extracellular domains but differs in molecular size from the surface ICAM. This soluble ICAM is produced by proteolytic cleavage of the surface ICAM. The soluble form is not the result of alternative splicing of the mRNA (Budnik *et al.*, 1996). The soluble ICAM has been detected in the circulation (Springer, 1990; Staunton *et al.*, 1994; Viac *et al.*, 1996).

Endothelial cells and lymphocytes respond to agents such as interleukin-1 (IL-1), TNF-α, IFN-γ and lipopolysaccharides (LPS) which can up-regulate the expression of ICAM-1 (Bevilacqua MP *et al.*, 1987, 1989; Stoolman, 1989; Springer, 1990; Etzoni, 1994; Klein *et al.*, 1994, 1995; Momosaki *et al.*, 1995). P- and E-selectins are also induced by LPS and TNF-α. Both selectins are induced in the endothelial cells of veins but only E-selectin is induced in arterial endothelial cells (Gotsch *et al.*, 1994). The induction of CAMs and selectins involves the transcription factor NFκB which controls the expression of the genes coding for the adhesion factors. Activation of human umbilical endothelial cells by IL-1β induces the translocation of NFκB to the nucleus and the induction of E-selectin and ICAM-1 expression, and this results in the enhancement of adhesion of tumour cells to the counter receptors on the endothelial surface (Tozawa *et al.*, 1995). In a complementary fashion, TNF and IL-1β induce the expression of genes coding for sialyl and fucosyl transferases which are involved in the synthesis of the oligosaccharide counter receptors (Majuri *et al.*, 1995).

The distribution of ICAMs in disease states

A differential distribution of ICAMs has been described between normal and disease states. In the chronic inflammatory condition of rheumatoid arthritis, for instance, ICAM-1 is expressed at higher levels in endothelial cells than in endothelial cells from normal subjects. ICAM-1 expression is also up-regulated in macrophages and lining cells. ICAM-3 is found in normal resting leukocytes but not in endothelial cells. This differential expression may suggest different roles for the ICAMs in the pathogenesis of rheumatoid arthritis and ICAM-1 may be associated with macrophage infiltration and tissue damage (Szekanecz *et al.*, 1994). Activated T-lympho-cytes infiltrating the synovial membrane show greatly increased affinity for ECM proteins and VCAM-1 and ICAMs (Postigo *et al.*, 1993). ICAM-3 is widely expressed in inflammatory dermatoses (Montazeri *et al.*, 1995). ICAM-1 expression in benign and malignant melanocytic lesions is similar (Denton *et al.*, 1992). Hepatocellular carcinomas have been found virtually invariably to express ICAM-1 but it is not detected on normal hepatocytes (Momosaki *et al.*, 1995). High levels of soluble ICAM-1 were detected in preoperative sera of patients with epithelial ovarian carcinoma compared with sera from patients with benign ovarian conditions. However, these ICAM levels did not correlate with International Federations of Gynaecology & Obstetrics (FIGO) stage or histological grade (Ferdeghini *et al.*, 1995). Neither has any association emerged between soluble ICAM-1 levels and progression of colorectal cancer (Reinhardt *et al.*, 1996).

It should be recognised, however, that the expression of cell surface and soluble ICAM is subjected to the operation of cytokines. It may be recalled here that TNF up-regulates the expression of ICAM-1 in the progression of malignant melanoma. Therefore the status of expression of cytokine receptor may provide additional clues to the involvement of ICAM in tumour progression. Consistent with this is the status of expression of two forms of soluble TNF receptors TNF-R1 and TNF-R2 in melanomas. Viac *et al.* (1996) have found TNF-R1 receptors only in the sera of patients with metastatic melanomas and not in sera from normal subjects. The TNF-R2 receptors have been found in both primary and metastatic melanomas.

Cancer cell adhesion to endothelial cells can be enhanced by interleukin-A, TNF-α and PMA, consistent with the ability of these agents to up-regulate ICAM expression (Steinbach *et al.*, 1996). Transfection of ICAM-1 gene into MCA-105 fibrosarcoma cells also enhances their adhesion to endothelial cell *in vitro* (Burno *et al.*, 1996). However, the *in vitro* demonstration of ICAM's ability to enhance adhesion is not supported by adhesion to vascular endothelium and invasion *in vivo*. For instance, transitional cell carcinoma of the bladder has revealed no differences between invasive and superficial types (Witjes *et al.*, 1995). ICAM expression in gastric carcinoma may be markedly different from benign gastric epithelium but the expression was not related to vascular invasion. No correlation has been found with disease relapse or patient survival but the ICAM integrin receptor LFA-3 strongly correlated with the state of dedifferentiation of the tumour and LFA-3 expression was conducive to adhesion to vascular endothelium and invasion (Mayer *et al.*, 1995). The picture differs quite markedly in renal cell tumours. ICAM-1 appears to be expressed in a majority of renal cell carcinomas and ICAM levels were also lower in cells from patients who were disease-free over 5 years than in tumours from patients where the disease had relapsed. Furthermore, the levels of soluble ICAM-1 were far lower in disease-free patients than in patients where the disease had progressed to the metastatic state (Santarosa *et al.*, 1995).

Yasoshima *et al.* (1996) isolated sub-lines from the human gastric carcinoma cell line AZ521 and selected a few cell lines which differed in metastatic potential upon growth in nude mice. Significantly, both ICAM-1 and LFA-1 showed reduced expression in highly metastatic lines compared with those with low metastatic ability. This is supported by the inverse relationship between ICAM-1 expression and the occurrence of liver metastases in gastric carcinomas (Ura *et al.*, 1996). However, if the postulate that ICAM expression promotes adhesion to and invasion of microvasculature is to be accepted one should find it expressed differentially between primary and metastatic lesions. This does not appear to be the case (Zhau *et al.*, 1996).

Thus, it seems imperative that factors which regulate ICAM expression and also the expression of other components of the system that participate in adhesive interactions are taken into account when judging the significance of its expression in relation to tumour progression.

VCAM-1 in cancer invasion

The adhesion of human melanomas to endothelial cells occurs by a preferential recognition of VCAM-1 and is mediated by the integrin $\alpha_4\beta_1$ VLA-4 receptor (Rice and Bevilacqua, 1989; Martin-Padura *et al.*, 1991). Invasive breast cancers invariably express ICAM-2 but show no detectable expression of ICAM-3 or VCAM-1 (Fox *et al.*, 1995c). ICAM-1 and MUC18 (a melanoma associated antigen, see page 121) have been found in both benign and malignant cutaneous lesions but VCAM-1 occurs in 79% of benign skin naevi and in 62% of primary melanomas <1.5 mm in depth compared with this, these ICAMs are expressed in only 6% of thicker melanomas. Also only 14% of lymph nodes metastases expressed VCAM-1 (Denton *et al.*, 1992). These authors have suggested therefore that the loss of ICAM-1 may lead to reduced adhesion and may be conducive to greater metastatic spread of melanomas.

The role of selectins in cancer dissemination

The cellular adhesion molecules, called the selectins, bind to carbohydrate antigens present on endothelial cells activated by cytokines. E-selectin, for example, has been shown to bind to the carbohydrate antigens sialyl Lewis (x) and sialyl Lewis (a) (Lowe *et al.*, 1990; Phillips *et al.*, 1990; Walz *et al.*, 1990; Takada *et al.*, 1991; Tiemeyer *et al.*, 1991). The selectins are known to be expressed in human tumours and this could enhance tumour cell adhesion to endothelial cells. Tumour cells may also activate other cellular elements, such as the platelets, and induce them to release factor which may in turn induce the expression of selectins by endothelial cells (Hakamori and Anderson, 1994). This would result in greater interaction and adhesion between tumour cells and the endothelial cells, thus facilitating the invasion of the microvasculature. Antibodies raised against E-selectin inhibit the adhesion of breast cancer cells to TNF-stimulated endothelial cells (Tozeren et al., 1995) and also inhibit invasion of endothelial cell layer in vitro (Okada et al., 1994). Interlukin-1 enhances the formation of lung colonies when A375M human melanoma cells are introduced into nude mice by the intravenous route. This increase in experimental metastasis is inhibited by antibodies to the IL-1 receptor (IL-r) and in vitro the IL-r antibodies have been found to inhibit the induction by IL-1 of E-selectin and VCAM-1 expression on endothelial cells (Chiviri et al., 1993). These findings argue strongly in favour of an important role for adhesion molecule in tumour cell extravasation from the microvasculature and in the adhesion processes leading to their anchorage in distant metastatic target organs.

It was shown some years ago that colon carcinoma cells recognise and bind to E-selectin of endothelial cells (Rice and Bevilacqua, 1981; Lauri et al., 1991). The expression of E- and P-selectins is far more intense in the tumour endothelium of peripheral regions of invasive breast cancer (Fox et al., 1995c). A pattern might possibly be emerging in the adhesion molecules and their counter receptors taking part in the tumour cell–endothelial cell interaction and adhesion. The E-selectin-mediated adhesion of several human epithelial tumour cell lines has been compared with that of leukaemic cell lines (Takada et al., 1991; Yago et al., 1993). The adhesion of epithelial cancers to cytokine-activated human umbilical endothelial cells appeared in these studies to be exclusively dependent upon E-selectin. Of the leukaemia cells, however, only three out of 12 cell lines studied showed E-selectin-mediated adhesion. The sialyl Lewis (a) antigen seemed to be used exclusively in the adhesion of six cell lines that were derived from pancreatic and colon cancers, and this antigen contributed significantly in the adhesion of a further six cell lines originating from lung and liver tumours. In the three leukaemic cell lines which showed E-selectin-dependent adhesion, sialyl Lewis (x) antigen was the adhesion counter-receptor. That the E-selectin/sialyl Lewis (a) interaction may operate in pancreatic cancer cells is supported by others (Iwai et al., 1993; Takada et al., 1993). However, Yago et al. (1993) found silayl (x) expression in 14 out of 15 epithelial tumour cell lines and sialyl (a) in only eight. They also stated that sialyl (x) is expressed exclusively in all leukaemia cell lines studied and these differences were reflected to some degree in the expression of α-(1,3)-fucosyltransferase genes. The possibility that E-selectin might be the major adhesion component in epithelial cancers is also illustrated by the higher serum level of soluble E-selectin in ovarian, breast and gastrointestinal cancers than in myelomas (Banks et al., 1993). However, no differences have been found in the levels of soluble forms of E-selectin, ICAM-1 or VCAM-1 in sera of bladder cancer patients and control serum samples (Griffiths et al., 1996).

Differential expression of the sialyl antigen may also correlate with metastatic ability. The endothelia associated with metastatic lesions of colon carcinoma have been reported to express E-selectin far more extensively than endothelia of corresponding primary tumours, and higher levels of soluble E-selectin may be found in sera of patients with metastases than in sera of patients with no metastatic spread (Ye et al., 1995). This has been confirmed by Wittig et al. (1996) who found similar levels of soluble E-selectin, 35 ng ml^{-1} and 40 ng ml^{-1} respectively, in normal subjects and in patients with primary neoplasm or patients showing local recurrence of the disease. But the levels were more than twofold greater in the sera of patients with metastatic disease.

The primary neoplasm may itself activate the endothelial cells and induce the expression of E-selectin. For instance, the MDA-MB-231 breast cancer cells can interact with and induce the expression of E-selectin by human umbilical endothelial cells *in vitro*. The induction process can be complemented by the addition of mononuclear cells to the culture medium. Furthermore, antibodies raised against IL-1β inhibit the induction of E-selectin expression (Narita *et al.*, 1995). This observation may be interpreted as suggesting that other adhesion factors besides E-selectin may be responsible for invasion and secondary spread from the primary tumour and, further, that the primary tumour may be heterogeneous with respect to the expression of factors, such as cytokines, that induce selectin expression and that these subpopulations of cells may be a factor conferring a selective ability for forming successful metastases. At the laboratory level, cell lines derived from a human colon cancer have shown marked differences in their adhesion to E-selectin-expressing endothelial cells, and this adhesive ability directly correlated with their metastatic potential (Sawada *et al.*, 1994). Cutaneous squamous cell carcinomaswhich possess a high potential for metastasis invariably express sialyl Lewis (a), unlike basal cell carcinoma with a lower metastatic potential (Groves *et al.*, 1993). Conversely, colon carcinoma-derived cells selected for high expression of sialyl Lewis (x) are able to metastasise to liver after intrasplenic injection far more efficiently than cells which express sialyl Lewis (x) at low levels (Izumi *et al.*, 1995). Looking at the other side of the coin, one could enquire whether the inability of tumours to metastasise is related to the expression of these carbohydrate antigens. It is now well known that gliomas rarely metastasise to extracranial sites. Martin K *et al.* (1995) compared the expression of the selectin-binding carbohydrate antigen, CD15, on glioblastomas and fetal astrocytes with that on tumours that had metastasised to the brain. It is interesting to note that the anaplastic astrocytoma and glioblastoma cells revealed the presence of CD15 only at low levels.

It may be that a degree of specificity of interaction is emerging in these adhesive contacts. Handa *et al.* (1995) found that cell lines from human solid tumours showed predominantly E-selectin-mediated adhesion to endothelial cells, whereas two leukaemic cell lines HL60 and U937 both bound via P-selectin. Handa *et al.* (1995) then transfected two cell lines (HRT18 and PC3) which did not express sialyl Lewis (x) or (a), and which showed no binding to P-selectin, with a cDNA clone coding for the P-selectin glycoprotein ligand-1 (PSGL-1). The PSGL-1 transfected cells were then able to bind to P-selectin and to E-selectin.

Neural cell adhesion molecule (NCAM) in differentiation and cancer

The neural adhesion molecule NCAM and *N*-cadherin have been studied intensively for their role in neurite regeneration and neuronal adhesion to other cells. NCAM-mediated cell interactions do not require Ca^{2+}, whereas N-cadherin is a Ca^{2+}-dependent adhesive protein (see page 103). NCAM, like other CAMs discussed above, also possesses immunoglobulin-like domains (Cunningham et al., 1987). Transfection of cDNAs coding for NCAM into cells which do not express these molecules enhances their intercellular adhesive properties (Edelman et al., 1987) and induces neurite regeneration and outgrowth (Doherty et al., 1989; 1990a,b). NCAM is found in fetal tissues and in neoplastic tissues, especially of neuroendocrine cells. The expression of NCAM mRNA is seen in association with the induction of neural differentiation in the presumptive neural ectoderm during early embryonic development (Kintner and Melton, 1987).

NCAM may occur as more than one isoform. Two transmembrane isoforms, NCAM-140 and NCAM-180, have been identified. In human sera NCAMs with molecular masses of 110–130 kDa and 150–180 kDa are present; both these lack the intracellular domains of NCAM-140 and NCAM-180. Apparently, the serum 110–130 kDa NCAM is found only in sera of normal subjects but, as far as these studies go, the 150–180 kDa NCAM has been found only in sera of cancer patients. The two isoforms found in sera differ by the presence in the larger isoform of α-(2,8)-linked N-acetylneuraminic acid, which is a characteristic feature of embryonal form of NCAM (Takamatsu et al., 1994). A 145 kDa isoform encoded by a 6.2 kb mRNA has been reported in small-cell lung carcinomas. This is identical to the ICAM isoform found in neuroblastoma, with the exception that a single base pair is altered without altering the amino acid residue (Saito et al., 1994). Human granulosa cells have been shown to possess isoforms with a 10-amino-acid insert in the extracellular domain of the 140 kDa NCAM and this insert may be deleted by alternative splicing of the message (Mayerhofer et al., 1994).

The interaction and adhesion of several human solid tumour cell lines is mediated by NCAM. Cell lines derived from human carcinomas show NCAM-dependent adhesion to human endothelial cells. NCAM appears to be able to promote the formation of adherence-type intercellular junctions and may cooperate with cadherin in their formation (Michalides et al., 1994). The adhesion of renal tumour cells to endothelial cells and heparan sulphate in vitro is inhibited by antibodies to NCAM (Zocchi et al., 1994). Zocchi et al. (1994) also transfected the renal epithelial cell COS7 with NCAM cDNA and confirmed the involvement of NCAM in the enhanced cell adhesion. These authors reported that NCAM expression is also associated with enhanced growth and that it is detectable in the actively proliferating regions of the tumour. However, rat glioma cells transfected with the 140 kDa isoform of NCAM behaved totally differently. These transfectants showed reduced migration on collagen. When they were injected intracerebrally the cells grew in a localised manner with no infiltration of surrounding brain tissue, which contrasts sharply with untransfected cells which showed pronounced local invasion (Edvardsen et al., 1994). In further contrast with the findings of Zocchi et al. (1994), NCAM-transfected rat glioma cells showed a reduction of growth rate. There is some support for the findings of Edvardsen et al. (1994) from Meyer et al. (1995) who have also described a distinct inhibition of migration on collagen I of cells transfected with the 140 kDa isoform of NCAM. However, the in vivo situation appears to be somewhat different. Thyroid carcinomas which express NCAM show a propensity for capsular invasion (Miyajima et al., 1996).

Furthermore, NCAM expression appears to be associated with perineural invasion in cancer of the bile duct, and, less prominently, also in cancer of the gall bladder (Seki *et al.*, 1993, 1995).

Lung cancers have been particularly well studied for the presence of NCAMs in the light of the neuroendocrine-related paraneoplastic properties of the various subtypes (see Sherbet, 1974; Minna *et al.*, 1982). NCAM is expressed in a high proportion (>75%) of small-cell lung cancers (SCLC) and only in a small proportion of non-SCLC specimens (Brezicka *et al.*, 1992; Pujol *et al.*, 1993); Roussel *et al.* (1994) found no NCAM expression in adenocarcinomas of the lung. Generally, CAMs may be differentially expressed in lung cancer subtypes. Thus, ICAM may be expressed in non-SCLCs but not in SCLCs (Schardt *et al.*, 1993), but NCAM may be found virtually ubiquitously in SCLCs and probably in some non-SCLCs (Table 8). Similarly, NCAM may be expressed in gastric carcinoids but not in adenocarcinomas (Sakamoto *et al.*, 1994).

The levels of NCAM in SCLC patients appear to relate to disease activity. Higher levels of NCAM occur where there is extensive disease compared with only localised disease (Jacques *et al.*, 1993; Ledermann *et al.*, 1994) and shorter disease-free survival (Segawa *et al.*, 1993). The presence of tumour cells in bone marrow aspirates of patients with SCLC can be detected by immunochemical staining for NCAM. Patients with NCAM-positive cells in bone marrow aspirates have shown shorter survival times than patients with NCAM-negative aspirates (Pasini *et al.*, 1995). However, the findings of Vangsted *et al.* (1994) are not in agreement with this. They found no differences in the amounts of NCAM in sera between localised or extensive disease. Although NCAM positivity in non-SCLC is reportedly expressed in only a small proportion of cases, it has been correlated with shorter survival times of patients (Pujol *et al.*, 1993). These studies imply an association of NCAM with highly aggressive disease. Mooy *et al.* (1995) studied a series of primary melanomas with different metastatic ability and also metastatic lesions, using an antibody, HNK-1, which recognises a common epitope occurring in NCAM isoforms. They found NCAM expression in all primary and metastatic tumours and the more aggressive primaries also showed more intense NCAM expression. Interestingly, they found reduced levels of NCAM in liver metastases, which may suggest that these metastatic deposits did not contain NCAM isoforms with the epitope recognised by HNK-1 antibody. However, it would be premature to attribute organ-specific metastasis to specific NCAM isoforms.

Table 8.   Differential expression of ICAM and NCAM by lung tumours

Lung tumour subtype	ICAM	NCAM
Small cell lung carcinoma	−	+
Squamous cell carcinoma	+	−
Large cell carcinoma	+	−
Adenocarcinoma	+	+ (some)

The basic features of NCAM function, especially its expression in relation to cell differentiation, the expression in cancers of an NCAM isoform characteristic of embryonal tissues and its differential expression in parallel with the expression of neuroendocrine properties of certain tumour types, makes the study of NCAM potentially rewarding. The ambivalent nature of the relationship between NCAM and invasion and metastasis serves only to recommend further studies of this aspect of NCAM function.

MCAM (MUC-18) expression in melanomas

MUC-18 is a 113 kDa glycoprotein expressed on the cell surface. The gene *MCAM* encoding MUC-18 is a member of the immunoglobulin family. The MCAM glycoprotein is an adhesion molecule bearing homology to other cell adhesion molecules such as NCAM and ICAM and also to the *DCC* gene product (see page 177), as well as to MHC-2 and MHC-1. MCAM is found in some mesenchymal tissues, e.g. smooth muscle cells, endothelial cells and Schwann cells but not in epithelial or haemopoietic cells. MCAM is found consistently in mesenchymal neoplasms of both smooth muscle and endothelial origin and bears obvious relationship to malignancy with the exception that, although it is expressed consistently in neurofibromas and schannomas, it is not found in malignant peripheral nerve sheath tumours (Shih *et al.*, 1996). Interestingly, MCAM is expressed in a subset of capillaries and tumour endothelia but it is not found in the endothelia of arteries or large veins (Sers *et al.*, 1994). MCAM is not found in normal melanocytes or in benign cutaneous naevi, but it is highly expressed in malignant melanomas and metastatic lesions. MCAM-transfected cells show enhanced adhesion to endothelial cells and this is inhibited by antibodies to the MCAM glycoprotein. The MCAM-transfected cells also show differential adhesion to laminin and increased invasive ability in *in vitro* assays. These alterations in adhesive and invasive behaviour are reflected in enhanced metastatic ability (Huang *et al.*, 1996). MCAM expression is up-regulated by transfection of melanoma cells by carcinoembryonic antigen (Grimm and Johnson, 1995) which is regarded as a good biomarker for total tumour burden (Sherbet, 1982). Huang *et al.* (1996) report that the MCAM transfectant cells also show enhanced expression of MMP-2, which might constitute the mechanism by which MCAM alters biological behaviour. The expression of MCAM is regulated by the transcription factor AP-2 which, incidentally, also regulates the genes coding for PAI, MMP-2, E-cadherin and insulin-like growth factors, and also the *bcl-2* and c-*kit* genes. Thus, a concerted expression of several adhesion factors and metalloproteinases may be involved in the regulation of the invasive and metastatic behaviour of melanomas. Furthermore, the presence of the glycoprotein in tumour endothelia has been linked with endothelial proliferation, suggesting a close liaison with angiogenesis (Sers *et al.*, 1994).

Another member of the family of immunoglobulin cell adhesion molecules is the basal cell adhesion molecule (BCAM). BCAM has the characteristic immunoglobulin domain structure and is closely related to MCAM (31% sequence homology) and to NCAM (Campbell *et al.*, 1994).

BCAM promotes cell–matrix adhesion, as may be expected from the amino acid sequence homology it shares with MCAM and NCAM. It may be expressed in several normal tissues, both fetal and adult, but is also associated with malignant transformation of some cell types. A uniform expression of BCAM has been described in epithelial cancers of the ovary, but it is not found in non-epithelial ovarian cancer, or in lymphomas, sarcomas and tumours of neuroectodermal origin (Garinchesa *et al.*, 1994).

9

Proteinases and their inhibitors in cancer invasion

It has long been recognised that normal biological processes of morphogenesis, differentiation, wound healing, angiogenesis, cell motility and the aberrant processes of cancer invasion and metastasis require the remodelling of the extracellular matrix (ECM). Remodelling of the ECM may consist of its degradation by means of excision and deletion of ECM components, regeneration of the ECM components and their spatial and temporal reorganisation. Several enzymes are known to be integral components of the ECM, others are secreted and may remain associated with the cell membrane. The proteolytic function of the enzymes are counter-balanced and regulated by appropriate protease inhibitors. These proteases and their inhibitors actively participate in determining the complex structure and biochemical characteristics of the ECM which lead to the expression of specific forms of biological behaviour. In order successfully to establish metastatic deposits, the adhesive ability of cancer cells has to be regulated. In the initial stage of dissemination, the release of cells from the primary tumours requires a decrease in intercellular adhesion. The cells that are released have to acquire the ability to adhere to, and penetrate the barriers presented in the form of the ECM, host tissue stroma and the vascular endothelium. The adaptability of the cell to enter into these interactions with the ECM and other cellular elements is provided by remodelling of the ECM. This process is aided by the proteolytic enzymes synthesised by the tumour cells. These may be secreted by tumour cells or they may remain associated with the cell membrane. The proteolytic activity is regulated by specific inhibitors and thus both the degradative enzymes and their inhibitors form

Table 9. Proteinases and their putative ECM targets

Proteinases	Function/targets of degradation
Serine proteinases	
Urokinase plasminogen activator (uPA)	Activation of plasminogen
Tissue-type plasminogen activator (tPA)	Activation of plasminogen
Plasminogen	
Plasmin	Laminin, type IV collagen
Thrombin	
Elastase	
Cathepsins	Collagens, laminin
Cathepsin D (aspartic proteinase)	
Cathepsins B, L (cysteine proteinases)	
Cathepsin G (serine proteinase)	
Cathepsin O2 (similar to cathepsins S and L)	
Integral membrane proteinases	Localised ECM degradation
Matrix metalloproteinases (MMP)	
MMP-1 interstitial collagenase	Degradation of interstitial collagen types I, II, III, VII
Neutrophil collagenase	Collagen I
MMP-2 (type IV collagenase, gelatinase) (two major forms)	Types I, II, III, IV, V, VII collagens, fibronectin
MMP-9 (type IV collagenase)	
MMP-3 (Stromelysin-1)	Types IV, IX collagens, laminin, fibronectin
MMP-10 (Stromelysin-2, transin)	Collagens III, IV, V, fibronectin
MMP-11 (Stromelysin-3)	
MMP-4	α_1-chain of type I collagen
MMP-5	Native 3/4 collagen fragments
MMP-6 Acid metalloproteinase	Cartilage proteoglycan
MMP-7 (pump-1)	Gelatin of types I, III, IV, V collagens, fibronectin

Collated from Liotta *et al.* (1981); Lah *et al.* (1989); Emonard and Grimaud (1990); Mackay *et al.* (1990); Chen (1992); Basset *et al.* (1993); Bromme and Okamoto (1995).

essential tools and may be seen as regulating the process of remodelling the ECM. Among the dramatis personae are serine proteases, cathepsins and matrix metalloproteinases (Table 9).

Urokinase in cancer invasion and metastasis

Urokinase (uPlasminogen-activator, uPA) is a serine proteinase which is secreted as a single-chain inactive proenzyme which is subsequently cleaved into two chains and these are held together by disulphide linkage. The pro-urokinase may be activated by other membrane-associated proteinases such as cathepsin B (Kobayashi *et al.*, 1993). Urokinase activity is detected predominantly in the cell membrane fraction, perhaps owing to the fact that the inactive chain A binds to specific membrane receptor and the chain B performs the catalytic function of conversion of plasminogen to plasmin (Vassalli *et al.*, 1985). Early studies have shown that urokinase and tissue plasminogen activator (tPA) are both found in breast cancers. Urokinase-specific receptors have been demonstrated in a number of human tumour cell types, such as breast and colonic cancers and A431 carcinoma cells (Stoppelli *et al.*, 1986; Needham *et al.*, 1987; Boyd *et al.*, 1988; Hollas *et al.*, 1991). The invasive ability of cancer cells is not related directly to the amount of urokinase synthesised or secreted by the tumour cells but depends upon the expression of the appropriate receptors (plasminogen activator receptors, PARs). Urokinase not only binds to specific PARs, but it also causes the cleavage of the receptor, leading to the internalisation of the receptor–PA complex (see Moller, 1993). The PAR is a highly glycosylated protein which is bound to the plasma membrane by means of a glycolipid domain, and it interacts with PA by means of an *N*-terminal domain. The receptor protein can bind urokinase and also the pro-urokinase and this binding is orientated in such a way that the inactive proenzyme is activated at the plasma membrane (Behrendt *et al.*, 1995).

The invasion of ECM by cancer cells can be prevented by blocking the urokinase receptors with antibodies against the urokinase A-chain (Hollas *et al.*, 1991). Plasminogen activator function is modulated by a glycoprotein inhibitor (PAI) which binds to PA covalently and inhibits its activity (Loskutoff *et al.*, 1986; Yagel *et al.*, 1988). Two forms of plasminogen activator inhibitors have been described: PAI-1 and PAI-2 (Kruithof *et al.*, 1987; Wun and Reich, 1987; Ye *et al.*, 1987). In view of the importance of ECM degradation in facilitating the invasive behaviour of cancers, much work has been carried out on the expression of plasminogen activators, their receptors and the PAIs in cancer invasion and metastasis.

The topographical distribution of PAs in tumours has provided good reasons to believe that they assist the tumour in the invasion of neighbouring tissues. It was demonstrated several years ago that the metastatic potential of B16 murine melanomas can be modulated by altering the uPA activity associated with these cells, and the level of uPA activity of B16 cells was reported to be directly related to their ability to form pulmonary deposits (Hearing *et al.*, 1988). An inhibition of the binding of endogenous PA to the PA receptors on the membrane can result in the inhibition of the invasive ability of tumour cells. Kobayashi *et al.* (1994) synthesised four peptides with amino acid sequences found in the growth factor-like domain of PA. The invasive behaviour and spontaneous metastasis of Lewis lung carcinomas could be inhibited by multiple intraperitoneal injections of these peptides. It is of considerable interest to note that they were unable to inhibit the development of lung metastasis in an experimental metastasis assay where Lewis lung carcinoma (3-LL) cells pretreated with the peptides were introduced into host mice by intravenous injection and the animals were also subsequently injected with the peptides. This experimental metastasis assay procedure bypasses the early stages of vascular invasion and it is therefore significant that the peptides failed to inhibit the formation of lung nodules in this assay. This reinforces the view that these early stages of invasion are markedly aided by PA.

The importance of a peripheral distribution of this enzyme is supported by the study of several tumour types. High levels of PA occur at the zone between normal colonic epithelium and adenocarcinomas (Buo *et al.*, 1993). Endometrial carcinomas show enhanced levels of urokinase compared with normal endometrium (Gleeson *et al.*, 1993). Gastric carcinomas also show high PA levels (Plebani *et al.*, 1995). PA receptors (PARs) to which PA can bind and discharge its proteolytic function, have been found in tissues from invasive breast carcinoma but not in normal breast tissue (Bianchi *et al.*, 1994). Malignant brain tumours such as the glioblastoma show high PAR content, and molecular hybridisation studies have shown a high level of expression of PAR mRNA at the invasive edge of tumours (Mohanam *et al.*, 1994). In most tumour types, the increase in PA is also associated with an increase of the PA inhibitor, PAI. Gleeson *et al.* (1993) also discovered that higher PAI-2 levels in endometrial cancers correlated with greater depth of invasion of the myometrium. One would have expected high levels of the inhibitor to be inversely related to degree of invasion. Obviously, it is the relative levels of PA and PAI, and not the PA content alone, that would determine the degree of invasion achievable and high levels of PAIs which tilt the balance in favour of PAIs could be expected to reflect a reduced invasive and metastatic ability.

Hachiya *et al.* (1995) have provided some experimental evidence in support of a role for the PAs in cancer invasion. These studies were carried out on the human breast cancer cell lines MCF-7 and MDA-MB-231 cells. The MDA cells produce more PA than the MCF-7 cells and, consistent with this, MDA cells have been found to be more invasive than the MCF-7 cells. Hachiya *et al.* (1995) then showed that the expression of both uPA and tPA is enhanced in the human breast cancer MCF-7 and MDA-MB-231 cell lines by treatment with oestrogen and at the same time a twofold increase in their invasive ability was also noted. That the PA production is regulated by oestrogen is indicated by the fact that if the cells are treated simultaneously with oestrogen and its antagonist tamoxifen, the increase in the invasive ability is blocked. Furthermore, treatment of the cells with progesterone and prolactin, which only marginally increase PA production, do not affect the invasive ability of the cells. TGF-β is also able to increase the PA production and invasion by MCF-7 cells, but in MDA cells the growth factor decreased PA production and also decreased the invasive ability. The other half of the equation is the expression of the inhibitor PAI, which should achieve an equilibrium with the PAs in relation to the degree of invasiveness associated with tumours. Mueller *et al.* (1995) transfected human melanoma cells capable of producing PA with PAI-2 cDNA and showed that this caused a total inhibition of soluble and membrane-associated PA, together with inhibition of the matrix degradation capability of these cells. When the transfected cells were introduced intravenously in severe combined immunodeficiency (SCID) mice, the PAI-2 expressing tumours grew as fully encapsulated tumours, whereas untransfected parental cell lines metastasised to lymph nodes and the lung.

The levels of production of PA and PAI not only reflect the invasive ability of tumours but have also shown correlation with tumour differentiation, clinical stage and metastastic status and therefore PA/PAI status has been investigated for its prognostic value. Higher urokinase levels have been found in gastric tumours with metastatic spread than in tumours without metastases (Plebani et al., 1995). Poorly differentiated gastric carcinomas contained more PA than well-differentiated tumours. PAI levels of endometrial cancers have been found to correlate positively with tumour stage, with stage II and III tumours showing far higher production of PAI-2 than stage I tumours (Gleeson et al., 1993). A direct correlation between urokinase levels and tumour grade has also been found in human gliomas. Higher-grade (grades 3 and 4) tumours showed four- to fivefold more urokinase than grade 2 gliomas and pilocytic astrocytomas (Hsu et al., 1995). Therefore, it is possible to read a meaningful correlation between tumour differentiation and stage and the levels of PA and PAI expression.

High urokinase levels have been reported to correlate with poor overall survival of breast cancer patients (Grondahl-Hansen et al., 1993; Janicke et al., 1993). Not only are high PA and PAI in primary tumours associated with increased risk of relapse and mortality, but in node-negative patients low levels of expression was significantly related to reduced risk of relapse. Janicke et al. (1993) found that 93% of patients with low PA and PAI showed disease-free 3-year survival compared with only 55% of patients with high PA and PAI levels. Urokinase may be a useful prognostic marker, especially for the subgroup of patients with oestrogen-receptor (ER)-positive and lymph node-negative tumours, but for patients with ER-negative tumours, the clinical outcome did not appear to be related to PA levels (Duffy et al., 1994). Urokinase receptors have been examined by Duggan et al. (1995). However, the levels of PAR did not correlate with tumour size, axillary nodal metastasis, or ER status. Although these authors noted some correlation of PAR status with prognosis, they believe that PAR status is not as powerful a prognostic marker as urokinase itself. Ganesh et al. (1994) regard high PA and PAI expression as strong prognostic indicators in colorectal cancer.

The functional pathway of ECM degradation by PA is believed to be the generation of plasmin, which is known to be capable of degrading the ECM components laminin and type IV collagen (Liotta et al., 1981; Mackay et al., 1990). The regulation of invasive behaviour of breast cancer cells by oestrogen appears to follow this pathway. Another functional pathway has been suggested by Mars et al. (1993) who show that PA activates the hepatocyte growth factor (HGF) (see page 92). HGF bears sequence homology to PA and occurs in the mitogenically inactive single chain form and in the active two-chain form. Mars et al. (1993) showed that PA cleaves the single chain HGF to generate the active two-chain form of HGF. They have confirmed this by demonstrating that HGF which is mutated at the cleavage site cannot be activated by PA. HGF is a powerful mitogen and can stimulate vigorous angiogenesis. Hildenbrand et al. (1995b) found that high urokinase levels correlated with the induction of angiogenesis and vascular invasion. This apparent new pathway of PA function mediated by HGF significantly increases the importance of PA as a mediator of cancer invasion.

Cathepsins in cancer invasion and progression

Cathepsins are lysosomal enzymes, but may be found associated with the plasma membrane in erythrocytes (Bernacki and Bosmann, 1972) and in macrophage endosomes (Diment et al., 1988). Several cathepsins are known and they are identified by a designatory letter, e.g. cathepsins D, B, etc. Cathepsin D is an aspartic proteinase, cathepsins B and L are cysteine proteinases and cathepsin G is a serine proteinase. Cathepsins are glycoproteins containing phosphomannosyl residues, which bind to mannose-6-phosphate receptors and are delivered to the lysosomes. Alterations of this system of delivery to, and localisation of, cathepsins in the lysosomes can occur in disease processes and as a normal biological process in some cell types. This results in their release or secretion and consequent subcellular and cellular damage. Cathepsins subserve a variety of physiological functions by means of their proteolytic activity and their physiological function is controlled by the regulation of their proteolytic activity.

Cathepsin D in cancer

Cathepsin D has been studied extensively for its perceived role of assisting cancer invasion and secondary spread. It is known to be regulated by intracellular pH, growth factors, hormones and by specific endogenous inhibitors (Goldberg et al., 1980; Barrett, 1984; Gallo et al., 1987; Touitou et al., 1988). In breast cancer, cathepsin D is secreted in the form of a 53 kDa precursor, the pro-cathepsin D (Morisset et al., 1986). Oestrogen and growth factors such as insulin-like growth factor I, EGF, bFGF stimulate the expression of cathepsin D in breast cancer cells (Cavailles et al., 1988, 1989). Paradoxically, its expression has been found, not infrequently, to be unrelated to steroid receptor status of tumours (Metaye et al., 1993; Scorilas et al., 1993; Rochefort, 1994).

   The expression of cathepsins D and B has been studied with great enthusiasm and much effort has been directed to relating cathepsin levels to histopathological and clinical features of tumours. This is illustrated by a broad spectrum of human tumours where cathepsin D has been found to be over-expressed or abnormally processed or secreted. Early studies and also more recent investigations with human neoplasms have shown an enhanced cathepsin D expression in hepatomas (Maguchi et al., 1988), thyroid dysplasias and carcinomas (Sinadinovic et al., 1989; Metaye et al., 1993), melanomas (Tsushima et al., 1989), gynaecological malignancies (Galtier de Reure et al., 1992; Nazeer et al., 1994; Scambia et al., 1995), gastric tumours (Matsuo et al., 1996) and carcinoma of the prostate (Kuczyk et al., 1994; Makar et al., 1994), bladder (Nakata et al.,

1994; Lipponen, 1996), colon (Adenis *et al.*, 1995) and of the breast (Rochefort *et al.*, 1990; Charpin *et al.*, 1993; Johnson MD *et al.*, 1993; Scorilas *et al.*, 1993). Elevated levels of pro-cathepsin D have been reported in the plasma of patients with breast cancer (Jarosz *et al.*, 1995).

The importance of cathepsin D in cancer invasion has been experimentally evaluated. Johnson *et al.* (1993) measured the *in vitro* invasive ability of nine clones of the human breast cancer MCF7 cell line and also the secreted cathepsin D, but found no correlation between them. Neither was the invasive ability of the cells inhibited by the aspartyl proteinase inhibitor pepstatin A. Transformed breast epithelial cells do not show any alterations in the expression of cathepsins D, B and L, even though they are capable of anchorage-independent growth and show increased invasive ability (Lah *et al.*, 1995). However, MDA-MBA-231 cells showing marked invasion *in vitro* have been found to be rich in vesicles that contain ECM material and cathepsin D (Montcourrier *et al.*, 1993, 1994). The *in vitro* invasion by glioblastoma cell lines is inhibited by antibodies raised against cathepsin D (Sivaparvathi *et al.*, 1996a). *In vivo*, the invasive behaviour of tumours may be linked to the degree of cathepsin D expression. For instance, the depth of myometrial invasion may relate to the level of the cathepsin content of endometrial adenocarcinomas (Nazeer *et al.*, 1994). Transitional cell carcinomas of the bladder showing muscle invasion express cathepsin D at a high level in the invasive zone (Lipponen, 1996). High cathepsin D immunoreactivity has been detected at the invasion front also in gastric tumours (Matsuo *et al.*, 1996).

It follows from the somewhat equivocal nature of the evidence concerning the involvement of cathepsin D in cancer invasion that its association with cancer progression would be also uncertain. Several studies of breast cancer advocate no specific role for this enzyme in the progression of the disease. Cathepsin D levels have shown no relationship to established prognostic factors (Ruppert *et al.*, 1994). Pro-cathepsin D levels correlate with total cathepsin D content, but pro-cathepsin D levels appear to have no prognostic value for overall survival or metastasis-free survival (Brouillet *et al.*, 1993). Similarly, no correlation has emerged between cathepsin D expression and tumour grade, steroid receptor status or nodal invasion (Charpin *et al.*, 1993; Scorilas *et al.*, 1993), although correlation with vascular and nodal invasion has been noted by others (Charpin *et al.*, 1993; Hahnel *et al.*, 1993). Hahnel *et al.* (1993) found localisation of cathepsin D at the tumour periphery and, furthermore, there was a marked association with high-grade infiltrating ductal carcinomas. Charpin *et al.* (1993) found that the enzyme levels are related to tumour grade and also to the proliferative index. High-grade prostate cancers show higher levels of the enzyme than low-grade tumours (Kuczyk *et al.*, 1994; Ross *et al.*, 1995), but Ross *et al.* (1995) found no correlation with tumour recurrence. In thyroid neoplasia, cathepsin D expression appears to be related to tumour size (Metaye *et al.*, 1993), but in pancreatic cancer there is no correlation with nodal invasion or metastasis to liver or lung (Nakata *et al.*, 1994). Thus, there is only qualified agreement as to the value of cathepsin D measurement in the clinical setting.

The ambiguity of the enzyme expression as an indicator of tumour progression stems partly from measuring the total levels of the enzyme without due cognizance of the possibility of differential expression of the cathepsins in tumours or the expression of individual cathepsin by different cellular elements composing the tumour. Some recent work on breast cancer amply illustrates this point. Escot *et al.* (1996) have reported distinct patterns of expression of mRNA of cathepsin D, MMP3 and uPA in breast cancers. They found cathepsin D mRNA in the epithelial component of the tumour but not in the fibroblasts, in contradistinction to MMP3 mRNA which was found in peripheral fibroblasts. Urokinase (uPA) mRNA was found in both cellular elements. These authors further made the point that it is the pattern of distribution of the three proteases that differentiates carcinomas from benign breast lesions. This appears to highlight the significance of cathepsin D present in epithelial tumour elements as opposed to that of the stromal component in tumour invasion. It should be recalled, however, that Tetu *et al.* (1993) assessed cathepsin D levels immunohistochemically and found that the enzyme occurs in both tumour and stromal cells. A striking feature of the work of Tetu *et al.* (1993) is the observation that cathepsin D levels of tumour cells were not related to prognosis, but that the presence of the enzyme in the stromal cells correlated with shorter metastasis-free survival, and it is the stromal enzyme levels that also correlated with poor tumour grade, aneuploidy and steroid receptor status. Tumour macrophages have been reported to show higher cathepsin D expression in advanced stages of endometrial adenocarcinoma (Nielsen and Nyholm, 1995). Host cell infiltrates possessing high amounts of cathepsin D have also been reported in transitional cell carcinoma of the bladder and in gastric carcinomas, especially in the peripheral invasive zone of the tumours (Lipponen, 1996; Matsuo *et al.*, 1996). However, Matsuo *et al.* (1996) did not see any relationship between cathepsin-positive inflammatory cells and the incidence of metastases. Nevertheless, these reports clearly implicate cathepsin D, produced by the infiltrating cells, in assisting the invasion of neighbouring tissues by tumour cells. Thus, there is a shift of emphasis from the cancer cell to the stromal cell, although there is a fundamental incompatibility in that host cell infiltration is usually inversely related to the aggressiveness of the tumour.

One must conclude, therefore, that despite the massive effort committed in the cause of this cathepsin, its importance in tumour invasion is still inconclusive and its value as a prognostic factor is ambivalent. As Mansour *et al.* (1994) have pointed out, the biological rationale for ascribing a role for cathepsins is impeccable, but they attribute the difficulties which seem to arise in the interpretation of the information to the methods of analysis. There is neither consistency in the methodology, nor in the design of clinical studies.

Cathepsin B in cancer invasion

Cathepsin B has been widely studied with regard to its possible function in cancer invasion and metastasis (see Sloane, 1990; Sloane *et al.*, 1990). The possible importance of this cathepsin was highlighted by the demonstration that the metastatic potential of B16 murine melanomas growing as subcutaneous tumours closely correlated with the levels of the enzyme (Sloane *et al.*, 1981, 1982). This correlation was subsequently confirmed in other murine tumours (Keren and LeGrue, 1988; Qian et al., 1989). Cathepsin B activity is associated with the plasma membrane and in endosomes derived from many forms of murine and human neoplasms (Sloane et al., 1990). Recently, elevated levels of cathepsin B have been reported in lung tumours (Ebert et al., 1994; Inoue et al., 1994), carcinoma of the pancreas (Nakata et al., 1994), prostate (Sinha et al., 1995), breast (Benitez-Bribiesca et al., 1995; Lah et al., 1995), stomach (Plebani et al., 1995) and gliomas (Rempel et al., 1994; Mikkelsen et al., 1995).

Cathepsin B is secreted by cells in the form of inactive pro-cathepsin B and is activated in the extracellular environment (Mort and Recklies, 1986). The inactive pro-cathepsin B is more stable in the extracellular environment than the activated form. Glioma cells secrete an inactive 42 kDa pro-cathepsin B which is activated by proteolysis to an active 29 kDa form (McCormick, 1993). This activation is mediated by other cathepsins, e.g. cathepsin G and the serine proteinases elastase and uPA (Dalet-Fumaron et al., 1993; Keppler et al., 1994). The activated cathepsin B is a broad spectrum endopeptidase (Barrett, 1984) and can be expected to degrade the ECM efficiently. Apart from this, cathepsin B can further assist ECM degradation by converting pro-urokinase into an active form (Kobayashi et al., 1993; Weiss et al., 1994). Another mechanism by which cathepsin B could promote cancer cell invasion has recently come to light. Mikkelsen et al. (1995) found that intense cathepsin B staining was associated with proliferation of endothelial cells in gliomas. A similar association of cathepsin B with the plasma membrane of endothelial cells has been found in carcinoma of the prostate (Sinha et al., 1995). The process of neovascularisation accompanying tumour development begins with a local dissolution of the basement membrane by proteolytic enzymes which are synthesised in endothelial cells in response to angiogenic stimuli such as the bFGF. Cavailles et al. (1988, 1989) had previously shown that the steady-state level of cathepsin D mRNA is enhanced by several growth factors, including bFGF. Interleukin-1 which is an inducer of angiogenesis can significantly increase cathepsin B levels in human chondrocytes (Meijers et al., 1994). Therefore, cathepsin B may also be involved in the dissolution of the basement membrane and promote tumour angiogenesis.

Consistent with the consensus view of a correlation between invasion and the degree of cathepsin B expression, the latter has also emerged as an important indicator of cancer progression. The cathepsins B and L occur in significantly higher levels in tumours of the head and neck compared with corresponding normal tissues (Kos et al., 1995; Budihna et al., 1996) but the levels of expression of the inhibitors stefins A and B were unaltered (Kos et al., 1995), suggesting that tumour tissue contains higher levels of the active forms of the cathepsins. Cathepsin B levels have been found to correlate frequently not only with tumour grade and lymph node metastasis, but clearly also with overall survival and disease recurrence. Luthgens et al. (1993) measured cathepsin B and the inhibitors stefins A and B in the bronchoalveolar lavage fluid (BALF) in lung cancer patients. Cathepsin B levels and that of the inhibitors were substantially higher in BALF from metastasis as compared with squamous cell carcinoma (SCC) and small cell lung carcinoma (SCLC). Some of the enzyme was in the form of a complex with the inhibitors stefins A and B but not with cystatin (see below). The amount of cathepsin B secreted by adenocarcinomas was also several-fold greater than SCC or SCLC. In adenocarcinomas, the over-expression of cathepsin B has been associated with basement membrane degradation and nodal invasion (Sukoh *et al.*, 1994). Besides advanced stage IIIA, IIIB tumours contained significantly higher amounts of cathepsin B than stage I tumours. The levels of cathepsin B were inversely related to 5-year overall survival figures. The favourable state of prognosis associated with low cathepsin B levels was also reflected in relation to the clinical stage. Thus, low cathepsin B content in stage I tumours was identified with 94% 5-year survival as opposed to only 45% of patients with high levels of cathepsin B. Low cathepsin B content indicated better prognosis also for advanced stages of the disease (Inoue *et al.*, 1994). A grade-related expression has also been encountered in gliomas and consistently higher proportions of cathepsin B-positive cells occurred in anaplastic astrocytomas and glioblastomas than in differentiated astrocytomas (Rempel *et al.*, 1994; Mikkelsen *et al.*, 1995; Sivaparvathi *et al.*, 1995). Rempel *et al.* (1994) found that cathepsin B transcripts as well the protein increased with tumour grade. Characteristically, invasive cells of glioblastomas tended to be cathepsin B-positive and involved in vascular invasion (Rempel *et al.*, 1994; Mikkelsen *et al.*, 1995). The over-expression of the proteinase could then assist subsequent metastatic extension of the tumour. For example, gastric carcinomas with metastatic spread contained more cathepsin B compared with carcinomas without metastasis (Plebani *et al.*, 1995). However, in pancreatic tumours, cathepsin B over-expression does appear to relate to invasive behaviour, without being indicative of metastatic spread. Thus, on the one hand, Ohta *et al.* (1994) found that invasive tubular adenocarcinomas of the pancreas stained more strongly than intraductal papillary adenocarcinomas, while, on the other, Nakata *et al.* (1994) saw no correlation between cathepsin B expression and dissemination of the tumour to lymph nodes, liver or the lung. Similarly, the association between enzyme expression and progression is unclear in breast carcinoma (Benitez-Bribiesca *et al.*, 1995; Lah *et al.*, 1995; Thomssen *et al.*, 1995). Thomssen *et al.* (1995) noted an association of over-expression of cathepsins B and L with early recurrence, despite a lack of correlation with vascular invasion and nodal metastasis.

It is often difficult to attribute specific functions exclusively to cathepsin B, since there may also be parallel contributions to the process of ECM degradation and promotion of local and vascular invasion by other enzymes or cofactors. This is illustrated by experiments using murine myeloma cells (P3X63Ag8.653) which secrete a pro-cathepsin (L) and possess high metastatic potential. However, when these cells were fused with spleen cells from animals immunised against cathepsin L, the hybridomas continued to secrete the pro-cathepsin and anti-cathepsin L antibodies, but they had lost their tumorigenic ability (Weber *et al.*, 1994). This essentially highlights the necessity of using a panoply of markers, as well as emphasising that it is crucially important that one takes into account the microenvironment of the cancer cell. Unlike cathepsin D, there is also a paucity of information on whether there is any heterogeneity in the expression of cathepsin B, and whether there is differential expression in the component cellular elements of the tumour. Frohlich *et al.* (1995) claim that cathepsin B is found exclusively in tumour cells. Rozhin *et al.* (1994) examined cathepsin B-containing vesicles in three pairs of cell lines differing in malignancy. These vesicles appeared to be located in the periphery of cells with greater malignancy and their translocation to the peripheral regions was induced by acidic pH in the pericellular region. In malignant cells this resulted in a gradual reduction in the amount of intracellular cathepsin B detectable, together with an increase in its secretion. Thus, the intracellular trafficking and secretion of cathepsin B may be an important feature of cells exhibiting invasive ability. Therefore, the current debate appears to support, albeit not overwhelmingly, the view that cathepsin B may be a major factor in cancer invasion, but further substantive evidence about its intracellular and topographical distribution will be essential to establish its function in cancer cell invasion.

Cathepsins L and H in cancer

Unlike cathepsins D and B, other cathepsins such as L, H and G have not received much attention from the scientific community. Initial studies do not appear to attribute to them any substantial part in cancer invasion and metastasis. That they may be implicated in the tumorigenic process is suggested by the induction of secretion of pro-cathepsin L, for instance, by the tumour promoter phorbol-12-myristate-13-acetate (PMA) (Heidtmann et al., 1993). But PMA is a highly versatile biological response modulator and is also known to induce the expression of matrix metalloproteinases (see page 137). The expression of cathepsin L has been found to be greater in gastric carcinomas with metastatic involvement compared with carcinomas without metastasis (Plebani et al., 1995). However, experiments using murine mammary carcinoma cell lines have revealed no differences in cathepsin L expression even when there might be substantial differences in in vitro invasion as well as in their metastatic potential (Morris et al., 1994). No significant differences have emerged in cathepsin L expression of human breast epithelial (MCF-10F) cells following neoplastic transformation by exposure to dimethylbenz(a)anthracene or by c-H-ras transfection (Lah et al., 1995). However, the expression of both cathepsins L and H is far higher in glioblastomas and anaplastic astrocytomas than in low-grade gliomas and normal brain tissue, and antibodies against these cathepsins also markedly inhibit the in vitro invasive ability of human glioblastoma cell lines (Sivaparvathi et al., 1996a,b). Cathepsin H expression is not altered in tumours of the head and neck, even though the expression of cathepsins B and L is greater in tumour tissue than in normal tissues (Kos et al., 1995). A differential expression of cathepsins is increasingly being reported but the evidence is far too tentative to seek correlations with the biological behaviour of tumours.

Cysteine proteinase inhibitors

The activity of serine and cysteine proteinases and also metalloproteinases is regulated by appropriate inhibitors. The proteolytic activity of cysteine proteinases is subject to control by inhibitors belonging to the cystatin superfamily. The cystatin family is divided into three subfamilies called the stefins, cystatins and kininogens (Barrett et al., 1986a; Barrett, 1987). Three stefins A, B and C have been identified. The stefins are single-chain approximately 11 kDa proteins. Stefin A (human) and cystatin-α (rat) occur in epithelial cells and polymorphonuclear leukocytes, whereas stefin B and cystatin-β show a ubiquitous tissue distribution (Davies and Barrett, 1984; Katunuma and Kominami, 1985; Barrett et al., 1986b). Cystatins are c.13 kDa proteins found in many biological fluids (Abrahamson et al., 1986; Barrett et al., 1986b). Cystatin inhibits the conversion of pro-cathepsin to the active form (Heidtmann et al., 1993; Ryan et al., 1995). The glycine-4 residue of cystatin A is highly conserved; truncation of the molecule including glycine-4 results in the loss of inhibitory activity. If this residue is replaced with residues with bulkier side-chains, the inhibitory activity of cystatin is reduced. When glycine-4 is substituted with residues bulkier than valine its inhibitory activity is totally lost (Shibuya et al., 1995a,b), possibly a consequence of steric hindrance to the binding of the inhibitor to the target enzyme.

Sloane et al. (1990) reviewed some of the literature where reductions in stefin levels have occurred with tumour progression and have speculated that this might be responsible for the enhanced levels of cyteine proteinase activity associated with tumour progression, as discussed above. The view that endogenous inhibitors may regulate the activity of proteinases, and thereby control cancer cell invasion, is amply supported by the abolition by the cysteine proteinase inhibitor E-64 of the in vitro invasion by EJ bladder carcinoma, and by the inhibition in vivo of vascular dissemination and formation of metastasis by EJ cells (Redwood et al., 1992). Stefins have been isolated from several forms of human cancer and stefin A, and not stefin B, appears to be responsible for the inhibition of cathepsin B activity in sarcomas and ovarian carcinomas (Lah et al., 1989, 1990). In lung cancers, cathepsin B is found in the bronchoalveolar lavage fluid, partly in complex with stefins A and B. Possibly, the levels of the active enzyme are regulated by the stefins, as suggested by the study of Kos et al. (1995) who found vast differences in cathepsin B activity associated with lung cancers, but the levels of stefins were unaltered. There is much evidence that stefin A expression inversely correlates with tumour progression and it has been regarded as a tumour suppressor (see Calkins and Sloane, 1995). Kininogens strongly inhibit the proteolytic activity of cathepsins L and H activity and, to a lesser extent, that of cathepsin B. The ascitic fluid from mice bearing sarcoma 180 contains a cysteine proteinase which appears to be a low molecular weight kininogen (Itoh et al., 1987; Sueyoshi et al., 1990). Cystatin A, which is the major form of cathepsin inhibitor in human squamous epithelia, is widely expressed throughout the epithelium of the normal uterine cervix, but a progressive loss of expression seems to occur from low-grade to high-grade cervical intraepithelial neoplasia (CIN) and virtually no staining is seen in epithelia and nuclei of poorly differentiated CIN III (Pollanen et al., 1995). Cystatin C has been found in the serum of patients with autoimmune diseases (Brzin et al., 1984).

Matrix metalloproteinases (MMPs) in cancer

In the pursuance of the theme of the important functions subserved by proteolytic enzymes in the remodelling of the extracellular matrix in normal physiological processes, and in pathogenesis, matrix metalloproteinases (MMP) have been accorded a prominent position and there has been sustained study of the facility with which they seem to promote tumour invasion and metastasis (Figure 14). A large family of metalloproteinases (see Table 9, page 124) and three inhibitors of metalloproteinases, called tissue inhibitors of metalloproteinases (TIMPs), have been identified and characterised.

Molecular organisation of metalloproteinases and their inhibitors

The members of the metalloproteinase family are closely related in structure of which the basic plan is provided in Figure 15. Four major domains can be identified: the translocation signal domain, the 'pro' domain which is involved in the maintenance of the enzyme in the latent form, the catalytic domain and haemopexin domain. The translocation signal domain is at the *N*-terminal end of the molecule which contains the peptide sequence that provides the signal for the translocation of the product to the endoplasmic reticulum. The MMPs are secreted in a pro-MMP form which are then activated by a mechanism called the cysteine switch followed by proteolytic processing. The 'pro' domain contains the conserved amino acid sequence PRCGXPDV and this sequence is involved in the maintenance of the enzyme in the pro-MMP form. The cysteine residue has been shown to be involved in the process of activation. The cysteine switch postulates that the *N*-terminal part of the molecule is folded in such a way that the cysteine residue interacts with the Zn atom of the catalytic site which includes the Zn^{2+}-binding domain. The disruption of this interaction is regarded as the first step in the activation of the pro-MMP (Nagase *et al.*, 1990; Springman *et al.*, 1990; Salowe *et al.*, 1992) resulting from the exposure of the active site of the enzyme (Vallee and Auld, 1990). This is followed by proteolytic cleavage of the PRCGXPDV peptide at the carboxyl end of the peptide. The activated MMP removes the 'pro' domain by autoproteolysis (Stetler-Stevenson *et al.*, 1989b) and is thus able to maintain the activated form. The fourth domain at the carboxyl end is the haemopexin domain/vitronectin-like domain which appears to be involved in the binding of the MMP inhibitors to the enzyme (Fridman *et al.*, 1992; Murphy *et al.*, 1992). The haemopexin domain occurs in all MMPs with the exception of MMP-7 (pump-1).

Three MMP inhibitors have been identified, of which TIMPs 1 and 2 have been cloned and fully characterised (Docherty *et al.*, 1985; DeClerck *et al.*, 1989; Stetler-Stevenson *et al.*, 1989a). A third member of the inhibitor family is TIMP-3 (Pavloff *et al.*, 1992). The TIMPs recognise and tightly bind to the MMP molecule. The cDNAs for both TIMP-1 and 2 code for 21 kDa proteins, but TIMP-1 is glycosylated and exhibits a 28 kDa molecular size in SDS polyacrylamide gel

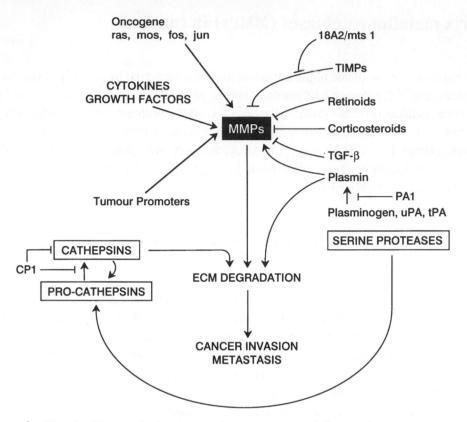

Figure 14.   The significant role that MMPs play in ECM remodelling and in cancer invasion and metastasis is depicted here. MMP expression is influenced by a variety of biological response modifiers, such as growth factors, cytokines, tumour promoters and oncogenes. MMP function is controlled by appropriate inhibitors (TIMPs) and modulated by retinoids and corticosteroids. Other proteinases, e.g. the serine proteinase associated with tumours, also affect MMP activity. Serine proteinases may be directly involved with ECM degradation in addition to achieving the same objective via activation of cathepsins.

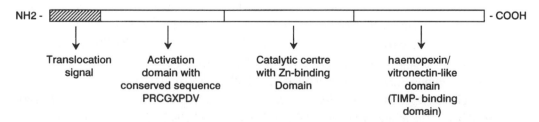

Figure 15.   The functional domains of matrix metalloproteinases. Based on Stetler-Stevenson *et al.* (1993).

electrophoresis. TIMP-1 contains 184 amino acids, as deduced from its cDNA (Carmichael *et al.*, 1986). It occurs in body fluids, and tissues which synthesise MMPs also produce the inhibitor (Herron *et al.*, 1986a,b). Their molecular structures are closely related. Especially characteristic is the occurrence of 12 cysteine residues which enter into six disulphide bonds and provide a distinct tertiary structure to the molecule and demarcate two major domains, each containing three disulphide linkages – the inhibitor domain, which is available for binding to the active site of MMPs, and a second domain which may be involved in forming complexes with pro-MMP molecules (Stetler-Stevenson *et al.*, 1989b; Williamson *et al.*, 1990; Kolkenbrock *et al.*, 1991).

Regulation of MMP synthesis

Several biological response modifiers have been shown to be capable of regulating the synthesis of MMPs. Emonard and Grimaud (1990) have reviewed the effects of these agents on MMP production (Table 10). Cytokines and growth factors have been shown to enhance the production of MMP-1 and MMP-3 and it appears that regulation occurs at the transcriptional level. The production of neutrophil collagenase is stimulated by phorbol esters.

An early event in the growth factor signalling pathway is the transient expression of the so-called immediate early response genes, c-*fos* and c-*jun*. The transcription factor AP-1 is a complex between the products of the immediate early response genes. The promoters of collagenase and stromelysin contain AP-1 recognition sites, which mediate the response to growth factors and cytokines. Both positive and negative regulation of MMPs is mediated through the AP-1 recognition site. Thus, the induction of stromelysin RNA by EGF requires the stimulation of both *fos* and *jun* (McDonnel *et al.*, 1990) and antisense c-*fos* RNA blocks this process (Kerr *et al.*, 1988; Schonthal *et al.*, 1983). The transcriptional activation of collagenase and stromelysin genes by phorbol esters and tumour necrosis factor is also mediated by the AP-1 recognition site (Angel *et al.*, 1987a,b; Brenner CA *et al.*, 1989). Conversely, retinoids and corticosteroids inhibit the synthesis of MMP-1 and MMP-3. Retinoic acid (RA) represses the transcription of the rat stromelysin gene. It has been shown that the RA–RA receptor complex represses transcription of the gene by blocking the AP-1 binding promoter element of the gene (Nicholson *et al.*, 1990). Glucocorticoid receptors are also potent inhibitors of AP-1 activity (Yang-Yen *et al.*, 1990). Similarly, inhibition of stromelysin gene expression by TGF-β is mediated by the AP-1 recognition sequence (Kerr *et al.*, 1990).

The regulation of MMPs and TIMPs function appears to be a highly coordinated process. TIMP-1 is expressed in a variety of cell types, e.g. macrophages (Campbell *et al.*, 1991; Shapiro *et al.*, 1991), fibroblasts (Stricklin and Welgus, 1983; Clark *et al.*, 1985; Murphy *et al.*, 1985; Overall *et al.*, 1989a) and endothelial cells (Herron *et al.*, 1986b; DeClerck *et al.*, 1989). Its expression is regulated by growth factors such as bFGF, TGF-β, EGF (Edwards *et al.*, 1987; Overall *et al.*, 1989b), TNF-α (Chua and Chua, 1990), interleukins (Murphy *et al.*, 1985; Le Febvere *et al.*, 1991; Lotz and Guerne, 1991; Maier *et al.*, 1993), and also by retinoids (Braunhut and Moses, 1994),

Table 10.   Inducers and inhibitors of metalloproteinases

Inducers of MMP expression	Target MMP
Cytokines	
Interferons α, β, γ	MMP-1,3
Interleukin-1 (Frisch and Ruley, 1987)	MMP-3
TNF	MMPs 1,2,3
Growth factors	
EGF (Matrisian *et al.*, 1985, 1986b;	
Edwards *et al.*, 1987)	Transin, MMP-1,2
bFGF (Edwards *et al.*, 1987)	MMP-1,3
PDGF (Bauer *et al.*, 1985)	MMP-1
NGF (Machida *et al.*, 1989, 1991)	Transin
Tumour promoters	
Phorbol myristate acetate (Brinckerhoff *et al.*, 1986)	Neutrophil collagenase, MMP-2,3
TPA (Angel *et al.*, 1987a,b)	MMP-2
1,25-$(OH)_2$-vit D_3	MMP-2
Oncogenes	
H-*ras* (Schonthal *et al.*, 1983; Matrisian *et al.*, 1985, 1986b)	
mos (Schonthal *et al.*, 1988)	
fos, *jun* (Kerr *et al.*, 1988; Schonthal *et al.*, 1983)	
Other agents	
Heat shock	MMP-3
Colchicine	
Calcium ionophores	
Inhibitors of MMP	
Retinoids	
Corticosteroids	
TGF-β	

Based on Emonard and Grimaud (1990), and references cited in the table and in the text.

phorbol esters (Clark *et al.*, 1985; Murphy *et al.*, 1985), glucocorticoids (Shapiro *et al.*, 1991) and steroid hormones (Sato *et al.*, 1991). These biological response modifiers may differentially modulate their synthesis. For example, glucocorticoids and tumour necrosis factor are known to decrease the production of MMPs but increase TIMP expression (Clark *et al.*, 1987). In rat ovarian granulosa cells, luteinising hormone (LH) and 12-O-tetradecanoylphorbol 13-acetate (TPA) can enhance the expression of the inhibitor and thus provide control over the proteolysis and remodelling of the follicular connective tissue associated with ovulation (Mann *et al.*, 1991). Thus, the regulation of MMP activity appears to be controlled not only by differential induction of proteinase and inhibitor expression, but also by compensatory modulation of expression of the appropriate inhibitor. In breast carcinoma cell lines, oestrogen is known to enhance invasive behaviour, accompanied by increased degradation of type IV collagen (Thompson *et al.*, 1988). In oestrogen-responsive T47D and MCF-7 cells, oestrogen does not alter the expression of MMP-2 but does down-regulate TIMP-2 expression by 50% (van den Brule *et al.*, 1992). The regulation of the MMP/TIMP may also be tissue specific and the overall proteolytic response may be governed by several factors. EGF is able to induce stromelysin (transin) expression in fibroblasts (Matrisian *et al.*, 1986b; Kerr *et al.*, 1988), but in PC12 cells only nerve growth factor and not EGF appears to be able to induce stromelysin expression (Machida *et al.*, 1989). In MRC-5 fibroblasts, bFGF and EGF stimulate both collagenase and TIMP expression but when TGF-β is present the latter modulates the overall balance between the collagenase and TIMP. It appears that TGF-β suppresses collagenase expression while, at the same time interacts with bFGF and EGF to promote excessive TIMP induction (Edwards *et al.*, 1987). This complex process of regulation of proteolytic activity is also exhibited by cancer cell apparently concomitantly with invasive and metastatic behaviour (see below).

Developmental regulation of MMPs

The remodelling of the ECM in early embryonic development involves several matrix metalloproteinases (MMP), such as collagenases and stromelysin whose expression can be seen to modulate with developmental processes (Alexander and Werb, 1989; Brenner CA *et al.*, 1989; Werb *et al.*, 1989), and this remodelling allows embryonic cells to participate in intercellular and cell–ECM adhesive interactions, which are so crucial in cell migration, growth and morphogenesis. Remodelling of the ECM is responsible for the release of cells that form the blastema in the regeneration of appendages in *Ambystoma* and this process appears to be mediated by MMPs whose expression is up-regulated in response to limb amputation (Yang and Bryant, 1994). The induction of differentiation of F9 embryonal carcinoma cells by exposure to retinoic acid or dibutyryl cAMP increases the expression of collagenase and stromelysin genes, and also that of the gene coding for an inhibitor, namely the tissue inhibitor of metalloproteinases (TIMP) (Adler *et al.*, 1990), thus emphasising the fact that the control of ECM remodelling may be achieved by the MMP–TIMP system.

The role of MMPs and TIMPs in cancer invasion and metastasis

The significant role played by proteolytic enzymes in the invasive behaviour of embryonic cells has been known for many years (see Sherbet, 1982, 1987). Embryonic trophoblast cells invade the uterine epithelium, the basement membrane, connective tissue and blood vessels in the processes of implantation and the development of the placenta; process which bear considerable analogy with the processes involved in the invasion and metastatic dissemination of cancer cells. The trophoblast cells adhere to the basement membrane and degrade it by the agency of the metalloproteinases, type IV collagenase and interstitial collagenase, and also serine proteases. The metalloproteinase activity associated with the invasive faculty of trophoblasts is controlled by the induction of TIMPs by TGF-β which is produced by the decidua (reviewed by Lala and Graham, 1990).

A direct correlation between invasive and metastatic ability and the production of MMPs by cancer cells was documented several years ago. Type IV collagenase was shown to be associated with the degradation of basement membrane collagen and with the invasive and metastastic potential of tumour cells (Liotta *et al.*, 1980; Turpeenniemi-Hujanen *et al.*, 1985; Nakajima *et al.*, 1987; Reich *et al.*, 1988; Murphy *et al.*, 1989). Cell transformation produced by exposure to chemical carcinogens has been known to produce alterations of stromelysin-2 gene transcripts (Matrisian *et al.*, 1986a; Ostrowski *et al.*, 1988; Matrisian and Bowden, 1990). Transformation of cells with the H-*ras* oncogene has similarly been shown to result in the secretion of collagen type IV, together with the gain of metastatic properties (Collier *et al.*, 1988). Oncogenic transformation by *ras* and *myc* genes often also generates phenotypes with metastatic ability, but this can be inhibited by the introduction of the E1A gene. Coincidentally, the introduction of the E1A gene also causes an inhibition of MMP (Bernhard *et al.*, 1995). Similar experiments on rat embryo cells transformed by *ras* and *ras* + *E1A* oncogenes, were also described by Sreenath *et al.* (1992) who confirmed a high level of production of stromelysins 1 and 2 by transformed cells with high metastatic potential compared with transformed cells of low metastatic potential. Antibodies raised against type IV collagenase inhibited the invasion *in vitro* of reconstituted basement membrane by A2058 human melanoma cells (Hoyhtya *et al.*, 1990), emphasising the role played by the MMP. It was found that TIMP-2 could inhibit this invasive and metastatic ability. Ponton *et al.* (1991) detected reduced expression of TIMP in metastatic variant cell lines derived from SP1 murine mammary adenocarcinoma compared with non-metastatic variant lines. Indeed, alteration of either component of the MMP–TIMP system would be expected to, and does, modulate the invasive and metastatic properties. Antisense RNA-induced TIMP down-regulate in Swiss 3T3 cells which are non-tumorigenic, conferred invasive properties on them (Khokha *et al.*, 1989). The *TIMP*-1 gene has been transfected into human gastric cancer cells, and upon subcutaneous implantation into nude mice, these transfectant cells have been found to possess greatly reduced ability to metastasise (Watanabe *et al.*, 1996). Albini *et al.* (1991) showed that alteration of the balance between MMP and TIMP-2, brought about by the addition of extraneous TIMP-2 or antibodies to MMP-2, affected the invasive ability of HT-1080 human fibrosarcoma cells. DeClerck *et al.* (1992) transfected an invasive cell type of rat embryos cells with TIMP-2 cDNA and demonstrated that TIMP-2 expression in the transfectants suppressed the invasive ability of these cells as well as inhibiting the formation of tumour nodules in the lung upon intravenous injection. Compatible with these observations, we have found a down-regulation of TIMP-2 expression in six invasive glioma cell lines tested compared with non-invasive cell lines and human fetal brain cells (Merzak *et al.*, 1994b). Curiously, in one non-invasive cell line, TIMP-2 was in fact found to be down-regulated, which provides further support to the view that a balance between MMP and TIMP needs to be achieved in the manifestation of a given degree of invasive behaviour. As noted above, the *ras* oncogene and the adenovirus E1A gene modulate the expression of MMPs. Compatible with this is the observation of the influence of the metastasis-promoting gene *18A2/mts1* (page 191) in relation to invasive behaviour. Merzak *et al.* (1994b) demonstrated that invasive glioma cells show high levels of *18A2/mts1* transcription and in parallel show a total down-regulation of TIMP-2. In contrast, the non-invasive glioma line and fetal brain cells do not have detectable levels of *18A2/mts1* transcripts but these cells do express TIMP-2. The implications of these observations to the invasive process is significant. We have postulated that *18A2/mts1* genes may confer invasive and metastatic properties by remodelling the ECM and presumably this is achieved through enhancing MMP activity by down-regulating the expression of the TIMPs.

With the vast amount of data available on the association between the MMP/TIMP system and the invasive and metastatic phenotype may be regarded by some as beyond debate. Nevertheless, there are important questions which have remained unanswered over the past decade. Ostrowski *et al.* (1988) noted no differences in the levels of MMP secretion between some primary tumours and their metastatic deposits. This suggests that the expression of MMP may be heterogeneous and further that the subpopulation of cells which metastasise may not produce MMPs. The expression of MMP-2 and MMP-9 has been reported in the plasma membrane of breast carcinoma cells, but a considerable variability in expression has also been described (Visscher *et al.*, 1994). These authors found no relationship between MMP expression and the clinical course of the disease, but the expression of TIMP-2 did relate to progression. Furthermore, they found that TIMP-2 activity was detectable in the stromal component of the tumours. The contribution of stromal cells to the proteolytic pool has been documented by others. Basset *et al.* (1990, 1993) found high expression of stromelysin-3 in stromal cells of breast cancer and stromelysin is expressed in this way in other tumours such as head and neck cancers (Muller *et al.*, 1993) and basal cell carcinomas (Wolf *et al.*, 1992). Kawami *et al.* (1993) found the expression of stromelysin-3, rather than type IV collagenase to correlate strongly with metastasis of breast cancer to the lymph nodes. They suggested that the MMP might be produced by stromal cells surrounding the cancer cell. MMP expression occurs at higher levels in the connective tissue stroma of colorectal carcinomas compared with adenomas and normal mucosal tissue and the most intense staining was found in the stromal component associated with neoplastic glands. The pattern of expression of TIMP was similar to that of MMP (Hewitt *et al.*, 1991). MMP-2 and also MMP-9 were expressed at significantly higher levels in transitional cell carcinoma of the bladder than in normal bladder tissue. Both MMPs were associated with invasive rather than with superficial tumours and were expressed chiefly in stromal tissue rather than in tumour cells (Davies B *et al.*, 1993). Presumably, the secretion of the proteinases by stromal cells might aid the dissemination of the metastasising subpopulation. In other words, the faculty of invasion and metastasis may be a paracrine phenomenon. Metastatic deposits themselves can disseminate and presumably, again, the paracrine phenomenon might account for this.

It is obviously of great significance to determine the intratumoral distribution of the proteinases, and whether the absence of MMP in metastatic deposits reported by Ostrowski *et al.* (1988) is a one-off event. It may be recalled, however, that the fraction of the tumour cell population producing MMPs, in this case type IV collagenase, has been found to correlate with nodal spread as well as with the presence of distant metastases (Grigioni *et al.*, 1986; Cioce *et al.*, 1991). A study of 186 cases of node-negative breast cancers revealed that the occurrence of a high proportion (>80%) of type IV collagenase (MMP-2) positive cells is associated with greatly increased local invasion and recurrence, but tumours with far lower MMP-2 positivity showed significantly higher incidence of distant metastases (Daidone *et al.*, 1991). These data seem to imply essentially that metastatic dissemination occurs as an event distinguishable from local invasion and recurrence. A further inference from this study is that local dissolution of basement membrane might be occurring around only a small proportion of tumour cells. This generates a further conundrum that a small subpopulation of cells might be responding to paracrine signals and begin to express proteolytic enzymes that will enable them to access the vascular compartment for dissemination.

The metalloproteinases, MMP-3, MMP-7 (pump-1), and MMP-10 have been studied in human gastric and colon carcinomas. Of these, only MMP-7 has been found to be expressed in a majority of these tumours and this expression appears to be restricted to tumour cells and is not found in stromal cells or lymphocytes (McDonnell *et al.*, 1991). After an investigation of the expression of MMP-2 in lung cancer cell lines, Zucker *et al.* (1992) concluded that factors other than MMP alone might be involved in the invasive and metastatic process. This is based on two important observations. They found that high levels of MMP-2 were associated with high tumorigenicity and invasive and metastatic potential of lung cancer cell lines. They then transfected these cells with K-*rev-1* which reverts them to a less malignant phenotype. Zucker *et al.* (1992) noted that the revertants produced MMP-2 at the same levels as the parent cell line, but possessed slightly lower invasive ability and a vastly reduced metastatic potential.

Even after more than a decade of studies, there is much uncertainty about many aspects of the expression of the MMP/TIMP system in relation to cancer invasion and metastasis. Undoubtedly, there has emerged a clear correlation between the expression and regulation of MMP activity and the invasive process, with MMP expression often prominent in the invasive zones of a tumour, or at the interface between tumour and stromal component of the tumour. Apparently, no stringent substrate specificity is exhibited by MMPs. Nevertheless, some MMPs have been claimed to be more tumour-associated or related to progression than others. The significance of these perceived specificities of association is not understood at present. No solid evidence is yet available about whether MMP expression constitutes an autocrine or paracrine function of the cancer cell and this is a very important question that needs to be addressed. The influence of other genes, such as those coding for growth factors and metastasis suppressor and dominant metastasis genes, on the possible modulation of MMP/TIMP, together with possible repercussions for the invasive and metastatic properties of the cancer cell, also needs to be studied in depth. Here again we have correlative conclusions rather than incisive experiments providing insights into the mechanisms of gene interactions. Not surprisingly, therefore, there have not been any significant studies of the importance of MMP/TIMP expression as a prognostic aid and presumably this reflects these uncertainties.

10

Oncogenes and cancer metastasis

Metastatic ability is a heritable property. Therefore, the progression of tumours to the metastatic state implies changes in the expression of genes. These differences in biological behaviour are not transient but are attributable to genetic alterations. The precise nature of the genetic changes undergone by tumours during progression in general or in the acquisition of metastatic potential are poorly understood (Weiss, 1990). The implication of genes as driving forces of invasive and metastatic behaviour raises the questions of which genes might be associated with the invasive and metastatic abilities of cancer cells and of how they might be regulated. A prime objective, therefore, is to identify these genetic changes.

Experiments aimed at elucidating the role of known oncogenes in the metastatic cascade using gene transfer techniques, or by comparing their structure and expression in primary and secondary tumours, have provided little direct support for a universal association between modulation of cellular oncogene expression and the acquisition of metastatic ability. Several oncogenes have been tested for their ability to confer invasive and metastatic abilities upon normal cells, and among these are the *ras* homologues, which have been studied rather extensively (see below). Comparatively less well studied oncogenes are *src* (Chambers and Wilson, 1985), *fes/fps* (Sadowski *et al.*, 1988), and *mos* (Gao *et al.*, 1988), and the S-100 family genes (Parker *et al.*, 1991, 1994a,b; Davies BR *et al.*, 1993), among others.

In general, it should be stated that although gene transfer experiments have provided some insight into cellular features that can be related to or occur in parallel with neoplastic transformation, only a few studies have made an unequivocal contribution to our understanding of the process of tumour progression. Often, this has been due to technical difficulties. For instance, there are two major *in vivo* assays for metastatic ability: the experimental metastasis model of intravenous injection of cells and measuring their lung colonisation, and the spontaneous metastasis model which measures different features of the metastatic cascade. The former, an extensively used assay, cannot provide a full picture of the spectrum of the associated events, since the introduction of cells directly into the vascular system obviously bypasses several early stages of the metastatic cascade. Furthermore, there seems to be little appreciation of genomic perturbations occurring as a consequence of transfection and stable integration of extraneous DNA into the cellular genome. Some years ago Kerbel *et al.* (1987) noted that $Ca_3(PO_4)_2$-mediated DNA transfer itself caused alterations in the biological behaviour of cells. They found that 17% of CBA/J mouse mammary adenocarcinoma cells transfected with pSV-*neo* carrying no known oncogene, showed lung colonisation. The Graham and van der Eb (1973) method of DNA transfer has consistently been used in a large number of studies and there does not appear to be much support for the view expressed by Kerbel and colleagues. It cannot be denied, however, that integration of extraneous DNA is liable to cause considerable perturbation in the genome of the recipient cells and it is possible that in Kerbel and colleagues' experiments plasmid integration may have occurred in areas of the DNA-harbouring genes liable to change the biological behaviour of cells.

It now appears that on occasions oncogenes might be cooperating with other genes, rather than function as candidate genes. It is interesting to note in this context, that transfection with *ras* enhances the expression of the S-100-related protein p9ka/42a (De Vouge and Mukherjee, 1992) which is the rat homologue of the murine *18A2/mts1* gene product. We know that some members of the S-100 family show cell cycle-related and metastasis-related expression, as discussed in a later section (see page 191). Furthermore, the activated *ras* gene induces expression of the surface glycoprotein CD44 (Hoffman *et al.*, 1993; Jamal *et al.*, 1994) which has been associated with increased metastatic potential. Thus, it seems possible that activation of other genes might be involved in certain events of metastatic dissemination.

Davies BR *et al.* (1993) transfected rat mammary epithelial cells with *p9Ka* gene. The *p9Ka*-transfected cells produced tumours at a higher frequency, with a reduced latent period, and showed a higher incidence of metastasis than untransfected parental lines. We transfected its murine homologue, the *18A2/mts1* gene, placed under the control of the dexamethasone-inducible mammary tumour virus promoter into B16-F10 murine melanoma cells and demonstrated an increase in lung colonisation by the transfectant cells, when the transfected gene is switched on. In these cells alterations were seen in the cytoskeletal organisation of the cells accompanied by the accumulation of a greater number of cells in the S-phase fraction (Parker *et al.*, 1994b). In both these studies the genes were transfected into either continuous cell lines or into transformed cells and it is suggested that these genes may be capable of altering the biological behaviour of cells only when they have undergone cellular transformation. It would be of considerable value to study the effect of transferring these genes into non-transformed cells or primary cell cultures, since such studies would enable one to distinguish between transforming genes and those associated with invasion and secondary spread of already transformed cells and this could allow one to establish whether they merely advance the stage of progression while not being able to achieve cell transformation on their own. There do not appear to be differences in the structure and expression of oncogenes between primary tumours and their metastases (Bos, 1985; Albino *et al.*, 1989; Rochlitz *et al.*, 1989) but the expression of certain oncogenes such as the *ras*, *c-erb*B2 and *myc*, among others, has been reported to change at different stages of tumour progression (D'Emilia *et al.*, 1989; King *et al.*, 1989; Ro *et al.*, 1989; Borg *et al.*, 1990; Field and Spandidos, 1990).

The *ras* oncogene in tumorigenesis

Increased *ras* expression has been described in several human tumours (Slamon *et al.*, 1984; Spandidos and Agnantis, 1984; Viola *et al.*, 1985, 1986). Egan *et al.* (1987) subsequently showed that *ras* expression level correlated with metastatic potential in 10T1/2 and NIH-3T3 cells. The relationship between *ras* gene expression and cell transformation has been studied by several groups. The *ras* proto-oncogene and also the mutant forms of the gene can produce cellular transformation upon transfection (Egan *et al.*, 1989). There are several other gene transfer experiments with *ras* (Chambers and Ling, 1984; Spandidos and Wilkie, 1984; Bondy *et al.*, 1985; Pozzati *et al.*, 1986; Collard *et al.*, 1987a; Chambers *et al.*, 1990), which have generally supported its role in achieving neoplastic transformation. However, transfection of human melanocytes by *ras* does not produce the morphological and cytogenetic changes which are known to characterise melanoma *in vivo* (Albino *et al.*, 1992). More recently Davies BR *et al.* (1993) found no conferment of tumorigenicity or metastasis on rat mammary epithelial cells transfected with the *ras* oncogene. A study of activating *ras* mutations in breast cancers and their metastases has revealed no differences in the incidence, suggesting that activating mutations of the oncogene may not be significantly involved in metastatic progression (Rochlitz *et al.*, 1989). This is consistent with the view expressed by Bos (1985) that *ras* activation is not an obligatory event in tumour progression, since activating mutations reveal no pattern of incidence or relationship to clinical or biological features of malignancy. However, the *ras* oncogene appears to stimulate endothelial cell motility (Fox PL *et al.*, 1994), which is essential for the formation of microvasculature that enables the tumour to disseminate to distant metastatic sites.

The members of the *ras* oncogene family have also received much attention in recent years on account of the diverse role the ras proteins play in the transduction of extracellular signals which affect cell proliferation, differentiation and the regulation of cytoskeletal dynamics. Ras proteins are membrane-bound guanine nucleotide-binding proteins. These are bound to GDP in the resting state. The release of GDP is promoted by an exchange factor and this leads to the formation of a complex with GTP. Signalling by ras protein is activated by GTP binding and inactivated by GTP hydrolysis. Mutations in the ras proteins lead to reduced GTPase activity and to constitutive binding to GTP, and consequently the *ras* gene appears to acquire oncogenic potential. Mutated oncogenic forms of *ras* have been reported in a variety of human cancers, e.g. carcinomas of the colon, pancreas, lung thyroid, lymphomas and myeloproliferative disorders. Although attempts have been made to assess the clinical significance of *ras* activation, there is no incontrovertible evidence of its association with disease stage or recurrence, although some studies have suggested that it may serve as a marker related to the malignant potential of tumours (Harada *et al.*, 1992). *Ras* mutation appears to be an infrequent event in bronchioalveolar adenocarcinoma (Rusch *et al.*, 1992) and of little clinical relevance in lung adenocarcinoma (Rodenhuis and Slebos, 1992). Gulbis and Galand (1993) have critically examined the question of whether ras protein expression can be regarded as a criterion of malignancy. Their study reveals that an insufficiency of information makes it difficult to determine whether ras expression can serve as a marker in tissues of the colon, lung, bladder, ovary, and neural and odontogenic tissues and their corresponding neoplastic counterparts. In other tissues, e.g. pancreas and stomach, the status of ras protein does not distinguish between malignant and corresponding normal tissues. However, in liver tumours, salivary adenocarcinomas and uterine carcinomas, the ras proteins are detectable only in malignant tissues.

There is little valuable information on *ras* activation status in gynaecological cancers. Some years ago Enomoto *et al.* (1990, 1991) reported that K-*ras* activation was not a characteristic of cervical carcinomas or ovarian epithelial tumours, with the exception of mucinous adenocarcinomas. Point mutations have been described in some endometrial carcinomas (Lester and Cauchi, 1990). A recent study by Carduff *et al.* (1995) indicates that although a small proportion (11.6%) of endometrial carcinoma shows point mutations of K-*ras*, there was no evidence of any correlation with stage, grade, depth of invasion or clinical outcome. It is possible that *ras* activation by mutation may be compounded by allelic deletions involving *p53* and other suppressor genes such as *nm23* (Imamura *et al.*, 1992). Such an accumulation of sequential genetic abnormality is known to be associated with other neoplasms such as colon carcinoma (see page 172).

Erb genes as predictors of cancer progression and prognosis

A family of genes have been cloned in recent years whose protein products belong to a family of receptor tyrosine kinases. The genes are called *erbB (erbB1,EGFr), erbB2 (neu/HER-2), erbB3 (HER-3) and erbB4 (HER-4)*. The products of this family of genes are transmembrane tyrosine kinases, each with a single transmembrane domain, a cysteine-rich extracellular domain and an intracellular catalytic domain. They act as receptors for a number of peptide growth factors such as EGF, TGFα and neuregulins. The binding of the ligands leads to dimerisation and autophosphorylation of the receptors. The activated receptors are then able to bind to proteins containing *src*-homology-2 (SH2) domains. The SH2 domain proteins recognise and bind to specific phosphotyrosine-containing sequences of the activated receptor (Moran *et al.*, 1990; Margolis *et al.*, 1992; Pawson and Schlessinger, 1993; Songyang *et al.*, 1993). These SH2-containing adaptor molecules then trigger downstream signalling pathways, ultimately resulting in gene activation. Because of the involvement of the *erb* family gene products in extracellular signal transduction, much work has been targeted upon these genes in order to see if they are implicated in neoplastic development and progression.

The *erbB2 (neu/HER2)* gene is located on chromosome 17p21. It codes for a 185 kDa transmembrane glycoprotein related to, but quite distinct from, the epidermal growth factor receptor (EGFr) (Padhy *et al.*, 1982; Schechter *et al.*, 1985; Bargmann *et al.*, 1986a; Hung *et al.*, 1986; Yamamoto *et al.*, 1986). The EGFr bears sequence homology with the *erbB1* product (Downward *et al.*, 1984). The *erbB2* gene is activated by a point mutation which results in the change of amino acid residue 664 from valine to glutamic acid (Bargmann *et al.*, 1986b) and this change is associated with its ability to transform cells (Stern *et al.*, 1986; Bargmann and Weinberg, 1988). Alterations in and amplification of this gene have been reported in a variety of human cancers such as carcinomas of the breast, bladder, colon, lung and gastric carcinomas.

Expression and amplification of erbB2 in breast cancer

Amplification of *erbB2* was studied extensively in breast and ovarian cancers and found to correlate with lymph node involvement and relapse-free survival, and also overall survival of patients (Slamon *et al.*, 1987, 1989). This relationship has not been borne out by some subsequent studies, such as those by Ali *et al.* (1988), Zhou *et al.* (1989) and Kury *et al.* (1990). The expression of the protein appears to be associated with tumour grade (McCann *et al.*, 1991; Tervahauta *et al.*, 1991). Studies using immunohistochemical methods show that *erbB2* protein expression does not differentiate between invasive and *in situ* breast carcinomas (Moe *et al.*, 1991; Porter *et al.*, 1991). McCann *et al.* (1991) detected no correlation between over-expression of *erbB2* protein and lymph node status. But McCann *et al.* (1991) have themselves stated that over-expression of the oncoprotein was significantly related to shorter disease-free survival. Furthermore, over-expression of the protein in node-positive patients was predictive of poor prognosis. Watatani *et al.* (1993) found *erbB2* amplification in all stages of breast cancer and also that amplification was linked to lymph node involvement. Tervahauta *et al.* (1991) also regarded low expression of the oncoprotein as predictive of longer survival. Recently, the results of a study of 942 invasive ductal carcinomas has been presented by Quenel *et al.* (1995) which confirms the prognostic value of c-*erbB2* expression. They found that it correlated not only with tumour grade but also very significantly with overall survival as well as relapse-free and metastases-free survival.

There have also been some attempts to examine whether the predictive value of c-*erbB2* expression can be increased by the simultaneous assessment of other prognostic factors. As alluded to earlier, *erbB2* protein is an EGFr-related protein. The co-expression of both these proteins was associated with poorer prognosis than when either protein was expressed alone (Osaki *et al.*, 1992). The expression of c-*erbB2* was not found to be associated with long-term (>8.5 years) disease-free survival. However, within a group of patients who showed tumour recurrence in less than 2 years after presentation, c-erbB2 amplification and expression was significantly associated with shorter survival (Pauley et al., 1996).

The data presented by Tiwari et al. (1992) shows erbB2 amplification in 17 out of a series of 61 primary breast cancers studied and, most importantly, 16 of these 17 patients presented with metastatic disease. A detailed investigation of micrometastases in the bone marrow of breast cancer patients has recently been carried out; it has revealed the presence of breast cancer cells in the bone marrow of 75% of patients who had overt metastases (M1 stage). Of much interest is the further observation that metastatic cells from the bone marrow of 48 out of 71 patients were positive for erbB2 expression (Pantel et al., 1993). However, an opposite view has been expressed that erbB2 aberrations may be an early event in the pathogenesis of breast cancer and co-amplification of this gene with other genes, e.g. c-myc and int-2 may also play an important part in breast cancer development (see Chen YH et al., 1995). It would appear that over-expression of the oncoprotein may occur in all stages of breast cancer, suggesting that it may play a role in breast cancer development if not obligatory for progression. However, its over-expression may be inversely related to clinical outcome.

The erbB2 gene expression in gynaecological cancers

Generally, one in three of epithelial ovarian cancers may show amplification of the erbB2 gene (Borrensen, 1992). Five to 68 copies of the gene have been encountered in 14% of carcinoma of the uterine cervix (Mitra et al., 1994). Whether gene amplification and/or over-expression of the gene product is related to the stage of the disease is unclear. There does not appear to be any relationship between the biological behaviour of ovarian cancers and their erbB2 expression status (Haldane et al., 1990; Zheng et al., 1991; Fajac et al., 1995). Mileo et al. (1992) found only sporadic amplification of the gene and found similar levels of gene expression in normal ovaries and ovarian tumours. Fajac et al. (1995) have reported >2.5-fold amplification in 9 out of 65 adenocarcinomas but not in benign and borderline tumours. Over-expression of c-erbB2 is reportedly associated with poor survival in advanced epithelial ovarian cancer (Berchuck et al., 1990). Amplification appeared to correlate with poor prognosis in univariate analysis but in multivariate analysis of stage, histological type, grade and residual tumour, gene amplification did not appear to be an independent marker of prognosis (Fajac et al., 1995). Borrensen (1992) confirms that ovarian cancers with erbB2 amplification and consequent over-expression of its product reflects more aggressive disease, accompanied by greater growth potential of the tumour and poor survival. In endometrial carcinomas over-expression of the gene was associated with advanced stage disease and the occurrence of distant metastases (Berchuck et al., 1991a). It may be pointed out, however, that only in 9 out of 95 carcinomas was erbB2 staining more intense than in normal endometrial samples. Three of these nine samples belonged to FIGO stage IA and B and the remaining six to stage IIIC and IVB with lymph node involvement and distant metastases. Whereas investigations of breast cancer have provided a sanguine picture of *erbB2* association with clinical outcome, such a picture has not emerged from the studies of gynaecological cancers described above. However, it should be borne in mind that there have been far fewer studies of gynaecological cancers than breast cancers and it would be premature to discard it as a marker of progression and prognosis of gynaecological malignancies.

erbB2 *expression in other forms of human cancer*

Work is less clearly focused upon other forms of human cancer. There is a study on nasopharyngeal carcinoma where *erbB2* expression seemed to relate to both overall as well as disease-free survival (Roychowdhury *et al.*, 1996). Underwood *et al.* (1995) have found *erbB2* amplification in 16 out of 89 patients with recurrent transitional cell carcinoma of the bladder, but found no amplification in non-recurrent or normal bladder tissues. Roughly half of the patients with recurrent disease showed characteristics of progressive disease, and of these one-third showed gene amplification. It is of considerable interest to note in this context that gene amplification was detectable only after disease progression to the invasive stage (Underwood *et al.*, 1995). No amplification of this gene has been encountered in carcinoma of the prostate (Latil *et al.*, 1994).

In summary, it would be safe to conclude that the current evidence overwhelmingly confirms the clinical predictive value of this oncogene, in terms of overall survival and of recurrence- and metastasis-free survival. Whether this applies with equal force to other tumour types than carcinomas of the breast is uncertain. Expression and amplification of *erbB2* currently appears to possess greater predictive value for breast than for ovarian carcinoma, but the possibility that its expression and/or predictive value may not be universally applicable should also be considered. The *erbB2* protein is expressed only in non-small cell lung cancer but not in small cell lung carcinoma and, moreover, its expression correlated with lymph node metastasis in squamous cell carcinomas but not in adenocarcinomas (Shi *et al.*, 1992). The significance of such differential expression is still unclear.

Experimental studies of the role of erbB *genes in cancer invasion and metastasis*

The evolution of the belief that amplification and over-expression of *erbB2* gene may be associated with tumour development and progression, and may be potentially valuable in the prediction of prognosis, has inevitably led to experimental studies aimed at assessing the influence of *erbB2* expression on the invasive behaviour and the metastatic potential of tumours and at elucidating the likely mechanisms of its involvement.

The *erbB2* gene was first identified as transforming gene *neu* in neuroblastomas induced by ethylnitrosourea (Schubert *et al.*, 1974; Shih *et al.*, 1981; Schechter *et al.*, 1984). An over-expression of the normal erbB2 and also the expression of genetically altered protein is able to transform human mammary epithelial cells and increase colony-forming efficiency and tumorigenicity in athymic mice (Pierce *et al.*, 1991). Yusa *et al.* (1990) transfected the activated c-*erbB2* gene into a clone of murine colon adenocarcinoma cell lines and noted an increase in their metastatic potential. *ErbB2*-transfected NIH-3T3 and Swiss Webster 3T3 (SW3T3) cells show an enhanced invasive ability, assessed by Matrigel invasion and enhanced lung colonisation upon introduction into host animals via the tail vein (Yu and Hung, 1991). Both transfectant clones showed lung colonisation in all injected animals, but none of the controls produced any lung colonies. Unfortunately, the controls did not include cells transfected with plasmid not carrying the mutated gene. Nevertheless, there is little doubt that introduction of the mutated gene markedly alters the behaviour of these cells. The adenovirus E1A gene products have often been shown to inhibit oncogene-mediated cell transformation. They can also reduce the transforming activity of *erbB2* gene (Yu *et al.*, 1991), in addition to negating or mitigating the enhancement of invasion and lung colonisation induced by *erbB2* transfection (Yu *et al.*, 1992a). Yu *et al.* (1992a) also attempted to understand the mechanisms involved in the E1A-mediated inhibition of invasion and lung colonisation. They found that *erbB2* transfectant cells showed greater adhesion to mouse lung endothelial cells than did the parental cells. The phenomenon of intercellular adhesion is mediated by several proteins, of these E-cadherin is believed to be a suppressor of the invasive ability. As discussed earlier (see page 103) in this book, the loss or reduction in the expression of E-cadherin has been linked with poor cellular differentiation and higher invasive potential. The over-expression of *erbB2* in human mammary epithelial cells results in the reduced expression of E-cadherin and α_2-integrin genes. Using an antibody that inhibits the phosphorylation of erbB2 protein, D'Souza and Taylor-Papadimitriou (1994) have been able to show that *erB2*-transfectants regain their ability to form three-dimensional structures in collagen gels together with up-regulation of expression of E-cadherin and α_2-integrin genes. This suggests that functional erbB2 protein may be linked with the regulation of these adhesive proteins. However, an extensive study including 226 infiltrating ductal carcinomas suggests that *erbB2* and E-cadherin expression may not be related (Palacios *et al.*, 1995a).

The ability to degrade the endothelial basement membrane is an essential requirement for the intravasation of tumour cells into the vascular system. The invasive ability of tumour cells is closely linked with their ability to secrete degradative enzymes (see page 123). Cell lines carrying transfected *erbB2* have also been shown to secrete degradative enzymes such as type IV collagenases at levels approximately tenfold greater than corresponding controls (Yu *et al.*, 1992a; see also Zhau *et al.*, 1996). These transfectants are also known to produce enhanced quantities of plasminogen activator (Gum *et al.*, 1995). E1A products partially reduced the adhesive properties of *erbB2*-transfectants, but reduced their invasive ability. These inhibitory effects of E1A on *erbB2*-mediated transformation, invasion and metastasis are compatible with the ability of E1A to down-regulate or repress *erbB2* expression (Yan *et al.*, 1991). Other pathways of *erbB2* inhibition have also been discovered. The suppressor gene *rb* (the retinoblastoma-susceptibility gene) has been shown to be able to suppress *erbB2*-induced transformation of cells by repressing *erbB2* transcription (Yu *et al.*, 1992b).

It is obvious from the above discussion that there are reasonable grounds for attributing a major role to *erbB2* gene in invasion and metastasis. The recent work of Zhau *et al.* (1996) has provided some further insights into how *erbB2* might influence the process. They transfected the gene into PC3 human prostate epithelial cells. A transfectant clone N35 showed enhanced growth rate and anchorage-independent growth in parallel with enhanced *erbB2* expression. They then tested clone N35 for its metastatic potential by subcutaneous and orthotopic implantation into the dorsal–lateral lobe of prostates of athymic mice. A striking difference was encountered in the metastatic spread, as assayed by these two methods. Upon subcutaneous introduction, the transfectant cells showed no change in their ability to form lung colonies, but they metastasised extensively when adminstered orthotopically. Subclones derived from tumours and metastases originating from clone N35 cells showed increased levels of type IV collagen and vimentin, but reduced levels of cytokeratin and ICAM-1. These results suggest that *erbB2* may not be a primary genetic factor capable of inducing invasion and metastasis, and that the alterations in the behaviour of the transfectants may result from secondary genetic changes. It is conceivable that orthotopic implantation might elicit responses from other transforming genes and the net effect might be a function of the cooperation between *erbB2* and other transforming genes.

erbB2 *oncoprotein expression and tumour proliferation*

Since the *erbB2* oncoprotein is an EGFr-related protein, there have been some attempts to examine possible correlations between levels of expression of this oncoprotein with tumour proliferation. The transduction of growth factor signals by tyrosine kinase-type receptors involves the transphosphorylation and/or activation of substrates, such as phospholipase C-γ and phosphatidylinositol kinases. The activation of these substrates results in the production of two second messengers, phosphatidyl 1,4,5-trisphosphate (IP$_3$) and diacylglycerol (DAG). IP$_3$ induces the release of Ca^{2+} from intracellular stores, and DAG activates protein kinase C. The phosphatidylinositol signalling pathway appears to be involved in signal transduction by *erbB2* protein. The *erbB2* oncoprotein possesses an intrinsic tyrosine kinase activity (Stubblefield and Sanford, 1987) and the ability to activate phospholipase C-γ (Peles *et al.*, 1991). Moreover, the *erbB* family oncoproteins are known to affect cell growth, together with changes in intracellular Ca^{2+} and phosphatidylinositol levels (Pimentel, 1987). The levels of *erbB2* protein and EGFr do not always relate to each other in a given tumour (Moe *et al.*, 1991; Osaki *et al.*, 1992), but they may independently relate to the proliferative state of the tumour. Poller *et al.* (1991) found that breast ductal carcinomas *in situ* which are immunoreactive for *erbB2* protein tended to possess higher DNA indices and generally a higher proportion of cells in the S-phase than *erbB2*-

negative tumours. Proliferative activity, as indicated by ^{3}H-thymidine labelling, was higher in tumours over-expressing *erbB2* than in tumours where its expression was within normal levels (Tommasi *et al.*, 1991).

Epidermal growth factor receptors in cancer

It was mentioned in the previous sections that the glycoprotein products of the *erb* gene family function as membrane receptors for growth factors. The growth of a variety of cancers is controlled and modulated by the binding of EGF to its specific receptor (EGFr). Therefore, there have been a large number of studies on EGFr status in breast cancer to determine whether EGFr expression is a marker for breast cancer progression and prognosis. The presence of EGF receptors has been regarded, on an empirical basis, as an indicator of clinical aggressiveness and higher metastatic potential of tumours. Thus, EGFr positivity in primary tumours is higher in patients with axillary node involvement or lymphatic invasion by the tumour than in node negative patients (Imai *et al.*, 1982; Sainsbury *et al.*, 1985a, 1987; Battaglia *et al.*, 1988; Spyratos *et al.*, 1990; Toi *et al.*, 1990; Hainsworth *et al.*, 1991). Metastatic tumours also have been reported to contain higher levels of EGFr than corresponding primary tumours (Sainsbury *et al.*, 1985a,b; Battaglia *et al.*, 1988). Furthermore, EGFr positivity correlates with poor differentiation and tumour grade (Sainsbury *et al.*, 1985c; Harris and Nicholson, 1988; Bolla *et al.*, 1990; Toi *et al.*, 1990; Hainsworth *et al.*, 1991). EGFr positivity is also regarded by many as the most important single predictor of prognosis, since it indicates poor relapse-free survival (Sainsbury *et al.*, 1987; Macias *et al.*, 1991; Nicholson *et al.*, 1991). The EGF receptor status of breast cancer appears to be closely related clinically to tumour progression and metastasis. Further evidence for a direct correlation of EGFr levels with metastatic potential has been provided by Radinsky *et al.* (1995). They found consistently higher (more than fivefold) levels of EGFr protein and also EGFr mRNA in cells of human colonic carcinoma with high metastatic potential than in cells with low potential for metastasis. Furthermore, EGFr positive cells produced a high incidence of liver metastasis upon inoculation into nude mice.

EGF and TGF-α (which can also bind to EGFr) are produced by a variety of human neoplasms and these can provide mitogenic stimulus to cells in an autocrine or in a paracrine fashion. EGFr is not only over-expressed in endometrial cancers but EGFr status also strongly correlates with histological grade and metastatic spread (Khalifa *et al.*, 1994). Higher levels of EGF/TGF-α or similar peptides have been reported in ovarian cancers than in corresponding normal tissues (Arteaga *et al.*, 1988; Kohler *et al.*, 1989). Ovarian cancers which express EGF receptors also show high cell proliferation (Henzen-Logmans *et al.*, 1994). According to Owens *et al.* (1991) a majority (88.5%) of ovarian cancers produced TGF-α and only 27.6% of tumours produced EGF. TGF-α shows much higher expression in endometrial cancer biopsies where there is myometrial invasion (Leake *et al.*, 1991). Cell lines derived from ovarian epithelial tumours have been shown to express genes coding for A and B chains of PDGF. These proteins have also been demonstrated in frozen section using antibodies against PDGF, but their receptors are not expressed (Versnel *et al.*, 1994).

Berchuck *et al.* (1991b) found a majority (82%) of ovarian cancers to express EGFr, while Scambia *et al.* (1992) placed EGFr positivity at a lower level (54%). Unlike for breast cancer, neither of these studies nor the earlier study by Bauknecht *et al.* (1988) have found any relationship between EGFr status and any clinical or pathological features of the tumour. Owens *et al.* (1991) investigated 150 consecutive patients with ovarian cancer and reported occurrence of EGFr in only 39.7% of the cases and this bore no relationship to stage of the disease; neither has a more recent study by van der Burg *et al.* (1993) found any correlation between EGFr status and *FIGO* stage. However, Scambia *et al.* (1992) have observed a tendency for omental metastases to be EGFr positive compared with the primary tumour. Furthermore, they have also suggested that in advanced disease higher EGFr expression could identify a subgroup which has poorer prognosis. Indeed, the median length of survival in patients with EGFr-positive tumours was 40 months compared with 26 months for the EGFr-negative group (Berchuck *et al.*, 1991b).

There is considerable evidence that EGF/TGF-α receptor function can be modulated by other factors such as steroid hormones, as shown in the case of endometrial cancers by Murphy (1994) who has argued, therefore, that constitutive expression or over-expression of the growth factor and/or its receptors might be an important element in the growth of endometrial cancers. This argument can be applied with equal force to other neoplasms. Among other factors known to affect EGFr function is the HPV16-E5 gene which amplifies the mitogenic signals from activated EGFr (Pim *et al.*, 1992). Furthermore, we know that high-affinity EGF receptors are linked with the cytoskeletal elements. It follows, therefore, that certain genes, such as the murine *18A2/mts1* gene, which promotes cytoskeletal depolymerisation (Lakshmi *et al.*, 1993) and *nm23* which is involved in the process of microtubule polymerisation, could decisively affect the transduction of signal by activated EGFr. In this context, it should be noted that human breast cancer cells which constitutively express the human homologue *h-mts1* are also high expressors of EGFr and contain large S-phase fractions (Sherbet *et al.*, 1995). Therefore, one can envisage situations where growth factor signals are amplified by genes such as *18A2/mts1* and HPV16-E5. Such deregulation of signal transduction can lead to aberrant growth which is so characteristic of cancers.

11

Developmental genes and their putative suppressor function

It was recognised many decades ago that developmental and neoplastic processes shared several features, and the range of these shared features has suggested that neoplastic transformation could be a pathological counterpart of normal differentiation and development, and further that it might result from inappropriate and misprogrammed gene expression (Markert, 1968; Sherbet, 1974). These concepts and ideas have been expounded at length by Sherbet (1982). Most salient among these is the invasive ability which tumour cells share with embryonic cells. Often cited as examples are trophoblast cells which invade the endometrium, and embryonic mesenchymal cells which are regarded as a highly invasive cell type. Much of this invasive ability is lost together with the acquisition of differentiated functions and organisation (Sherbet, 1970). In contrast, neoplastic development is characterised by loss of organisation and acquisition of motility. A process reminiscent of metastatic deposition also occurs in embryonic development, e.g. in the migration and secondary distribution of the neural crest-derived argentiffin cells in the primitive gut and its derivatives, and the distribution of chromaffin cells, again a neural crest derivative, as paraganglionic chromaffin bodies (Sherbet, 1982). The genesis of paraneoplastic syndromes involving the ectopic and inappropriate synthesis of hormones can be related to the degree of differentiation of the tumour (Sherbet, 1974).

The identification and cloning of genes which participate in tumorigenesis has led to their designation as 'oncogenes', which, with the benefit of hindsight, may be described as inappropriate nomenclature. The unrelenting pursuit of their mode of function in carcinogenesis has revealed that several so-called oncogenes also show development-related modulation of expression. Recently, several genes that control differentiation and embryonic development have been identified and some of them also function as tumour suppressor genes. The finest examples are the *wnt* family of genes and Wilms' tumour gene *wt-1*, which merit a detailed discussion of their normal function and their participation in neoplasia.

wnt genes in cell differentiation and neoplasia

The *wnt* family of genes comprises several members which figure prominently in embryonic development, differentiation and pattern formation, as well as in neoplastic transformation and tumorigenesis. Many *wnt* genes are expressed in developing and in adult nervous systems. In P19 embryonal carcinoma cells, retinoic acid induces neural differentiation and together with this characteristic changes also occur in the profile of expression of nine *wnt* genes. The *wnt-1* gene is not expressed in undifferentiated P19 cells. It is expressed in early neuroectodermal differentiation, together with the loss of expression of the SSEA-1 antigen which is a characteristic feature of undifferentiated P19 cells. Furthermore, *wnt-1* itself appears to induce the expression of other members of the family (Smolich and Papkoff, 1994). Expression of *wnt-1* may be induced by a factor, described as the wnt-1 inducing factor (WiF-1). A region of the *wnt-1* promoter appears to contain a binding site for WiF-1. This factor is not detectable in undifferentiated P19 cells. Also, Wif-1 is not detectable in P19 cells induced to differentiate into mesodermal derivatives by dimethylsulphoxide (Starnaud and Moir, 1993). This seems to suggest that *wnt-1* expression can directly commit these cells to the neural differentiation pathway and, possibly, that other *wnt* members might be involved with the induction of mesodermal differentiation. This view is supported by some preliminary work in *Xenopus*, where presumptive ectoderm isolated from embryos injected with X*wnt*-8 RNA at the gastrula stage of development, could be seen to differentiate into mesoderm (Sokol, 1993).

    The expression of *wnt* genes shows a temporal and a spatial relationship with identifiable stages of embryonic development, especially the development of and pattern formation in the central nervous system (CNS). The differentiation of the CNS begins in the embryonic disc, which is composed of the epiblast and the hypoblast (Figure 16, see page 158). An initial identifiable feature of the beginning of morphogenesis is the formation of the primitive streak in the midline of the clear area of the epiblast which is termed the area pellucida. The primitive streak is formed by cell migrations occurring in the area pellucida and with the continued cell migrations towards the primitive streak it becomes narrower, elongates anteriorly and subsequently develops a median groove and the terminal Hensen's node. Cells migrate and invaginate along the primitive streak groove and form the mesoderm and the endoblast (Rao, 1994). The axial polarity of the embryo is now established. Following this process of gastrulation, one can note the formation of the neural plate, the development of the neural groove and the formation of the neural folds. The neural folds then fuse along the midline to form a neural tube. During further development, morphogenesis of the brain becomes evident in the form of the prosencephalon (forebrain), the mesencephalon (the midbrain) and the rhombencephalon (the hindbrain).

There have been many studies aimed at establishing whether *wnt* genes show any patterns of expression which can be related to these early developmental stages. These have been carried out starting with the earliest discernible stages of chick embryo development. A newly discovered member of the family, *Cwnt-8c*, for instance, may be expressed in the primitive streak and Hensen's node of the chick embryo (Hume and Dodd, 1993); these authors also showed that injection of exogenous *Cwnt-8c* mRNA induced duplication of the embryonic axis and dorsalisation of mesodermal tissue, i.e. the gene possesses the potential to determine the formation of the neuro-axis. *Cwnt-8c* expression may be restricted during neurulation to certain regions of the hindbrain (Hume and Dodd, 1993). Subsequently, Hollyday *et al.* (1995) reported the activity of at least six members of the *wnt* gene family in the central nervous system of chick embryos. The expression may be spatially restricted to different sections of the developing neural tube; yet, temporally, there can be an overlap of expression of different genes. Thus, *wnt-1* and *wnt-4* are initially expressed in the neural plate region corresponding to the presumptive mesencephalon, whereas *wnt-3* is found in the presumptive rhombencephalon. These genes then show overlapping expression when distinct subdivisions become apparent in the closed neural tube. Thus *wnt-1*, 3a and 4 show overlapping expression in the posterior diencephalon, a subdivision of prosencephalon, and in the rhombencephalon and spinal cord. The earlier work by Parr *et al.* (1993) has suggested that the *wnt-3*, -3a and -7b expression pattern may relate to the subdivisions of the prosencephalon. Admittedly, there are obvious differences in the described patterns, but these studies do underline a basic fact that these genes are actively involved not only in the determination of the embryonic axis, but also in both neuro-ectodermal differentiation and pattern formation.

The *wnt* genes also play a role in the differentiation of limb buds. Mouse embryo forelimb primordia show a uniform expression of *wnt-3*, -4, -6 and -7b and gradients of expression of specific genes have also been found (Parr *et al.*, 1993). However, a different set of *wnt* genes have been reported to be involved in pattern formation in the chick embryo limb bud (Dealy *et al.*, 1993). *wnt-4* and *wnt-5a* have been implicated in cell proliferation and differentiation of murine mammary gland (Olson and Papkoff, 1994).

The nature and function of wnt proteins

The *wnt* genes code for proteins which are secreted as glycosylated proteins of 35–42 kDa molecule size. The wnt proteins carry conserved structural features and may exhibit similar biological and biochemical properties. Sequence homology has been reported between wnt proteins derived from different species. The *wnt-4* and *wnt-11* genes from chicken encode proteins comprising 351 and 354 amino acid residues respectively, and both have 24 cysteine residues shared with other wnt proteins. Chicken wnt-4 and wnt-11 have been reported to bear

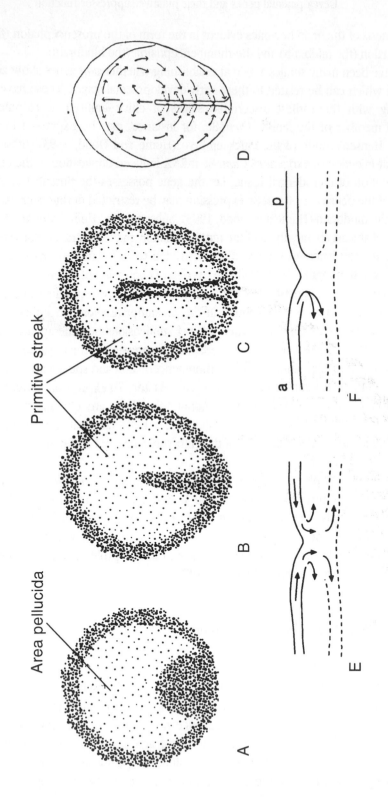

Area pellucida

Primitive streak

A

B

C

D

E

F

a

p

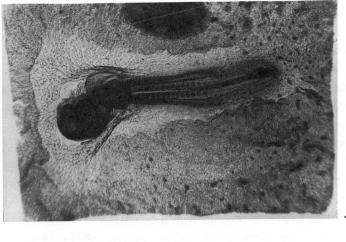

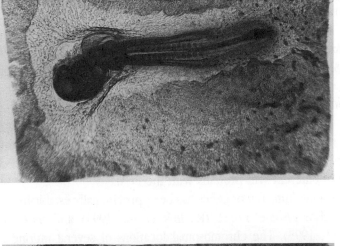

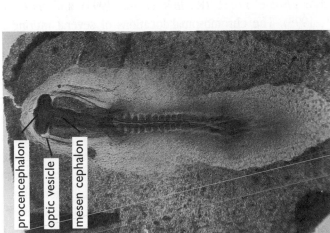

I

procencephalon
optic vesicle
mesen cephalon

H

area pellucida
neural tube
neural fold

G

Figure 16. The beginnings of morphogenesis are illustrated here with examples from chick embryo development. A, B and C represent the embryonic blastoderm, composed of the epiblast and the endoblast. The central clear area is called 'area pellucida'. Here the primitive streak forms as a consequence of cell migrations occurring in the epiblast (D). The cell movements are shown in the cross-section (E) and sagittal section (F) of the blastoderm. In (F) a and p indicate the anterior–posterior polarity of the blastoderm. These cell migrations also cause the primitive streak to elongate in an anterior direction and to form a median groove. Cells continue to migrate and invaginate into the primitive groove and form the primary mesoderm. The primary mesoderm then induces the presumptive neuroectoderm above to differentiate into neural tissue and form the neural axis. G shows a later stage of development where the neural grove is formed, and this folds and fuses along the midline to form the neural tube. H and I show the morphogenesis of the brain. A–C, E and F reproduced with permission from Rao (1994).

partial sequence homology with *Xenopus* wnt-4 and mouse wnt-11 (Tanda *et al.*, 1995). Murines wnt-11 and wnt-12 show 38% and 49% homology, respectively, in certain regions of the protein, with other murine wnt proteins (Adamson *et al.*, 1994).

The wnt proteins associate tightly with the extracellular matrix upon secretion, but they may be released into the culture medium upon treatment with suramin (Blasband *et al.*, 1992; Papkoff, 1994). These findings have been confirmed by Smolich *et al.* (1993) by transfecting seven *wnt* genes into AtT-20 cells and characterising the products of the exogenous genes. However, there are indications that wnt proteins may be released spontaneously into the culture medium (Bradley and Brown, 1995). Barras and McMahon (1995) found that murine wnt-1, -3a, -5a, -5b, -6 and -7b are released into the culture medium by suramin, but treatment with heparin releases only wnt-1, -6, and -7b, which suggests that there might be differences with regard to the association of different wnt proteins with the ECM.

The chromosomal location of some human *wnt* genes has been provisionally established: e.g. *wnt-*3 has been mapped to chromosome 17q21 (Roelink *et al.*, 1993) and *wnt-*5A to chromosome 3p21 (Clark *et al.*, 1993). The chromosomal locations of several murine *wnt* genes are also known.

Mammalian wnt-1 has been found to be homologous to wg protein encoded by the *wingless (wg)* gene and the *arm* (armadillo) gene, which are segment polarity genes of *Drosophila*. The *arm* and *wg* genes exert similar effects on embryonic development (Peifer *et al.*, 1991). The *arm* gene is a component of signal transduction pathway of the *wg* gene and it is regulated by *wg* (Riggleman *et al.*, 1990). Similarly, in vertebrates, β-catenin and plakoglobin (homologues of the *Drosophila* arm protein) are components of the signal transduction pathway of the *wnt* gene and both the arm protein and β-catenin are associated with cell–cell adherence junctions in epithelia and Ca^{2+}-mediated cell–cell adhesion (Hinck *et al.*, 1994; Peifer, 1995) (see Figure 13, page 104). *wnt* expression enhances the accumulation of β-catenin and plakoglobin and the binding of β-catenin to cadherin which mediates cell adhesion. Expression of wnt protein parallels that of E-cadherin and α-N-catenin in embryonic mouse brain (Shinamura *et al.*, 1994). In PC12 cells, *wnt* expression correlates with enhanced steady-state levels of plakoglobin and alterations in its intracellular distribution. E-cadherin expression is elevated in these cells, together with the stabilisation of its binding with β-catenin, and this results in Ca^{2+}-mediated cell–cell adhesion (Bradley *et al.*, 1993; Hinck *et al.*, 1994). In the light of these findings, one can justifiably conclude that the *wnt* genes may play a significant role in modulating the behaviour of cells, e.g. cell motility and invasive behaviour in the context of tumorigenesis.

wnt *genes in cell proliferation, transformation and tumorigenesis*

Cell differentiation and proliferation are integral but mutually exclusive components of growth, development and morphogenesis. The demonstration that *wnt* gene expression may modulate cellular behaviour by altering cellular adhesion has inevitably raised questions concerning the possible implications of their expression for cell proliferation, neoplastic transformation, invasion and tumorigenesis.

As stated before, several *wnt* genes are expressed in the proliferation and differentiation of murine mammary glands. C57MG mammary cells respond to mitogenic stimulation by growth factors such as EGF, FGF and TGF-β, but their partial transformation by *wnt*-1 can substitute for these growth factor signals. Furthermore, *wnt*-4 and -5a, which are normally expressed in these cells, are down-regulated by FGF or partial transformation by *int*-2. A transformation of cells by the oncogene *neu* completely suppresses the transcription of *wnt*-4 and -5a (Olson and Papkoff, 1994). Expression of *wnt*-1 suppresses the ability of rat PC12 phaeochromocytoma cells to respond to neurite growth factor (NGF) (Shackleford *et al.*, 1993a). That induction of proliferation can be achieved by wnt proteins is indicated by the experiments reported by Bradley and Brown (1995), who demonstrated that conditioned medium obtained from a mammary cell line which expresses *wnt*-1 can induce proliferation and transformation of cells.

Both *wnt* genes and their *Drosophila* homologues are efficient inducers of cell transformation. The *wg* gene of *Drosophila* can transform and induce proliferation in mouse mammary epithelial cells, and RAC311c mammary cells carrying the *wg* gene have been found to be tumorigenic (Ramakrishna and Brown, 1993). The ability to transform cannot be uniformly attributed to all members of the *wnt* gene family. According to Wong *et al.* (1994), *wnt*-3a and *wnt*-7a possess high transforming ability. *wnt*-2, *wnt*-5b and *wnt*-7b were less efficient than *wnt*-3a and *wnt*-7a. At the end of this spectrum *wnt*-4 and *wnt*-5a, which are expressed in the normal state, have no transforming ability (Wong *et al.*, 1994; Bradley and Brown, 1995). The expression of these genes has been examined recently in human cancer and cancer-derived cell cultures. There are reports of differential expression of *wnt* genes in human breast cancer cell lines and tumour tissue. The *wnt*-3, -4, -7b genes have been found in cell lines and in tumour tissue, and *wnt*-2, in addition, has been found in tumour tissue alone. *wnt*-2 and -4 expression was found to be 10–20-fold higher in fibroadenomas than in normal breast tissue or in carcinomas, and in a small proportion of tumours *wnt*-7b was expressed at 30-fold higher levels in tumours than in normal or benign breast tissue (Huguet *et al.*, 1994). It has emerged, from another study from the same laboratory, that *wnt*-5a expression is considerably up-regulated in benign proliferative conditions and invasive breast cancer tissue compared with normal breast tissue (LeJeune *et al.*, 1995). Clearly, the expression of some of these genes correlates with proliferative capacity, but further studies are required to assess the implications of the levels of their expression for progression to invasive and metastatic stages of the disease, since in the study described by LeJeune *et al.* (1995), *wnt*-5a expression did not relate to any established markers of malignancy such as lymph node metastasis and EGF receptor status.

Possibly, several *wnt* gene combinations may be involved in cellular transformation and *wnt* genes may cooperate with other oncogenes to transform cells. Experiments with bitransgenic mice, with *wnt*-1 and *int*-2 (FGF family gene), have shown that mammary tumours appear in bitransgenic, especially male, mice carrying both genes at a far higher frequency than in either parent line. Whereas all bitransgenic males developed mammary tumours within 8 months, only 15% with wnt-1 alone and none carrying int-2 alone developed tumours (Kwan et al., 1992). Further evidence that wnt-1 might cooperate with FGF family genes, int-2 and hst, to accelerate mammary tumorigeneis has been provided by Shackleford et al. (1993b).

Cell transformation by wnt genes can occur as a paracrine phenomenon. Cells expressing wnt-1, although not themselves transformed, can induce transformation of target cells grown in co-culture (Jue et al., 1992). Similarly, RAC311c mammary epithelial cells carrying the wnt-1 homologue wg gene are able to transform cells grown in co-culture (Ramakrishna and Brown, 1993). Parkin et al. (1993) believe that the paracrine effects can be mediated by membrane-bound wnt proteins. However, the possibility that the transformation of target cells in co-culture may be due to wnt proteins released from effector cells cannot be ruled out.

Activation of wnt genes

There are suggestions that wnt family genes and int proto-oncogenes may be transcriptionally activated by MMTV insertion mutations (Sarkar et al., 1994; Sarkar, 1995). Sarkar (1995) found that out of 79 tumours derived from different genetic backgrounds 31 showed insertional mutations in wnt-1, and only 14% of the tumours contained int-2 mutations. Activation of wnt-1 can conceivably enhance expression of other wnt genes as downstream events (Smolich and Papkoff, 1994). Starnaud and Moir (1993) attempted characterisation of the wnt-1 promoter of P19 embryonal carcinoma cells. These cells can be induced to differentiate along the neuroectodermal pathway by exposure to retinoic acid but, in contrast, they differentiate into mesoderm when treated with dimethylsulphoxide (DMSO). Starnaud and Moir (1993) have identified a 230 bp region of the promoter from positions -278 to -47 5' upstream of wnt-1 sequence which appears to be involved with retinoic acid-mediated transcription. This region contains a GC-rich binding site for a nuclear protein which has been called the wnt-1 inducing factor (WiF-1). This factor is detectable in P19 cells treated with retinoic acid and not those treated with DMSO. WiF-1 is a 65 kDa protein which appears to function as a GC-box-binding transcription factor. The wide spectrum of differential expression of the wnt genes may be an indication of their regulation in a temporal and spatial programme, possibly mediated by different transactivating factors.

With the demonstration that wnt genes are actively associated with cell proliferation, the possibility that they may be subject to regulation by p53 has been examined. In wnt-1 transgenic mice that are p53 deficient (p53−/−) tumours appear earlier than in hosts which carry normal p53 alleles (Donehower et al., 1995). This observation clearly implicates p53 in a regulatory role in the induction of proliferation and tumorigenesis by the wnt gene.

Wilms' tumour gene *wt1* in embryonic development and neoplasia

Incidence and pathogenesis of Wilms' tumour

Wilms' tumour is a paediatric nephroblastoma, with an incidence rate of 1/10 000 live births. Wilms' tumour occurs both sporadically and in a familial fashion, although only 1% of tumours show a familial history (see Tay, 1995). It is associated with aniridia, genito-urinary malformation and mental retardation (Miller *et al.*, 1964; Ricardi *et al.*, 1978). The total syndrome has therefore been described as the WAGR syndrome. Three basic components can be identified in Wilms' tumour and these are the blastema, immature epithelium and stroma, and the genesis of the tumour is a result of aberrant differentiation of nephric stem cells consequent upon loss of suppressor effects normally exerted by tumour suppressor genes associated with its pathogenesis.

Chromosomal deletions associated with the WAGR syndrome

Some years ago, an interstitial deletion of chromosome 11p13 was reported to occur as constitutive abnormality in a small group of patients with the WAGR syndrome (Ricardi *et al.*, 1978, 1980; Francke *et al.*, 1979). This deletion has been confirmed subsequently using short-term cultures of tumour tissue (Reeve *et al.*, 1984; Scott *et al.*, 1985; Kumar *et al.*, 1987). Loss of DNA at chromosome 11p13 was demonstrated in Wilms' tumour suggesting that the Wilms' tumour gene (*wt1*) occurs within this band (Fearon *et al.*, 1984; Koufos *et al.*, 1984; Orkins *et al.*, 1984; Reeve *et al.*, 1984). The *wt-1* gene has been mapped to 11p13 (Call *et al.*, 1990). The WAGR may be a reflection of the contiguity of genes at the 11p13 locus (Porteous *et al.*, 1987). Indeed, the WAGR genes occur between the catalase gene and the gene coding for the β-subunit of follicle stimulating hormone (FSH-β) (Figure 17). The Wilms' tumour gene is found 700 kb centromeric to the aniridia gene named *PAX6*. The region showing deletions associated with mental retardation occurs p-terminal to the *PAX6* and the region which shows abnormalities in association with genito-urinary malformations occurs centromeric to the Wilms' tumour gene (Turleau *et al.*, 1984; Glaser *et al.*, 1986, 1987; Gessler *et al.*, 1989a,b; van Heyningen *et al.*, 1989). The Wilms' tumour gene spans less than 345 kb (Rose *et al.*, 1990). Wt33, the longest cDNA cloned, is approximately 2300 bp long (Call *et al.*, 1990).

Often, allelic loss in Wilms' tumour is also associated with chromosome 11p15 (Mannens *et al.*, 1988, 1990; Wadey *et al.*, 1990). It has also been found that tumours from WAGR patients

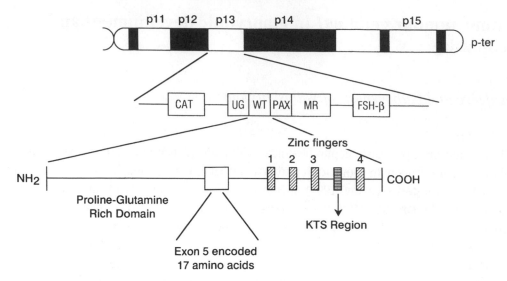

Figure 17.   The organisation of WAGR locus at 11p13. Based on references cited in the text.

with chromosome 11p13 deletions can also show loss of heterozygosity at 11p15 (Henry *et al.*, 1989; Jeanpierre *et al.*, 1990). These observations suggest that a second gene, which leads to a predisposition to form Wilms' tumour, occurs at 11p15. Indeed, sporadic Wilms' tumours do show loss of heterozygosity at this locus (Reeve *et al.*, 1989). The chromosome 11p15 region also represents the Beckwith-Wiedemann syndrome (BWS) locus. Patients with BWS show loss of heterozygosity at this locus and frequently develop Wilms' tumour with loss of heterozygosity at 11p15 (Waziri *et al.*, 1983; Turleau *et al.*, 1984; Henry *et al.*, 1989; Mannens *et al.*, 1990). The oncogene H-*ras* also occurs at this chromosomal region, and Wilms' tumours have been reported to show allelic loss of H-*ras* (Reeve *et al.*, 1984). Baird *et al.* (1991) screened six Wilms' tumours showing loss of heterozygosity at 11p13 for *ras* mutations, but no sequence mutations were found. Cowell *et al.* (1993) did not detect any mutations of the gene from tumours which had 11p13 deletions. Neither were mutations found in the zinc finger region of wt1 most prone to mutate frequently. Considering that only a small, although not insignificant, proportion of Wilms' tumours show *wt1* abnormalities, it would be reasonable to assume that other genes may also be involved in the predisposition to Wilms' tumour development. As stated above, chromosome 11p15 is often deleted in Wilms' tumours. To this locus a second Wilms' tumour gene (*wt2*) has now been assigned. There are other genes mapped to this region: e.g. insulin-like growth factor II (Reeve *et al.*, 1985; Scott *et al.*, 1985) and FSH *β*-subunit, and these cannot be excluded from possible participation in the pathogenesis of the tumour. A third Wilms' tumour susceptibility gene (*wt3*) is believed to be located on chromosome 16, in the light of the frequency of allelic loss associated with this locus in Wilms' tumours (Maw *et al.*, 1992; see also Tay, 1995).

Wilms' tumour gene function in development and differentiation

The *wt1* gene shows a definable pattern, both temporal and spatial, of expression in the developing kidney. Its expression is first detectable in the intermediate mesenchyme lateral to the coelomic cavity of 13-somite early 9-day embryos, then in the urogenital ridge (early mesonephric tubules). The uninduced metanephric mesenchyme shows *wt1* expression by 11 days and soon this is followed by enhancement of its expression in the induced mesenchyme of the kidney and markedly in the nephrogenic condensations; later in the development of the kidney, it is restricted to the glomeruli (Armstrong *et al.*, 1993). No expression is found in the proximal or distal tubules and loop of Henle. The genital ridge, fetal gonad and mesothelium are other major sites of *wt1* expression. No expression is found in fetal heart, skin, adrenal gland, stomach, liver, eye or muscle (Pritchard-Jones *et al.*, 1990). The suppression of myogenesis during kidney development may also be a normal function of *wt1* (Miyagawa *et al.*, 1994).

Molecular bases of wt1 function

The changes in the pattern of expression of the gene during embryonic development is compatible with the notion of switching differentiation from mesenchymal to epithelial cells. The wt1 protein suppresses transcription of genes encoding several growth factors, e.g. PDGF-A (Wang *et al.*, 1992), IGF-II (Drummond *et al.*, 1992), TGF-β1 (Dey *et al.*, 1994). The expression of growth factor receptors also appears to be modulated by *wt1* (Werner *et al.*, 1994; Englert *et al.*, 1995). Furthermore, wt1 also contains the DNA-binding sequence found in the transcription factor induced by nerve growth factor (Milbrandt, 1987). It is conceivable, therefore, that its inactivation could lead to unregulated cell proliferation and aberrant differentiation, leading to tumorigenesis.

A variety of stimuli that regulate cell growth, e.g. growth factors and inducers of cell differentiation are transduced by the expression and regulation of transcription factors, which are encoded by oncogenes such as *myc*, *myb*, *fos* and *jun*. Another family of genes is known, vis., the *early growth response* (Egr) gene family and this includes five transcription factors, Egr1, Egr2, Egr3, Egr4 and the wt1 protein. These transcription factors are related by virtue of the presence of highly homologous zinc finger domains that participate in binding to DNA. The sequence of the wt1 protein does indeed show that it can function as a DNA-binding factor. wt1 is a *c.*53 kDa protein with a proline and glutamine rich *N*-terminal domain and four Kruppel-type zinc finger domains situated at the c-terminal end (Gessler *et al.*, 1990). A lysine–threonine–serine (KTS) region occurs between zinc fingers 3 and 4. Alternative splicing of wt-1 pro-mRNA results in the generation of wt1 isoforms in which exon 5 and the KTS regions may be excluded. Alternative splicing at exon 5 is only seen in mammals, but splicing at the KTS regions occurs in a wide range of species (Kent *et al.*, 1995). The nucleotide sequence of wt1 is conserved among several species, with both the zinc finger regions and transregulatory domain exhibiting marked similarity.

In analogy with the occurrence of proline-rich regions in several DNA-binding proteins and the *Kruppel* gene product, wt1 has been suggested as a sequence-specific DNA-binding protein and regulator of genetic transcription. The zinc-finger domain recognises the DNA sequence 5'-GCG(G/T)GGGCG-3' (Rauscher *et al.*, 1990). This represents the binding site for Egr-1, which is a transcription factor (NGF1-A) encoded by a gene which is induced by nerve growth factor (Milbrandt, 1987). wt1 has now been shown to repress the expression of IGF-II gene through this Egr1-binding element represented by nucleotides -87 to -65 of the IGF-II P4 promoter (Lee and Kim, 1996). The repressor function of wt1 has been attributed to the proline-glutamine rich region of the protein and if this region is fused with zinc finger domain of Egr-1, Egr-1 converts into a transcriptional repressor (Madden *et al.*, 1991). Since both Egr1 and wt1 bind to the same DNA-binding element, the relative concentration of the activating and repressor proteins might be significant in determining the direction of regulation.

Hamilton *et al.* (1995) state, however, that considerations of the mechanisms of zinc finger interactions with DNA suggest the occurrence of a recognition site larger than the 9 bp Egr-1 binding site. They showed that wt1[-KTS] showed very high affinity to a 12 bp sequence GCG-TGG-GCG-(T/G) (G/A/T) (T/G). Nakagawa *et al.* (1995) have identified a 10 bp sequence, 5'-GCGTGGGAGT-3' from murine genomic DNA to which wt1 binds with high affinity. Mutations in the zinc fingers II–IV abolished the binding to this motif, whereas mutations in the zinc finger I only reduced the binding. Thus, although Egr-1-like genes may be involved in growth regulation, wt1 may function by binding to higher affinity recognition sites than the Egr-1 motif.

The presence of splice isoforms of wt-1 may have a functional significance. Egr-1 site is known to occur in the promoters of several genes and wt1 can therefore bind to these promoters. However, the KTS isoform can bind to promoter 3 of human insulin-like growth factor 2, the (tccn)n of the transcription initiation site of PDGF-A, in which the Egr-1 consensus sequence has been identified. The KTS+ isoform, on the other hand, shows far less binding affinity. An abnormal balance between the two isoforms results in severe developmental abnormalites. The wt1 point mutations occurring in the Denys–Drash syndrome could be exerting their effects by generating such an isoform imbalance (see Little *et al.*, 1995). A significant proportion of Wilms' tumours also show wt1 isoforms lacking the 17 amino acid region encoded by exon 5 (Simms *et al.*, 1995). Splice variants resulting from exclusion of the exon 5 encoded 17 amino acid region also exhibit major differences in their ability to function as transcriptional regulators. Reddy *et al.* (1995) have reported that the wt isoform which contains the 17 residues encoded by exon 5 was a more powerful activator of transcription that the isoform without these 17 amino acid residues. It is therefore worthwhile reiterating that an imbalance in the expression of the isoforms may be associated with developmental abnormalities and tumorigenesis.

Alternative splicing of the wt protein appears to influence its intracellular distribution. The wt KTS+ isoform shows nuclear localisation with splice factors whereas the wt KTS− isoform localises with transcription factors (Charlieu *et al.*, 1995). Using antibodies raised against wt1 and splicing complexes (snRNPs, small nuclear ribonucleoprotein particles), it has been shown that wt1 co-localises with snRNPs (Larsson SH *et al.*, 1995) and may indeed be associated with complexes containing snRNPs called coiled bodies (Carmo-Fonseca *et al.*, 1992). Thus, an intriguing aspect of wt1 function is its ability to subserve two distinct functions, namely regulating gene transcription and acting as a splicing factor. The demonstration that wt1 associates with snRNPs does not *per se* justify designating it as a splicing factor, although it could be regulating the splicing process.

Inactivation of wt1 suppressor function

The inactivation of wt1 function may be seen as a consequence of genetic abnormalities of the gene. It is believed that up to 10-15% of Wilms' tumours may carry point mutations (Coppes *et al.*, 1993; Gessler *et al.*, 1994). Mutations occur in the coding sequence of the gene, but not in the *wt1* promoter (Grubb *et al.*, 1995). Somatic mutation appears to be an early event. Nephrogenic nests are regarded as the precursors of Wilms' tumour. In two cases of Wilms' tumour where a somatic mutation was detected, an identical mutation has been found in the nephrogenic nests (Park *et al.*, 1993). It has been reported that >95% of Denys–Drash syndrome patients carry *wt1* mutations (Coppes *et al.*, 1993). These occur in the zinc finger domain of *wt1*. Patients with Denys-Drash syndrome who develop Wilms' tumour, suffer from renal failure and show male pseudohermaphroditism and gonadal dysgenesis. These mutations totally abolish the DNA-binding ability of wt1 protein (Little *et al.*, 1995).

Although major mutational events appear to be associated with the zinc finger domain, exon 7 mutations also have been found. Gessler *et al.* (1993) reported an exon 7 single-nucleotide deletion in the second allele of the *wt1* gene in a WAGR patient. An insertional mutation has been described in a WAGR patient where a 14 bp sequence, a tandem duplication of an upstream exon sequence, is inserted in the intron part of the splice donor of exon 7 (Santos *et al.*, 1993). These authors have argued that this mutation may result in the abnormal processing of the *wt1* pre-mRNA and produce a non-functional protein. Large deletions at the 3' end of the gene result in the generation of truncated transcripts for wt1 protein lacking the fourth zinc finger (Algar *et al.*, 1995). In Denys-Drash syndrome, non-sense mutations can result in the formation of wt1 protein lacking two zinc fingers and this abnormal wt1 possesses no DNA-binding ability (Little *et al.*, 1995).

Cell proliferation in Wilms' tumour

The cellular components of Wilms' tumour show marked differences in proliferative activity. Delahunt *et al.* (1994) assessed this by measuring the expression of proliferating cell nuclear antigen (PCNA) and silver-staining nucleolar organiser region (AgNOR). They found that the blastemal and epithelial components showed far greater proliferative ability than the stromal component and there was also an indication that the proliferative activity, as determined by these methods, might be related to prognosis of the disease.

Several oncogenes are regulated by wt1, and among them are c-*myb*, *bcl*-2 and c-*myc* (Hewitt *et al.*, 1995; McCann S *et al.*, 1995), which are associated with the proliferation and differentiation of immature haemopoietic cells. Several genes encoding growth factors and/or their receptors are also known to be regulated by wt1. Among these is IGF-II which is over-expressed in Wilms' tumour (Waber *et al.*, 1993) and this growth factor may provide an autocrine stimulus for growth. This could be a result of the induction of IGF-II receptors by *wt1* expression. Stable transfection of *wt1* into RM1 cells induces the expression of these receptors and this is enhanced if *wt1* carries a mutation in the transactivation domain (Nichols *et al.*, 1995). For a dissenting view, one should cite the lack of inverse correlation between expression of *wt1* on one hand and the growth factor genes *IFG-II* and *PDGF-A* genes on the other (Langerak *et al.*, 1995). The expression of IGF-I receptor (IGF-Ir) is greater in Wilms' tumour compared with normal kidney tissue, and *IGF-Ir* mRNA is inversely related to the levels of *wt1* mRNA (Werner *et al.*, 1994). Werner *et al.* (1995) determined the activity of *IGF-Ir* gene promoter fragments in reporter gene constructs in two cell lines. One of these is G401, a Wilms' tumour-derived cell line where *wt1* expression is not detectable, and a human embryonic cell line 293 in which high levels of *wt1* mRNA are detectable. They found far higher levels of endogenous IGF-I receptor mRNA in the G401 compared with those in cell line 293. They also transfected G401 cells with a *wt1* expression vector and found that expression of the exogenous *wt1* inhibited proliferation of the transfectant cells, together with a reduction in the levels of *IGF-Ir* gene transcripts. From this work it is also obvious that the gene is able to control anchorage-independent growth, which is a characteristic feature of the transformed phenotype. Another growth factor receptor whose expression is modulated by *wt1* is the epidermal growth factor receptor (EGFr), which has been regarded as a marker of poor prognosis in certain human cancers (see page 153). *wt1* can also down-regulate the expression of EGF receptors. It seems to repress transcription of the *EGFr* gene by binding to two TC-rich repeat sequences. In the developing kidney, the decline of EGFr expression has been linked to *wt1* expression (Englert *et al.*, 1995). Microinjection of *wt1* mRNA apparently can block the entry of cell into the S-phase induced by serum stimulation, and this block can be removed by an over-expression of cyclin E-CDK2 and cyclin D1-CDK4 complexes, suggesting that wt1 might be controlling the progression of the cell cycle (Kudoh *et al.*, 1995).

It would be therefore of considerable interest to see if proliferation-related genes such as *p53*, *rb* and *mdm2* cooperate with *wt1* in determining the growth characteristics of Wilms' tumours. A preliminary study showed that the retinoblastoma susceptibility gene (*rb*) and the *ras* oncogene may not be altered in Wilms' tumour (Waber *et al.*, 1993), but more extensive studies are required to support this conclusion.

Since Wilms' tumours often show abnormalities associated with chromosome 17, there have been several studies which have been aimed at elucidating the possible relationships between wild-type and mutant *p53* in the regulation of the function of the wt1 protein as a transcription factor. wt1 modulates transcription of PDGF-A gene by binding to the Egr-1 element which occurs in the PDGF-A promoter. But this has been found to be dependent upon *p53* status, in the sense that wt1 and PDGF-A are co-expressed where mutated but not wild-type *p53* occurs. This has led to the suggestion that wt1 acts as a transcriptional activator in the absence of *p53* or in the presence of the mutated gene and as a transcriptional suppressor when wild-type p53 is present (Rodeck *et al.*, 1994). Nichols *et al.* (1995) also state that induction of IGF-II by *wt1* may be related to the presence of mutated *p53*. Consistent with the perceived stabilisation of p53 by cellular proteins (see page 28), wt1 has been reported to form a complex with p53. This interaction causes both proteins to transactivate their respective target genes. wt1 expression also seems to enhance the steady-state levels of p53 protein attributable to stabilisation and an enhancement of its half-life (Maheswaran *et al.*, 1993, 1995). Thus, there are clear implications of an interaction between wt1 and p53 for the control of cell proliferation.

Expression of wt1 *may be related to prognosis of Wilms' tumour*

The emergence of a possible link between *wt1* expression and the expression of growth factors and their receptors, together with *p53* mutation status and cell proliferation, has inevitably led to the study of *wt1* expression as a marker for tumour progression and possibly in assessing prognosis of the disease. Whereas in some studies Wilms' tumours showed no associated *p53* abnormalities (Waber *et al.*, 1993), others have found interesting correlations between *wt1/p53* expression and disease progression. Malkin *et al.* (1994) reported a low level of *p53* mutation (two out of 21). These two mutations were in exons 6 and 9 and they resulted in amino acid substitutions. Both tumours in which they were found were in advanced stage. Bardeesy *et al.* (1994) screened a large number of Wilms' tumours for *p53* mutations and mutations of this gene were found in eight out of 11 anaplastic tumours.

There is very little information about whether *wt1* expression correlates with invasive behaviour of tumours. Bladder cancers which show loss of heterozygosity at a high frequency at the *wt1* locus as well as at 11p15 might be ideally suited for this type of study because these tumours occur as invasive or superficial tumours that are clearly distinguishable in histology and a small proportion of superficial tumours may recur as invasive tumours. Judging by its involvement in cell proliferation, differentiation and morphogenesis, it may be expected that the gene might bring about secondary changes in cell adhesion properties and preliminary studies do indicate that expression of the gene modulates the levels of several extracellular matrix components (Peringa *et al.*, 1994).

Does wt1 *expression relate to prognosis in other human tumours?*

Information concerning *wt1* expression is now available for a number of tumour types. Investigations of ovarian cancers have revealed frequent deletions at 11p13, but without any apparent abnormalites or loss of heterzygosity of the *wt1* gene. In these tumours the gene may be expressed in a large proportion of tumours (Bruening *et al.*, 1993), but the level of expression can be highly variable (Viel *et al.*, 1994). The *wt1* gene is not involved in colorectal carcinomas (Cawkwell *et al.*, 1994) or primary brain tumours associated with Wilms' disease (Rainov *et al.*, 1995). *wt1* expression has been detected in seven out of nine melanomas, but not in normal melanocytes (Rodeck *et al.*, 1994). In a study of bladder cancers loss of heterozygosity at the *wt1* locus occurred in seven out of 14 cases and less frequently (two out of seven) at the 11p15 region containing the IGF-II gene (Shipman *et al.*, 1993).

Wt1 gene transcripts are not detectable in non-small cell lung carcinoma cell lines and lung cancer tissue (Amin *et al.*, 1995). Loss of heterozygosty at the *wt1* locus was found in five of 53 cases of non-small cell lung cancer and this was associated significantly with advanced tumour stage and nodal spread. Loss of heterozygosity (LOH) correlated with nodal involvement in the squamous cell carcinoma subtype and patients with tumours with LOH at 11p13 showed poorer survival than those without LOH at this locus (Fong *et al.*, 1994). Bepler and Garciablanco (1994) have identified three other regions at 11p13 and 11p15 which suffer somatic loss associated with these tumours, suggesting that these genetic loci might harbour suppressor genes that might be involved with their pathogenesis.

The expression of *wt1* is detectable in a majority of cases of malignant mesotheliomas (Amin *et al.*, 1995) but this may be variable (Langerak *et al.*, 1995). Although the wt1 protein is known to act as transcriptional repressor of IGF-II and PDGF-A, Langerak *et al.* (1995) found no inverse relationship between *wt1* expression and the levels of *IFG-II* and *PDGF-A* gene transcripts, nor was cellular morphology related to *wt1* expression.

The expression of *wt1* in acute myelocytic leukaemia (AML) has been studied by Brieger *et al.* (1994) who reported that *wt1* expression is detectable in 41 out of 52 untreated AML patients. In contrast, a majority of patients in complete remission had lost all *wt1* expression and, interestingly, in three out of four cases where there was recurrence, expression of the gene was detected before relapse. According to Menssen *et al.* (1995) the wt1 protein can be found only on the nuclei of leukaemia blast cells but not in normal CD34+ progenitors, and blast cells from 12 out of 20 leukaemia patients showed *wt1* expression, together with strong immunofluorescence for wt1 protein. Thus, *wt1* expression could serve as a marker for malignant blast cells.

12

Tumour suppressor genes

The basic concept that neoplastic transformation of cells and their progression to the metastatic state may be a result of the abrogation of control mechanisms of cell proliferation, intercellular adhesive and invasive behaviour of normal cells has been in vogue for over two decades. The idea of suppression of malignancy was articulated by Harris *et al.* (1969) and Knudson (1971). Harris *et al.* (1969) demonstrated that fusion of tumour cells with normal cells resulted in suppression of tumorigenicity. Some hybridomas appeared to regain tumorigenic potential and this reacquisition was related to chromosomal loss. Sidebottom and Clark (1983) then found that metastatic ability could be similarly suppressed by cell fusion. Knudson (1971) provided further evidence for the occurrence of a suppressor gene from epidemiological studies on retinoblastomas. This subsequently led to the identification and cloning of the retinoblastoma susceptibility gene (*rb*) (Friend *et al.*, 1987) and to the development of the concept of tumour growth inhibition by the rb gene product and that the lifting of this control by deletion or mutation of both gene copies results in the development of tumours. The characterisation of tumour suppressor genes is based on the identification of genetic deletions or alterations of specific chromosome loci associated with tumour incidence or with a predisposition to tumour development. The presence of a putative suppressor gene is revealed by one of three ways: the loss of function of the gene accruing from a mutation in one of the alleles and the loss of the second allele by deletion of the relevant region of the chromosome; the occurrence of mutations in both alleles; or by homologous deletion of both alleles. The subsequent discovery that *p53* and *rb* function as tumour suppressor genes and that their inactivation causes profound deregulation of cell proliferation, which often leads to tumorigenesis, has inevitably led the search for metastasis suppressor genes.

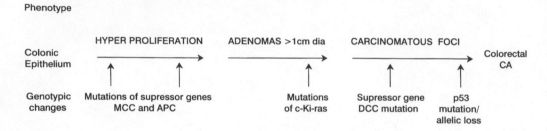

Figure 18. Genetic changes associated with the development and progression of colon cancer. Based on Bos *et al*. (1987), Forrester *et al*. (1987), Baker *et al*. (1989), Nigro *et al*. (1989), Fearon *et al*. (1990), Fearon and Vogelstein (1990), Remvikos *et al*. (1990), Kinzler *et al*. (1991a,b), Nishisho *et al*. (1991), Shirasawa *et al*. (1991), and other references cited in the text.

Progression of colorectal neoplasia

The pathogenesis of colorectal cancer has provided a most suitable model for analysis of the genetic events occurring in colonic epithelium leading to a hyperproliferative state and formation of adenomas, with their further growth and progression leading to the formation of overt colorectal carcinomas. These events are summarised in Figure 18. It can be seen that specific genetic changes may be associated with particular tumour phenotypes. There is an initial phase of hyperproliferation of the colonic epithelium which leads to the formation of adenomas, and this is associated with mutations of the suppressor genes *APC* (adenomatous polyposis coli) and *MCC* (mutated in colonic cancer). This is followed by a growth period characterised by mutations in the c-Ki-*ras* gene and subsequent progression into the development of carcinomatous foci. This phenotypic change is associated with mutations in *DCC* (deleted in colon carcinoma), and mutations of the suppressor gene *p53* occur as late events, culminating in the formation of overt colorectal carcinoma. Thus the process of neoplastic progression from normal mucosa to the development of benign polyps progressing further to frank carcinomas not only involve several genetic events but the appearance of the carcinoma is a cumulative effect of these genetic changes.

The car *gene in colon cancer*

Pullman and Bodmer (1992) have cloned a gene (*car*) which appears to be able to regulate cell adhesion. The *car* gene was cloned from cells from a colon cancer cell line selected for their ability to adhere to collagen. They reported that cells with reduced ability to bind to extracellular matrix regain the ability when transfected with *car*. This gene is located on chromosome 16q. Pullman and Bodmer (1992) have argued that since there is a high incidence of allelic loss on 16q in the *car* region in breast and prostatic cancers *car* might function as a candidate tumour suppressor gene.

APC *and* MCC *genes in colonic tumours*

In familial adenomatous polyposis (FAP) the patients develop numerous benign adenomatous polyps which, if left untreated, progress into carcinomas. The *APC* gene, which is located on chromosome 5q21 (Bodmer *et al.*, 1987), has been identified as causing FAP. The *APC* gene and the *MCC* gene, also present at the same locus, are both believed to act as suppressor genes (Kinzler *et al.*, 1991a,b). Mutations of the *APC* gene, leading to a loss of its suppressor function, have been implicated in FAP (Groden *et al.*, 1991; Joslyn *et al.*, 1991; Kinzler *et al.*, 1991a; Nishisho *et al.*, 1991). Both germ-line (>150) and somatic (>300) mutations have been reported in colorectal adenomas and carcinomas from FAP and non-FAP patients (Miyaki *et al.*, 1995). The suppressor function has been confirmed by transfecting a full-length normal *APC* gene into colon cancer cell lines. Some of the clones carrying the exogenous normal gene have been found to exhibit altered cell morphology and suppression of tumorigenicity when implanted in nude mice (Groden *et al.*, 1995). The association of *APC* mutations with the progression of adenomas is supported by the finding that their detection increases with the size of the adenomas. Mutation frequency also tends to be higher in tubulovillous and villous adenomas, which are prone to frequent malignant transformation, than in tubular adenomas which only infrequently undergo malignant changes (De Benedetti *et al.*, 1994).

The mechanisms by which APC protein functions and suppresses the neoplastic process are currently being investigated with much fervour. The mutations of *APC* are predominantly truncating mutations and it has been suggested that the mutated protein can associate with the wild-type APC protein, but this is not supported by the work of Oshima *et al.* (1995). Alternatively, APC protein may associate with cellular proteins, which might affect their function. Su *et al.* (1995) showed that proteins encoded by a novel gene called *EB1* interacted with the APC protein, both *in vitro* and *in vivo*. The truncated APC protein may be unable to function appropriately. For instance, it is associated with cytoplasmic microtubules and the *C*-terminal region, which is frequently deleted in cancer, is required for the interaction of the APC peptide with microtubules, and the protein may be an essential component in the assembly of microtubules (Munemitsu *et al.*, 1994). APC protein has been found to co-localise with α-catenin in intestinal epithelium, especially along the lateral cytoplasmic membrane (Miyashiro *et al.*, 1995). The association with catenins, which in turn are linked to actin cytoskeletal elements, implicate APC proteins in cellular adhesion. It should be remembered, however, that α-catenin gene also occurs on chromosome 5 and therefore a co-expression with APC protein might be expected. The introduction of chromosome 5 into PC3 prostate cancer cells results in the re-expression of α-catenin in these cells and can suppress their tumorigenicity. However, this can occur only if the cells are able to express E-cadherin at the same time (Ewing *et al.*, 1995) (Figure 13).

β-catenin is another E-cadherin-associated protein and the gene has been assigned to chromosome 3p22 (Trent *et al.*, 1995). The 3p22 region is also frequently affected in human neoplasia. Therefore, one would expect to see some relationship between APC and E-cadherin expression, both of which appear to function as suppressors of malignancy (see page 104). Both E-cadherin and the APC protein compete for binding to β-catenin and the *N*-terminal domain of β-catenin mediates the binding of its complexes with E-cadherin or the APC protein, to the cytoskeleton (Hulsken *et al.*, 1994). Furthermore, wild-type APC protein appears to reduce β-catenin levels by promoting its degradation. The mutant APC protein lacks this ability to regulate β-catenin levels and this has been attributed to the loss of the central region of the APC protein (Munemitsu *et al.*, 1995). This is liable to alter the adhesive and cohesive properties of epithelial cells, and these may indeed be reflected as changes in biological behaviour.

APC isoforms

The *APC* gene has 15 exons. In addition to the transcript which encodes these, several mRNA isoforms have been detected and these are produced by alternative splicing of coding as well as non-coding regions (Horii *et al.*, 1993; Oshima *et al.*, 1993; Sulekova *et al.*, 1995; Xia *et al.*, 1995). These isoforms have been found to be differentially expressed and often in a tissue-specific manner. This has led to the suggestion that the splicing mechanisms themselves might be tissue-specific (Horii *et al.*, 1993). The multiple isoforms may be transcribed into APC proteins differing in biological properties. For instance, the APC isoform transcribed from cDNA lacking exon 1 does not contain the heptad-repeat which is required for the formation of protein homodimers (Thliveris *et al.*, 1994). The manifestation of atypical FAP phenotypes, reduction in APC severity, and the variability in the onset of disease, etc., may also be an attribute of the incidence of different APC isoforms (Samowitz *et al.*, 1995; van der Luijt *et al.*, 1995).

APC/MCC gene abnormalities in other human neoplasms

Although studies of colonic tumour progression have highlighted the role of the *APC* gene, it has been also implicated in the pathogenesis of other human tumour types. Mutations of *APC* has been detected in six out of 30 gastric adenomas, together with the deletion of the second allele in three tumours leading to a complete inactivation of the gene (Tamura *et al.*, 1994). In primary breast carcinoma, loss of heterozygosity (LOH) has been reported to affect *APC* exons 11 (nine out of 35 cases) and 15 (four out of 34 cases) and *MCC* exon 10 in seven out of 40 samples (Medeiros *et al.*, 1994), but the frequency of *APC* mutations might be low (Kashiwaba *et al.*, 1994). LOH has been found in 25% of oral squamous cell carcinomas (Largey *et al.*, 1994). LOH involving markers near the gene at 5q21 was found in 10 out of a group of 20 epithelial ovarian cancers (Weitzel *et al.*, 1994). A similar frequency of LOH, but not mutations of the *APC* gene, has been described in another study (Hayashi *et al.*, 1995). A high frequency (29%) of LOH at the *APC/MCC* locus was found in non-small cell lung cancer. In this study, LOH at 5q21 correlated significantly with poor patient survival, and in a most frequently affected tumour subtype LOH was also associated with tumour spread to mediastinal and/or hilar lymph nodes (Fong *et al.*, 1995b).

In contrast to the above, neither LOH at 5q21 nor mutations of *APC* in breast carcinomas showed any relationship to any clinical or pathological features (Kashiwaba *et al.*, 1994). *APC* appears to be unaffected in oesophageal and papillary thyroid carcinomas (Curtis *et al.*, 1994; Ogasawara *et al.*, 1994). In oesophageal cancers, truncating mutations have been discovered in the *APC* mutation cluster region (Powell *et al.*, 1994), namely codons 1286-1513. However, in view of the low frequency at which these occurred and the high rate of LOH reported at 5q, Powell *et al.* (1994) have suggested that other genes may be involved in allelic deletions and the pathogenesis of these tumours.

It is not known if *MCC* mutations occur in sporadic colorectal cancers; nor is it clear if *MCC* mutations are associated with FAP condition. Although LOH of *APC* and *MCC* may both be involved with the early stages of carcinogensis, they might follow different pathways in influencing the cell phenotype. There is a suggestion of this in the observation by Hsieh and Huang (1995) who found that loss of heterozygosity for *APC* occurred in three out of 15 differentiated gastric carcinomas, but none occurred in undifferentiated tumours. In contrast, LOH for *MCC* was found in undifferentiated but not in differentiated neoplasms.

The DCC *gene in colon cancer*

The suppressor gene *DCC* is involved in the late stages of the pathogenesis of colorectal neoplasia. It has been been mapped to a region on chromosome 18q21.3 that is frequently deleted (Fearon *et al.*, 1990; Fearon and Vogelstein, 1990). The *DCC* is a large complex gene containing 29 exons and encompassing 1.4 Mb (Cho KR *et al.*, 1994). It is highly expressed in normal colonic mucosa and many other tissues, including the brain and neural crest-derived cellular elements, but its expression is greatly reduced in colonic carcinomas. Presence of the DCC protein has been demonstrated immunohistochemically in normal colonic epithelium and in reticuloendothelial cells from human thymus, tonsil and lymph nodes (Turley *et al.*, 1995). A homologue of the *DCC* gene, called *XDCCα*, has been isolated from *Xenopus*, and the protein product of this gene appears to be developmentally regulated. Its expression is detectable at developmental stages 19-46 and is localised to the developing brain (Pierceall *et al.*, 1994b).

The suppressor function of *DCC* is restored when the gene is re-introduced or additional copies of chromosome 18 are introduced into tumour cells. Klingelhutz *et al.* (1995) transfected a full-length cDNA clone of *DCC* into HPV-transformed human epithelial cells and obtained suppression of tumorigenicity. Similarly, the introduction of chromosome 18 into endometrial carcinoma cell lines has resulted in a reduction of their tumorigenicity in nude mice together with an increase in gene expression (Yamada *et al.*, 1995b).

As stated previously, the development of frank carcinomatous foci in villous adenomas is characterised by allelic loss of the *DCC* gene, rather than the growth of the adenomas (Froggatt *et al.*, 1995) and, not surprisingly, much attention has been focused upon whether *DCC* abnormalities correlate with metastatic potential. LOH on chromosomes 17p, 18q (containing the *DCC* locus) and 22q, but not 5q (containing the *APC/MCC* locus), have been reported to occur far more frequently in advanced colorectal carcinomas than in intramucosal carcinomas. LOH on 17p (the *p53* gene occurs at 17p13.1) correlated with vascular invasion, but 18q LOH was related to lymphatic spread and incidence of hepatic metastases. Thus loss of *DCC* expression was found in five samples of metastatic tumour and five out of seven advanced primary carcinomas which had metastasised to the liver. In contrast, only five out of 15 carcinomas which showed no hepatic involvement exhibited a loss of *DCC* expression (Iino *et al.*, 1994). This indeed shows a strong relationship between loss of *DCC* in the primary cancers and their potential to metastasise. The potential role of this gene in conferring metastatic ability on the tumours is further confirmed by the observation that LOH on chromosome 5q (which contains the *APC* gene) did not correlate with the ability of the tumours to invade and metastasise (Iino *et al.*, 1994). Compatible with this view, DCC protein is found in differentiated cells of the intestinal epithelium, but it is lost in colorectal tumours that do not differentiate into mucus-producing cells (Hendrick *et al.*, 1994).

Mutations of *DCC* are not restricted to colonic neoplasia. Allelic losses on chromosome 18 and *DCC* mutations have been reported in several other human cancers. The aberrations affecting the *DCC* gene have been studied in gynaecological cancers. Deletions of the chromosomal region including the *DCC* locus have been reported in 26% of endometrial cancers, and loss of *DCC* expression has been seen in tumour samples and also in tumour-derived cell lines (Gima *et al.*, 1994; Enomoto *et al.*, 1995). The gene is expressed in normal endometrium, cervical epithelium and normal ovarian tissue, but expression is markedly reduced in the corresponding cancers. Furthermore, the expression of the gene may be down-regulated more markedly in advanced ovarian cancers than in early stages (Enomoto *et al.*, 1995). LOH at the *DCC* locus is not only very frequent in breast cancer, but appears to occur in invasive disease (Kashiwaba *et al.*, 1995). The involvement of *DCC* aberrations in breast cancer has been confirmed in another study, but LOH on another locus close to the *DCC* locus also takes place, suggesting the presence of more than one suppressor gene in this region of the chromosome (Huang *et al.*, 1995). Association of LOH with invasive behaviour has been encountered in bladder carcinoma (Brewster *et al.*, 1994b). Allelic loss of the gene in oesophageal cancers tends to occur in poorly differentiated tumours and shows a marked association with distant spread of the tumours (Miyake *et al.*, 1994), although Shibagaki *et al.* (1994) have found no *DCC* involvement in their series of oesophageal carcinomas. Allelic deletions occur at a high frequency in germ cell tumours. The expression of *DCC* is detected in normal testes, but it is reduced in germ cell tumour cell lines and tumour tissues (Murty *et al.*, 1994). LOH is found in non-small cell lung cancers but this does not appear to be related to the stage of the disease (Fong *et al.*, 1995b).

The *DCC* is now known to be altered in non-Hodgkin's lymphoma (Younes *et al.*, 1995), tumours of the head and neck (Rowley *et al.*, 1995), and gastric tumours (Barletta *et al.*, 1993) but none have been reported to date in some others, such as pancreatic tumours (Barton *et al.*, 1995).

The DCC protein is a cell adhesion molecule

The *DCC* gene encompasses approximately 1.4 Mb of DNA and contains 29 exons (Cho KR *et al.*, 1994). It encodes a transmembrane glycoprotein of the immunoglobulin family containing 1447 amino acid residues which shows significant homology to the neural cell adhesion molecule (N-CAM) (Fearon *et al.*, 1990; Hedrick *et al.*, 1994; Reale *et al.*, 1994; Cho and Fearon, 1995) (see also page 118). The extracellular domain which has approximately 1100 residues has four immunoglobulin-like domains and six fibronectin type III-like domains. Alternative splicing of *DCC* transcripts has been detected and protein species 175–190 kDa are transcribed (Reale *et al.*, 1994). The DCC protein also appears to share with N-CAMs the ability to stimulate neurite outgrowths in non-neuronal cells. The cytoplasmic domain of the protein is essential for stimulating neurite extension (Pierceall *et al.*, 1994a). The DCC glycoprotein is abundant in brain tissue and neural crest-derived cells and not infrequently found in low levels in other normal tissues (Reale *et al.*, 1994). Hedrick *et al.* (1994) demonstrated its presence in the axons of the central and peripheral nervous system. Pierceall *et al.* (1994b) isolated a homologue of the human *DCC* gene, called *XDCCα*, from *Xenopus*. The gene encodes a protein which has 1427 amino acid residues and bears >80% sequence homology with the human protein. As in the human protein, XDCCα also contains four immunoglobulin-like domains and six fibronectin type III-like domains in the extracellular domain and has 325 amino acid residues in the cytoplasmic region of the protein.

BRCA1 tumour suppressor (breast and ovarian carcinoma susceptibility) gene

A putative tumour suppressor gene called *BRCA1* has been identified and mapped to chromosome 17q21. This gene has been found to confer susceptibility to breast and ovarian cancer, since it has been associated with more than 45% of inherited breast cancers without ovarian cancer and 80% of families with breast and ovarian cancers (Easton *et al.*, 1993). Germline mutations of this gene appear to link the gene with this state of predisposition to cancer development (Miki *et al.*, 1994; Szabo and King, 1995). To date, 63 germline mutations have been detected and these are distributed across the entire coding region of the gene (Xu and Solomon, 1996). The *BRCA1* gene has been recognised as a classical suppressor gene, in the light of the data on the loss of its heterozygosity in familial cancers. This suggests the possibility that somatic mutations may also occur in breast and ovarian tumours. Somatic mutations have in fact been reported in about 10% of sporadic ovarian tumours (Merajver *et al.*, 1995) but, in general, somatic mutations of *BRCA1* have not been regarded as a critical event for the development of breast and ovarian cancer in the absence of germline mutations (Futreal *et al.*, 1994). Sporadic breast cancers do not carry *BRCA1* mutations (Friedman *et al.*, 1994; Miki *et al.*, 1994; Hosking *et al.*, 1995: Shattuck-Eidens *et al.*, 1995).

It should be unnecessary to emphasise that there may be other suppressor genes at chromosome 17q21 that might be potential participants in the neoplastic process; *BRCA1* spans 100 kb of genomic DNA (see Xu and Solomon, 1996) of the 17q21 region. Friedman *et al.* (1995) have cloned 22 genes – some novel genes and others already identified or homologues of known genes – from a 650 kb section of 17q21. They have also identified several mutations of these genes in tumours or *BRCA1*-linked families, but undetectable in controls. It has been possible to confer tumorigenicity and the capacity for anchorage-independent growth on breast cancer cells by transferring into these cells chromosome 17 not containing the *BRCA1* region (Theile *et al.*, 1995). Gao *et al.* (1995b) investigated the loss of heterozygosity at five microsatellite loci encompassing the *BRCA1* region in prostate cancer. They found 45% and 40% LOH at the D17S855 *BRCA1* intragenic locus and at D17S856, respectively, but far fewer cases were LOH-positive for other loci, suggesting that *BRCA1* and genes occurring between these two microsatellite loci might be involved in the pathogenic process. Tangir *et al.* (1996) reported a deletion at a locus approximately 60 kb centromeric to *BRCA1* gene in epithelial ovarian cancer, again suggesting that suppressors other than *BRCA1* may be involved.

The characteristics and intracellular distribution of BRCA1 protein

The *BRCA1* codes for a protein containing 1863 amino acid residues with two zinc-finger domains at the *N*-terminal region and an acidic *C*-terminal domain, suggesting that it may function as a transcription factor (Miki *et al.*, 1994; Vogelstein and Kinzler, 1994). A 220 kDa nuclear phosphoprotein considered to be a putative BRCA1 protein has been detected in normal cells and in cell lines derived from a variety of human tumours, including breast and ovarian tumours (Chen YM *et al.*, 1995). The BRCA1 protein is localised mainly in the nucleus of rodent cells and human breast cancer cells (Rao *et al.*, 1996) but it has been detected also in the cytoplasm in breast cancer biopsies. Occasionally, in some tumour cell lines, the protein has been found in both nucleus and the cytoplasm, or subpopulations have been identified that have the protein at either nuclear or cytoplasmic site (Chen YM *et al.*, 1995). However, the protein expressed in cells stably transfected with *BRCA1* gene has been found to be a 190 kDa protein (Holt *et al.*, 1996). Furthermore, using antibodies raised against the BRCA1 protein, Jensen *et al.* (1996) have demonstrated that BRCA1 is indeed a 190 kDa protein.

From the search for functional homologues for the BRCA1 protein, it has emerged that BRCA1 protein bears many similarities to proteins of the granin family. Granins are calcium-binding acidic proteins found in the trans-Golgi network and secretory granules. Their secretion results from the activation of cyclic AMP and they are regulated by oestrogen (Gorr *et al.*, 1989; Huttner *et al.*, 1991; Thompson *et al.*, 1992). Recently, Jensen *et al.* (1996) reported the existence of a perfect granin consensus sequence from amino acids 1214–1223 of the BRCA1 protein. The MDA-MB-468 cells show unusually high levels of the 190 kDa BRCA1 protein. This is found predominantly associated with membranes, with smaller amounts in the nucleus and the cytoplasm. Jensen *et al.* (1996) showed that the protein is secreted into the conditioned medium in which these cells are grown. BRCA1 also appears to be hormonally regulated (Gudas *et al.*, 1995b; see below). However, granins are said to be involved in the packaging and processing of peptide hormones (Huttner *et al.*, 1991). Although the function of granins themselves is still to be established, it is uncertain whether the BRCA1 suppressor protein is functionally homologous to granins. It is interesting to note that the BRCA2 protein also possesses the granin consensus motif (Jensen *et al.*, 1996).

The germline mutations invariably result in the production of a truncated BRCA1 protein (Szabo and King, 1995) that may be functionally impaired. Several BRCA1 peptides of different molecular sizes may be expressed in varying levels in normal and in tumour cells (Gudas *et al.*, 1996; Rao *et al.*, 1996). Two distinct mRNA transcripts of *BRCA1* occur in normal and in immortalised human mammary epithelial cells (Gudas *et al.*, 1996). Xu *et al.* (1995) had previously identified a new 5′ exon and reported the occurrence of two mRNA transcripts differing in respect of this new first exon. The significance and function of these *BRCA1* transcripts and their relationship to the several forms of BRCA1 proteins detected are yet to be elucidated.

The biological properties of the BRCA1 protein

Although the full identity and function of the BRCA1 protein is yet to be established, there are indications that it may function as a negative regulator of tumour cell proliferation and growth and alterations in its expression may accompany tumour progression. Thompson *et al.* (1995) demonstrated that inhibition of expression of *BRCA1* using antisense oligonucleotides resulted in the acceleration of proliferation of normal and also malignant epithelial cells. Similarly, the inhibition of the expression of endogenous BRCA1 protein in NIH3T3 cells transfected with antisense *BRCA1* RNA, not only accelerated growth of the transfected cells, but the cells also showed anchorage-independent growth and enhanced tumorigenic ability (Rao *et al.*, 1996).

Further experimental evidence has been provided by Holt *et al.* (1996) in respect of the growth inhibitory role of the BRCA1 protein. They transfected the wild-type *BRCA1* gene into breast and ovarian cancer cells and found that it inhibited the *in vitro* growth of both breast and ovarian cancer cells, but not that of lung or colon cancer cells. Transfection of mutant *BRCA1* did not inhibit growth of breast cancer cells. The growth of ovarian cells was not affected by *BRCA1* with mutation in the 5'-region, but was inhibited by mutations in the 3'-region. The wild-type, but not the mutant, gene inhibited tumour formation by MCF-7 human breast cancer cells in nude mice. Finally, Holt *et al.* (1996) also obtained inhibition of growth of established MCF-7 tumours in nude mice, upon intraperitoneal treatment of the animals with viral vectors carrying the wild-type *BRCA1* gene. Thus, there is adequate evidence to support the view that the BRCA1 protein functions as a suppressor of proliferation and tumour growth.

The BRCA1 *gene in embryonic development*

The *BRCA1* gene appears to play a significant part in embryonic development and differentiation. Studies using *BRCA1* knock-out mice have demonstrated that interference with the normal expression of the gene produces marked developmental abnormalites. Boyd *et al.* (1995) showed that *BRCA1* (+/−) mice do not show tumours, but embryos of *BRCA1* (−/−) mice die before birth and develop conspicuous neural tube defects. Hakem *et al.* (1996) have confirmed that *BRCA1* (+/−) embryos develop normally, but noted that *BRCA1* (−/−) mouse embryos die early in embryogenesis prior to gastrulation, apparently due to a total failure of mesoderm formation. In embryonic development, the primary mesoderm is formed during the gastrula stage by the invagination of epiblast cells through the primitive groove and the newly formed mesoderm interacts with and induces the differentiation of neural tissue from the presumptive neural ectoderm (see page 158). Therefore, any abnormalities in the formation of the mesoderm would inevitably lead to interference with the process of induction of neural tissue differentiation and consequently to neural tube defects.

The expression of the mouse homologue of the BRCA1 protein has been described by Lane *et al.* (1995). A definite pattern of expression has been found in relation to the terminal differentiation of tissues of ectodermal and mesodermal lineage. The gene is expressed in differentiating epithelial cells of several organs. The alveolar and ductal epithelial cells of the mammary gland show *BRCA1* expression and during pregnancy there is an increase in the level of gene transcripts, suggesting that gene expression may be related to functional differentiation (Lane *et al.*, 1995). The work of Marquis *et al.* (1995) also strongly suggests a role for *BRCA1* in cell differentiation. They found high expression in proliferating cell types undergoing differentiation in response to ovarian hormones. Indeed, the levels of both *BRCA1* transcripts and the protein are regulated by oestrogen and progesterone in human breast cancer cells. Both show reduction in levels upon withdrawal of oestrogen from cell cultures of MCF-7 and Bt20T cells. The expression of *BRCA1* is restored by β-oestradiol and this is accompanied by the expression of markers indicating the transition of cells into the S-phase (Gudas *et al.*, 1995b). The expression of the *BRCA1* mRNA may be cell cycle-related: in synchronised human breast epithelial cells, *BRCA1* mRNA expression has been found to be high in the exponential growth phase, but it decreases upon withdrawal of growth factors. The level of expression increases in the late G_1 phase prior to entry of the cell into the S-phase of the cell cycle (Gudas *et al.*, 1996). Conceivably, the hormones switch the cells from proliferation to the differentiation pathway and the *BRCA1* gene may be implicated as a regulatory factor in this process.

BRCA1 *mutations and tumour progression*

Since germline mutations result in the production of truncated BRCA1 proteins one should contemplate the possibility that this could lead to deregulation of cell proliferation and thus be reflected in cellular features that form a part of the pathological assessment of tumours. *BRCA1*-related hereditary breast cancers tend to be aneuploid and show higher rates of proliferation (Eisinger *et al.*, 1996; Marcus *et al.*, 1996) and germline mutations of the gene may be reflected in tumour grade (Eisinger *et al.*, 1996) indicating an aggressive phenotype. This is also suggested by the observation that the transition of breast tumour *in situ* to invasive stage is accompanied by a decrease in *BRCA1* expression (Thompson *et al.*, 1995). Furthermore, loss of heterozygosity at the *BRCA1* and *BRCA2* loci are far more frequent in liver and brain metastases than in the corresponding primary breast cancers (Hampl *et al.*, 1996). There is therefore a reasonable body of evidence implicating *BRCA1* in tumour growth, invasion and progression to the metastatic state.

DPC/BRCA2 tumour suppressor genes

Pancreatic carcinomas have shown a consistent loss of heterozygosity at chromosome 13q12 often described as the DPC (deleted in pancreatic carcinoma). The DPC region at 13q12.3 encompasses approximately 250 kb. The DPC region lies within the 6-cM region that contains the *BRCA2* breast cancer susceptibility gene, representing the loss of two loci. Two *DPC* genes, *DPC1* and *DPC2*, have been mapped to this region (Schutte *et al.*, 1995a,b). This has placed in perspective the LOH described in approximately one-quarter of pancreatic cancers (Hahn *et al.*, 1995) and the comparable levels of LOH occurring in breast cancer (Sato *et al.*, 1990; Devilee *et al.*, 1991b; Thorlacius *et al.*, 1991). The *DPC* genes and *BRCA2* have been considered as the prime targets of deletion in these cancers and regarded as tumour suppressor genes.

Another locus which is subject to consistent and high level of allelic loss is chromosome 18q (Hahn *et al.*, 1995). Approximately one-third of pancreatic cancers show homozygous deletion at 18q21.1. The target of this deletion has been identified as *DPC4* (Hahn *et al.*, 1996a,b). The *p16/ink4* located at chromosome 9q21 (Kamb *et al.*, 1994) (see page 66) is also frequently deleted in pancreatic cancer (Caldas *et al.*, 1994) and this gene has been called, albeit somewhat unhelpfully, *DPC3*. In a series of 36 pancreatic carcinomas, the frequencies of homozygous deletion of *p16/ink4* and *DPC4* were 42% and 39%, respectively (Caldas *et al.*, 1994; Hahn *et al.*, 1996a) and the frequency of deletions found at one or more of *DPC1,2/BRCA2*, *p16/ink4* and *DPC4* loci was 64% (23 out of 36) (Hahn *et al.*, 1996b). The relatively high frequency of inactivation of *DPC4* in pancreatic cancers (48%) compared with breast and ovarian cancers, at only 10% reported by Schutte *et al.* (1996), advocates a possible close association of *DPC4* inactivation with the pathogenesis of pancreatic carcinomas rather than with other forms of human cancer, although, admittedly, it would be premature even to speculate on this aspect.

A functional role for *DPC4* has been deduced on the basis of its sequence similarities to the *Drosophila melanogaster* gene *mad* and the *Caenorhabditis elegans* genes *sma* homologues of the *mad* gene (Hahn *et al.*, 1996a). The *mad* gene codes for a TGF-β-like protein. It is possible that, in analogy to the function of TGF-β as an inhibitor of cell proliferation (see page 64), the DPC4 protein may function as a negative regulator of cell proliferation.

13

Metastasis suppressor genes

The development of metastases is an aftermath of the interplay and cumulative function of a number of changes in the spectrum of biological properties of the cell and for this reason invasive and metastatic behaviour of tumours may be regulated by more than one gene. Nevertheless, the search for a candidate metastasis gene has made unrelenting progress in the past few years.

There are several investigations of note in this area. Subtraction hybridisation has allowed Dear *et al.* (1988, 1989) to identify two genes, the *WDNM1* and *WDNM2* in rat mammary adenocarcinoma DMBA 8 cell lines. These genes have been reported to be expressed at levels 20-fold higher in non-malignant tumours compared with their malignant counterparts. Initial Northern analyses have led to the identification of two *WDNM1* transcripts (Dear *et al.*, 1988) generated by alternative splicing of a single exon (Dear and Kefford, 1991). The predicted amino acid sequence of the spliced version shows strong homology with a family of proteins that includes inhibitors of human antileukoprotease (Seemuller *et al.*, 1986) and red sea turtle proteinase inhibitor (Kato and Tominaga, 1979). The secretory leukoprotease inhibitor (CLPI) is a 12 kDa protein (Abe *et al.*, 1991) which can inhibit the degradation of ECM proteins, e.g. by neutrophil elastase (Llewellyn-Jones *et al.*, 1994). Therefore, one could envisage that the WDNM1 protein, by analogy with its putative homologue, might function as a metastasis suppressor protein by preventing ECM degradation caused by tumour-associated proteinases. On the negative side, it should be recognised that despite the apparent tissue-specific expression of the CLPI gene, it is also expressed in several forms of human cancer (Garver *et al.*, 1994). This would be incongruous with a putative tumour suppressor function for the

WDNM1 protein. Glucocorticoids have been shown to up-regulate the transcription of the CLPI gene (Abbinantenissen *et al.*, 1995), and this could provide a means to test whether the leukoprotease inhibitor affects metastatic ability in experimental systems and, further, to test if *WDNM1* expression can be modulated by glucocorticoids. The second gene, *WDNM2*, identified and found to be down-regulated in metastasizing tumours has been reported to code for an enzyme involved with the reduction of quinones and redox dyes in the cell (Dear *et al.*, 1989).

Another report has recently appeared which indicates the occurrence of a putative suppressor gene on chromosome 11. This demonstration was by means of introduction of human chromosome 11 into a highly metastatic rat prostate cancer cell line. The introduction of this chromosome appeared to suppress the metastatic ability of these cells without affecting *in vivo* growth or tumorigenicity of the cells (Ichikawa *et al.*, 1992). It may be recalled that chromosome 11 contains genes such as the Wilms' tumour gene *wt1* and WAGR-associated genes, cyclin D1 and the cyclin-dependent kinase inhibitor *kip1* gene, as well as a host of fibroblast growth factor family of genes. However, Ichikawa *et al.* (1992) have further demonstrated that the metastasis suppressor ability resides with chromosome region 11 p 11.2–13, excluding the Wilms' tumour locus in the suppression of metastasis.

The putative metastasis suppressor function of the *nm23* gene

nm23 *gene expression in metastasis*

A putative metastasis suppressor gene (*nm23*) has also been described in murine melanoma (Steeg *et al.*, 1988a,b, 1990), reportedly expressed at low levels in the highly metastatic K-1735 melanoma compared with corresponding cell lines with low metastatic ability. Subsequently, two human homologues of the murine *nm23* gene – *nm23*-H1 (Rosengard *et al.*, 1989) and *nm23*-H2 (Stahl *et al.*, 1991) – have been cloned. These are located on chromosome 17q21.3. There are several studies in the literature which suggest a high expression of *nm23* gene or its product the NDP (nucleoside diphosphate) kinase is consistent with low metastatic potential. There are, however, an equal number of studies which do not bear out the inverse relationship between *nm23* and metastatic potential of cancers.

After the initial reports of the metastasis suppressor property of the *nm23* gene, much work has been focused upon its expression in human tumours. The interest in its potential use in the clinical context has been of such magnitude that except for the study by Steeg *et al.* (1988a,b) there has been only one report using an animal tumour model (Caligo *et al.*, 1992). This latter study confirmed the inverse relationship originally reported by Steeg *et al.* (1988a,b). Recently, there have been several studies on a variety of human tumour types. In a short series of human breast tumours, high levels of *nm23* expression were found in tumours where there was no metastatic involvement of the lymph nodes (Bevilacqua G *et al.*, 1989). Hennessy *et al.* (1991) studied a larger series of 145 tumours and have confirmed the inverse relationship between *nm23* expression and lymph node involvement. Low *nm23* expression was associated with poor differentiation and the absence of oestrogen receptors (ER). In a much smaller series of breast cancers, Albertazzi *et al.* (1996) have been unable to confirm this direct relationship between *nm23*-H1 expression and oestrogen receptor status. The metastasis suppressor effect of *nm23* expression was not clear-cut; they found that 10 out of 18 patients with *nm23*-positive tumours had nodal metastasis, and seven patients out of nine with *nm23*-negative showed nodal involvement. They reported, further, that *nm23*-positive tumours segregated into roughly equal ER-positive and ER-negative groups, but *nm23*-negative tumours tended to be more ER-negative than ER-positive. Ura *et al.* (1996) reported reduced *nm23* expression in gastric cancers with lymph node or hepatic metastases compared with primary tumours without metastases. A recent report by Florenes *et al.* (1992) has shown that in patients with melanoma developing metastases in the first two years after diagnosis, lower *nm23* messenger RNA levels were detected compared with patients with less aggressive tumours. Caligo *et al.* (1994) have reported that levels of *nm23* transcripts were higher in tumours of patients who showed disease-free survival of more than 24 months compared with tumours from patients with less than 24 months disease-free survival; but these authors also found lower *nm23* transcript levels in benign naevi than in melanomas.

The metastasis suppressor function of the gene has also been studied using experimental systems. Transfection of the *nm23* gene into the highly metastatic cell line K-1735 appears to reduce both tumorigenicity and metastasis (Leone *et al.*, 1991b). In high *nm23*-expressing transfectant clones, a 90-96% reduction in pulmonary metastasis has been reported by these authors. In another experimental model, *nm23* has apparently not displayed any metastasis suppressor ability. Thompson *et al.* (1993) investigated two cell lines, MIII and MCF7/LCC1 which were isolated from the human breast cancer cell line MCF-7. These cell lines possessed markedly enhanced metastatic ability in nude mice, but showed no loss of *nm23* expression.

Although in some tumour types and under certain experimental conditions *nm23* has behaved like a metastasis suppressor gene, in others the expected inverse relationship between gene expression and malignancy has not been observed. For example, *nm23* is expressed in all thyroid tissues, such as multinodular goitres, adenoma and carcinomas and the levels of expression were comparable in these. Indeed, in advanced (stage IV and anaplastic) carcinomas the expression was twofold greater as compared with stage I-III tumours and multinodular goitres (Zhou *et al.*, 1993). In neuroblastomas high levels of *nm23* expression were associated with advanced stages of the disease (Hailat *et al.*, 1991). Keim *et al.* (1992) found significantly higher levels of the nm23 protein in advanced (stages III-IV) neuroblastomas compared with early stage (I-II) disease. Haut *et al.* (1991) reported that *nm23* expression increased in the early stage of the development of colon cancers and remained at a high level in metastatic disease, but recent work has shown an association between allelic deletions of *nm23*-H1 with progression of colorectal carcinoma (Cohn *et al.*, 1991). In a study by Ayhan *et al.* (1993) colorectal carcinomas over-expressed the *nm23* gene compared with non-neoplastic tissue. Increased *nm23*-H1 (in 33 out of 41) and *nm23*-H2 (in 28 out of 41) expression has been reported by Myeroff and Markowitz (1993) in the absence of mutations in colonic cancers. However, there are several reports that *nm23* expression is down-regulated in metastatic tumours. Thus, Ayhan *et al.* (1993) reported that metastatic tumour in the lungs and liver showed reduced *nm23* expression compared with the corresponding primary carcinomas. A similar situation appears to exist in human gastric cancers, where higher *nm23* expression has been seen in primary gastric carcinomas than in corresponding normal mucosa, but 52% of secondary tumours showed reduced *nm23* levels compared with the primary carcinomas (Nakayama *et al.*, 1993). Both H1 and H2 homologues of *nm23* have been found over-expressed in ovarian carcinoma tissue compared with benign tumours. However, within stage III carcinomas, the expresssion of the gene may be lower in tumours with lymph node metastasis, and stage IV has shown lower gene expression than stage III tumours (Mandai *et al.*, 1994). Kapitanovic *et al.* (1995) also found marked differences in *nm23* expression between 73 benign and 54 malignant ovarian cancers. Furthermore, they have claimed that carcinomas that had metastasised contained significantly less nm23 protein than those that had not metastasised. Ferrandina *et al.* (1996) found *nm23*-H1 expression in 62% of human ovarian cancers, but the expression was not related to tumour grade or stage, nor was any relationship evident between *nm23* expression and lymph node involvement. However, they did note that far more *nm23*-negative tumours were EGFr-positive. These studies may be seen as providing some qualified support for its putative suppressor function in ovarian cancers. A loss of chromosome 17 has frequently been associated with gynaecological cancers, but the possibility that progression may have been due to the loss of functional *p53* which is located on this chromosome rather than to the loss of *nm23* cannot be excluded. However, allelic loss at 17q23-ter is strongly associated with high-grade ovarian carcinomas (Lowry and Atkinson, 1993). Therefore, it is possible that there might be genetic repercussions of this on the expression of *nm23* located at 17q21.3.

It is difficult to rationalise some of the observations which essentially reflect a situation where tumour development is apparently aided by *nm23*, but it is then down-regulated to promote metastatic spread. It is possible that *nm23* expression in the primary tumours is heterogeneous and that the *nm23*-negative subpopulations could be successfully forming metastases. There is now evidence which suggests that *nm23* may be co-regulated with other genes which have the ability to promote metastasis (Parker *et al.*, 1991; Parker and Sherbet, 1992b).

Alternative explanations have been sought to explain the many inconsistensies seen in the expression of *nm23* in relation to metastatic progression. One of these is possible allelic deletions, as reported by Cohn *et al.* (1991) for colorectal carcinomas. Previously, Leone *et al.* (1990) had reported allelic loss of *nm23* in lung and renal carcinoma. Genetic changes in *nm23*-H1 either in the form of a deletion in the coding sequence or allelic deletion was found by Wang L *et al.* (1993) to be associated with four out of eight colorectal adenocarcinomas with lymph node metastasis, but no molecular alterations were found in a further 12 tumours which had no metastatic involvement. Florenes *et al.* (1992) examined whether the differences in *nm23* expression could be related to allelic deletions. They studied the loss of heterozygosity in the relevant area of chromosome 17q in 24 matched pairs of tumour tissue and peripheral blood cells. Of 13 cases informative for the *nm23*-H1 locus only two (15%) showed a deletion of one of the alleles. In both these cases LOH was also observed for *D17S74* which is close to the *nm23* locus. In colorectal carcinomas, three out of 20 informative cases showed LOH (Ayhan *et al.*, 1993). However, Campo *et al.* (1994) found the loss of *nm23*-H1 but not that of *p53* (locus 17p13) was significantly related to shorter disease-free and overall patient survival. In human prostatic carcinoma, only one out of 21 high-grade stage cancers showed LOH at the *nm23*-H1 locus (Brewster *et al.*, 1994a).

Most intriguing is a recent report by Caligo *et al.* (1994) that breast tumours with *nm23*-H1 allelic deletion were less invasive to axillary lymph nodes. Furthermore, these authors have found that 40% of tumours with *nm23*-H1 allelic loss also showed allelic loss for pYNZ22, a marker for 17p13.3 (the locus of the *p53* suppressor gene). These recent reports thus strongly emphasise the degree of divergence of observation.

Another postulate implicates possible molecular changes in *nm23*, e.g. deletion or substitution mutations and gene amplification, being associated either positively or negatively with malignant progression. Leone *et al.* (1993) reported that in childhood neuroblastomas amplification of *nm23*-H1, but not H2, occurred in six out of 18 cases of stage III and IV tumours. Genomic amplification of *nm23*-H1 was associated with increased gene expression and reduced patient survival. Direct sequencing of *nm23*-H2 in a stage IV tumour has suggested a mutation of leucine to valine at position 48.

nm23/NDP kinase in human cancers

The *nm23* story now shifts to the study of the protein products, namely the NDP kinases encoded by the *nm23*-H1 and -H2 genes, which is probably more enlightening and conclusive than studies which concerned the expression of and abnormalities associated with the genes. The *nm23* gene product has been found to be identical to nucleoside diphosphate (NDP) kinase (Gilles *et al.*, 1991). In fact, the NDP kinase isoenzyme forms A and B from erythrocytes are identical to deduced sequences from *nm23*-H1 and *nm23*-H2 genes respectively (Rosengard *et al.*, 1989; Stahl *et al.*, 1991) and these exhibit similar NDP kinase activity (Urano *et al.*, 1992). In the wake of this identification of the nm23 protein, there have been several studies in which NDP kinase levels of a variety of tumours have been measured and attempts have been made to correlate these with clinicopathological features of the tumour and prognosis of the disease.

Leone *et al.* (1991b) also examined the expression of the *nm23* protein in metastatic deposits of *nm23*-transfected melanoma cell lines. They described a heterogeneous distribution of the protein in 75% of metastatic deposits with *nm23* protein expression predominantly in the invasion zone of the deposits. A total of 10% of the metastatic nodules examined showed low *nm23* protein expression and in another 15% there was no correlation between the expression of *nm23* protein and metastasis development. For the first group, Leone *et al.* (1991b) appear to suggest that loss of the transfected *nm23* gene may have occurred after the invasive phase and, for the second group, earlier than the invasive phase. It would have been of great value to compare the expression and distribution of the *nm23* protein in the primary tumours with those in the secondary tumours, especially in the metastases where low protein expression was seen. The situation regarding its role in the invasion phase is, to say the least, uncertain. As we have argued elsewhere (see page 200), the nm23/NDP kinase may be expected to inhibit invasion, which is contrary to what Leone *et al*. (1991b) appear to be suggesting. Compatible with our view is the demonstration by Kantor *et al*. (1993) that transfection of murine and human cells with *nm23* inhibits invasion *in vitro* in response to serum and other growth factors, but *nm23* does not appear to inhibit invasion of unstimulated cells.

Low NDP kinase expression has been correlated with reduced survival in patients with infiltrating ductal breast carcinomas (Barnes *et al*., 1991). A recent study by Royds *et al*. (1993) supports the findings of Barnes *et al*. (1991). In hepatocellular carcinomas NDP kinase levels were lower in the primary tumour where metastatic spread had occurred. Furthermore, the enzyme levels were lower in the metastatic deposits than in the primary tumours (Nakayama *et al*., 1992). All these investigations are supportive of the metastasis suppressor role for the NDP kinases, but much experimental evidence can be cited which suggests that they may not be relevant *per se* to the process of metastasis. In pulmonary adenocarcinomas NDP kinase was expressed independently of tumour pathology and patient survival (Higashiyama *et al*., 1992). High levels of NDP kinase expression occur in several solid tumour types and also in some benign tumours. NDP kinase immunostaining may be found in non-invasive and in invasive ductal breast carcinomas with or without lymph node involvement (Lacombe *et al*., 1991). Kobayashi *et al*. (1992) reported that NDP kinase staining was intense in a majority of intraductal components of human breast cancers compared with normal breast epithelium. A majority of invasive components also express the *nm23* protein at levels comparable with that of normal epithelium. Another study by Sawan *et al*. (1994) determined the NDP kinase A (*nm23*-H1) expression in 198 breast carcinomas. Of these 81% were NDP kinase positive. They found that the NDP kinase expression was not related to disease relapse or patient survival. Neither was the expression of NDP kinase related to other prognostic factors such as tumour grade, oestrogen and progesterone receptor status or p53 expression. In pancreatic tumours, positive staining for nm23/NDP kinase was associated with higher lymph node metastasis and perineural invasion and also with shorter overall survival and relapse-free survival (Nakamori *et al*., 1993). The levels of nm23 proteins did not correspond with the high *nm23* transcript levels found in gastric cancers with metastasis to regional lymph nodes (Muta *et al*., 1994). The *nm23* protein levels show no inverse correlation with the progression of oligodendrogliomas from the benign to the malignant type. Thus, the protein was detected in non-proliferative normal brain tissue and increased amounts of it appear in tumours with more pronounced cell proliferation. However, 76% of the malignant form of the tumour, glioblastoma contained no *nm23* protein (Pavelic *et al*., 1994). In colorectal cancer *nm23* protein expression showed no relationship to tumour size, grade, Duke's stage, metastatic spread or patient survival (Ichikawa, 1994). Thus, the inverse correlation between *nm23* gene expression and indicators of poor prognosis and the postulate that this gene functions as a metastasis suppressor has not been borne out by studies at the protein expression level. This may suggest the existence of post-transcriptional control mechanisms and therefore further studies of the expression of the products of both H-1 and H-2 genes are imperative. There has also been a suggestion that nm23/NDP kinases may have other biochemical properties. An acid-stable phosphorylation of serine-44 has been reported and the level of this phosphorylation rather than NDP kinase activity is now suggested to correlate with metastasis suppressor function (Macdonald *et al.*, 1993). This has therefore raised the question whether the empirical negative correlation between *nm23* and metastatic potential reported previously is an effect of the gene *per se* or an indirect effect associated with some other feature of the metastatic phenotype.

Leone *et al.* (1993) found that not only reduced *nm23* expression but also mutations in the gene can lead to tumour aggressiveness. Consistent with this Wang L *et al.* (1993) have reported genetic alterations constituting either allelic deletions or deletions in *nm23*-H1 coding sequences in some colorectal adenocarcinomas. Whether genetic changes in *nm23* will explain the erratic behaviour of the gene in human tumours remains to be seen. There is bound to be a burst of activity in the detection of possible mutations in this gene. Our overall assessment from review of the current literature is that the putative suppressor role of *nm23* needs to be re-examined and that the use of its expression as a marker of progression is premature, if not unwarranted. However, one should consider the possibility that other genes such as the murine *18A2/mts1* and its homologues might act in concert with this suppressor gene in bringing about the phenotypic properties of invasiveness and metastasis. There are sound reasons for believing this to be a viable hypothesis, as will be discussed in Chapter 14.

14

Dominant metastasis-associated genes

The search for metastasis-associated genes expressing as a dominant trait has proceeded alongside the exploration for suppressor genes, albeit at a torpid pace. The natural candidates were oncogenes, which have been studied extensively as they were identified and cloned. However, there has been no unequivocal demonstration of the involvement of known oncogenes in cancer spread. Differential screening of cDNA libraries of non-malignant and corresponding malignant tumour cell lines has revealed a number of differentially expressed genes, including those coding for fibronectin (Schalken *et al.*, 1988), and the protease transin (Matrisian *et al.*, 1986a,b). These have been alluded to earlier.

mta1 gene expression in mammary carcinoma and adenocarcinoma cell lines

Toh *et al.* (1994, 1995) isolated 10 differentially expressed genes using the 13762 rat mammary adenocarcinoma model. One of the clones, designated *mta1* has been studied in detail by these authors. *mta1* is expressed at a low level in several organs, with the exception of testes where its expression is very high. The gene shows markedly greater expression in metastatic tumours compared with non-metastatic ones. For instance, a fourfold higher expression is found in the highly metastatic MTLn3 cell line than in the non-metastatic cell line, MTC4. The levels of transcripts of the human homologue of *mta1* were examined in human tumours. A marked increase in the transcription of the gene was noted in association with increase in the invasive and metastatic abilities of MCF7 and MDA breast cancer cell lines. The ratio of expression for MCF7 (non-metastaic) : MCF7/LCC1 (invasive) : MCF7 (LCC2) (metastatic) was $1:2:4$ and for MDA-MB-468 (non-metastatic) : MDA-231 (metastatic) $1:4$ (Toh *et al.*, 1995). The full-length transcript of *mta1* encodes a protein with 703 amino acid residues. The sequence of the clone was found to be novel. There is a proline-rich stretch of sequence at the *C*-terminal domains, which shows homology with the SH3 domain-binding motif. This observation is significant, for one can envisage a potential function for the *mta1* protein. A group of non-receptor intracellular kinases have been identified which have been found to bind to activated growth factor receptors. These signalling proteins contain non-catalytic domains known as *src* homology (SH) domains and transduction of growth factor signals involve interaction of SH domains with activated growth factor receptors. Activation of these receptors can also lead to the phosphorylation of phospholipase C (PLC) and PLC-γ. PLC-γ can interact with cytoskeletal structures and its targeting may be mediated by SH3 domains (reviewed by Sherbet and Lakshmi, 1997). Therefore, the *mta1* protein might contain the necessary elements that might allow the protein to be targeted to cytoskeletal elements and provide a possible mechanism for its apparent association with invasion.

The role of murine 18A2/mts1 homologues and other S-100 proteins in cancer progression

The structure and function of S-100 family proteins

The S-100 proteins were first reported to occur in abundance in nervous tissue (Moore, 1965). They are a family of low-molecular-weight acidic proteins formed of homo- or hetero-dimers of α and β subunits which show 58% sequence homology (Isobe and Okuyama, 1978, 1981) and contain multiple copies of Ca^{2+}-binding regions with a common structural motif known as the EF hands. The EF hands bind calcium selectively and with high affinity. Typically, the EF domain consists of a loop of 12 amino acids flanked by two α-helices. The S-100 family proteins have a variant loop of 14 amino acids. The EF-hand proteins may take part in Ca^{2+} signalling and control processes which are Ca^{2+}-dependent. Some EF-hand proteins interact with other cellular proteins in a Ca^{2+}-dependent manner and regulate their biological activity.

The structure and organisation of S-100 family genes

The S-100 family genes exhibit a common intron–exon organisation. S-100β has three exons and two introns. The first exon codes for the 5′-untranslated region and the second and third exons each encode an EF-hand (Allore *et al.*, 1990). The genetic organisation of the human homologue, *h-mts1*, of the murine *18A2/mts1* gene, has been described in some detail by Ambartsumian *et al.* (1995). This has four exons interspersed with three introns of 232, 657 and 720 bp. The first and second exons of 54 bp and 49 bp, respectively, are non-coding exons, and exons three and four with 136 bp and 165 bp, respectively, contain the coding sequences for the mts1 protein. This organisation of the *h-mts1* is similar to that found in another member (S-100D) of the family. The mouse homologue, along with a majority of S-100 family genes, however, contain only three exons (Engelkamp *et al.*, 1993). Ambartsumian *et al.* (1995) have also reported the occurrence of two alternatively spliced variants of the *h-mts1* cDNA and also that alternative splicing occurs within the 5′ untranslated region of the original *h-mts1* transcript. The second non-coding exon mentioned above is found only in the variant form. This insertion, nevertheless, retains the main open reading frame (ORF) for the mts1 protein, without creating a new longer ORF (Figure 19). In contrast, we have recently detected the expression of a shorter *h-mts1* transcript in some breast carcinomas (Albertazzi *et al.*, 1996).

The significance of the occurrence of splice variants is currently being debated. Alternative splicing has been regarded as a widespread mechanism in the regulation of gene function (Green, 1991; Maniatis, 1991). It has been suggested also that the mutually opposing functions of genes in cell proliferation and differentiation and apoptosis may involve alternative splicing of pre-mRNAs as a molecular mechanism (Mikulski, 1994). Similarly, the antagonistic functions of proto-oncogenes and suppressor genes may be seen as a consequence of alternative splicing of a parental gene (Calin, 1994). This implies that splice variants may be functionally different, if not invariably antagonistic to one another. If this were the case, one would expect a differential expression of variants in different tissues and possibly also modulation of expression of individual splice variants with tumour development and progression. Ambartsumian *et al.* (1995) found that the *h-mts1* and *h-mts1(v)*, the variant form, are differentially expressed in human tissues. The *h-mts1(v)* variant is prominent in the colon but not in the liver and there is also a semblance of the variant in fetal liver. The *h-mts1* splice variants also show marked variation in tumour cell lines. They may be equally represented in some tumour cell lines, while a variant may predominate in others. However, it would be premature to speculate whether the pattern of expression is related to the histogenetic origin of tumours.

Transcriptional regulation of S-100 family genes

The promoter region of S-100β contains several potential regulatory elements, e.g. the cAMP responsive element and AP2 (Allore *et al.*, 1990). The calcyclin promoter region also contains an AP-1-like binding sequence, which, in competition assays, showed no binding by AP-2, AP-3 or NF1 transcription factors. In neuroblastoma cells induced to differentiate using retinoic acid, calcyclin mRNA levels increase together with the binding of AP-1-like transcription factor (Bottini *et al.*, 1994).

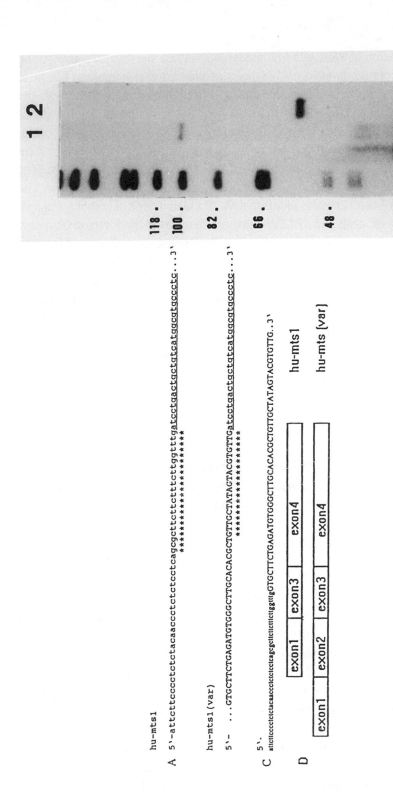

Figure 19. The generation and characteristics of alternatively spliced variants of *b-mts1*. Reproduced with permission from Ambartsumian *et al.* (1995).

e transcriptional regulation of *18A2/mts1* homologues has been investigated recently. The king region of the mouse homologue has been sequenced and homology has been d with promoter regions of rat fibrinogen and human prethrombin, and also with the elements of SV40 (Tulchinsky *et al.*, 1990, 1992). Its transcription may indeed be controlled by *cis*-regulatory elements, although Tulchinsky *et al.* (1992) found no *cis*-acting control elements in the 5′ regions of the gene. Subsequently, Tulchinsky *et al.* (1993) have identified a 16-nucleotide *cis*-acting transcription regulatory element in the first intron of gene which shows a high degree of homology to the enhancer element of the CD delta gene. The promoter region of the *18A2/mts1* contains motifs that show a high degree of homology to p53-binding negative regulatory elements and AP1-like enhancer elements in the 3′ region (Parker *et al.*, 1994a). This evidence, albeit preliminary in nature, indicates that the pathways of function of S-100 genes are under the control of transcription factors. Upon failing to find any *cis*-acting control elements in the promoter region of the gene, Tulchinsky *et al.* (1992) argued that the control of its expression may occur at a different level. The possibility of DNA methylation in this processs has been envisaged. The methylation of the first exon and the first intron has been implicated in the repression of transcription (Tulchinsky *et al.*, 1995).

The expression of S-100 proteins in cell proliferation, differentiation and neoplasia

The S-100 family of proteins now occupy a pre-eminent position with the discovery that some of the S-100 genes are associated with a variety of biological processes such as cell cycle regulation, cell differentiation and tumour progression. They interact with cytoskeletal structures and alter cell shape and motility. Glial cells of the brain are known to express S-100β predominantly (Kahn *et al.*, 1983; Kato and Kimura, 1985). S-100β is also found in Schwann cells; melanocytes and chondrocytes express both S-100α and β, but muscle cells express only S-100α (Takahashi *et al.*, 1984; Haimoto *et al.*, 1987). S-100β takes part in neuronal development and it is identical to the neurite extension factor (Kligman and Marshak, 1985). In glial cell cultures, inhibition of S-100β produces changes in cellular morphology, cytoskeletal organisation and cell proliferation (Selinfreund *et al.*, 1990). Other functions such as regulation of protein phosphorylation, ATPase, adenylate cyclase and aldolase activity have also been attributed to S-100 proteins (Donato, 1991). The gene coding for S-100β has been assigned to chromosome 21q22 (Duncan *et al.*, 1989) and therefore it has been implicated in the neurological abnormalities associated with Down's syndrome (Allore *et al.*, 1988).

Calcyclin or 2A9, which shows a 55% sequence homology to S-100β, has been reported to exhibit not only cell cycle-related expression but it is also over-expressed in human myeloid leukaemias and some breast cancer cell lines (Calabretta *et al.*, 1986; Murphy *et al.*, 1988). In human melanomas, expression of the calcyclin gene has been found to correlate with metastatic potential (Weterman *et al.*, 1992). Calcyclin RNA expression was higher in metastatic lesions. Immunohistochemical staining has revealed the presence of higher proportions of cells strongly staining for calcyclin in the vertical growth phase of primary melanoma (Weterman *et al.*, 1993). S-100β is expressed in large amounts in neuroectodermal tumours but it is not detectable in several cell lines derived from carcinomas of the colon, breast, lung and ovary (Marks *et al.*, 1990). S-100 protein-expressing dendritic cell (S-100DC) infiltration has been recorded in transitional cell carcinoma of the bladder and the extent of S-100DC infiltration found to be related to tumour grade and its invasive behaviour (Inoue *et al.*, 1993).

A cell proliferation-related gene, *18A2*, was cloned by Jackson-Grusby *et al.* (1988). The 18A2 mRNA was found to show homology to known calcium-binding proteins and was expressed in a wide variety of normal tissues (Jackson-Grusby *et al.*, 1988). This gene, subsequently called *mts1*, has been found to be expressed strongly in haemopoietic cells of both murine and human origin (Grigorian *et al.*, 1994). A dominant metastasis-associated gene (*mts1*) was reported to be highly expressed in highly metastatic murine tumours and human tumours grown as xenografts (Ebralidze *et al.*, 1989, 1990), and it is identical to the *18A2* gene belonging to the S-100 family. This gene was independently cloned by other groups, e.g. *42a* from PC12 cells following stimulation by nerve growth factor (Masiakowsi *et al.*, 1988), p9Ka from rat myoepithelium-like cells (Barraclough *et al.*, 1984), and pEL98 from Balbc/3T3 cells (Goto *et al.*, 1988). The *18A2/mts1* homologous product derived from bovine retina has a M_r of approx. 11 000 (Polans *et al.*, 1994). Ebralidze *et al.* (1990) found that the *18A2/mts1* protein shows 55% sequence homology to S-100β in the Ca^{2+}-binding domains. Some investigators have preferred to call the murine *18A2/mts1* and its homologues as *CAPL* (Engelkamp *et al.*, 1993). The product encoded by the gene has been called metastasin 1 (Grigorian *et al.*, 1993) and calvasculin (Watanabe *et al.*, 1992), although in the light of the spectrum of activities in which this product is implicated, neither of these appellations would seem appropriate.

Here, the mouse homologue of the gene is referred to as *18A2/mts1* and the human homologue as *h-mts1*. This nomenclature also serves to distinguish these genes from the putative multiple tumour suppressor *MTS1* gene frequently inactivated or mutated in human tumours (Kamb *et al.*, 1994). The p16/ink4 is a product of this multiple tumour suppressor *MTS1* gene and it inhibits the cyclin D–cdk4 kinase (Serrano *et al.*, 1993). The role played by this gene has been discussed in some detail in a previous section (see page 66).

The mouse homologue *18A2/mts1* is highly expressed in highly metastatic variants of the B16 melanoma but not in low metastasis variants (Parker *et al.*, 1991). The expression of this gene is altered by agents which modulate invasion and metastasis by B16 tumours. Thus, retinoic acid inhibits metastasis by B16 melanomas and also reduces the expression of the *18A2/mts1* gene. In contrast, α-melanocyte-stimulating hormone which enhances metastatic behaviour, up-regulates the *18A2/mts1* gene expression (Parker *et al.*, 1991). Davies BR *et al.* (1993) transfected benign rat mammary epithelial cell lines with the *p9Ka* gene, which is the rat homologue of the murine *18A2/mts1* gene. The transfectants showed higher tumour incidence and greater ability to metastasise than the untransfected control cells. We recently transfected the murine B16-F10 melanoma cells with the *18A2/mts1* placed under the control of the dexamethasone-inducible mammary tumour virus (MMTV) promoter. We found that switching on the expression of transfected *18A2/mts1* gene by exposure of the transfectant cells to dexamethasone induced a sevenfold increase in lung colonisation by these cells indicating a causal relationship between *18A2/mts1* expression and lung colonisation (Parker *et al.*, 1994b). Meanwhile, Grigorian *et al.* (1993) transfected anti-sense *mts1* constructs into a highly metastatic cell line, CSML-100, and tested the effects of the expression of the anti-sense message on the metastatic ability of the transfected cells. Cells expressing high levels of the anti-sense message were injected subcutaneously and were found to develop into tumours which were poorly metastatic to the lungs. Thus, *18A2/mts1* expression indubitably enhances the metastatic potential of cancers. Albertazzi *et al.* (1996) recently studied a series of human breast carcinomas and has shown that *b-mt1* expression strongly correlated with the presence of metastatic tumour in the lymph nodes. Furthermore, tumours which expressed *b-mts1* were generally oestrogen/progesterone-receptor negative. The expression of *b-mts1* is quite obviously indicative of aggressive disease. Possibly, therefore, the expression of this gene may be a useful prognostic factor, although much further work needs to be done in this area. Albertazzi *et al.* (1996) also found a shorter variant *b-mts1* transcript in some breast cancer specimens. Whether this is an alternatively spliced variant and whether its presence is related to tumour aggressiveness is currently being investigated.

The members of the S-100 family of genes, with the exception of S-100β, have been found to occur as a tight cluster on chromosome 1q21 (Dorin *et al.*, 1990). Thus, four members occur in a head-to-tail series 5'-S100E-CAPL-S100D-CACY-3'. Two further members, S-100L and S-100α have been linked to the gene cluster, by pulse-field gel electrophoresis, within a 450 kb DNA tract (Engelkamp *et al.*, 1993). It is interesting to note that S-100β, which shares sequence homology with S-100α, has been localised to chromosome 21q22 (Duncan *et al.*, 1989) and thus stands out as an aberrant member of the family. The *b-mts1* gene was provisionally assigned to chromosome 7q21 by Lakshmi *et al.* (1991). Therefore, one should consider the possibility of a pesudo *b-mts1* gene occurring on either location.

In this context it should be noted that chromosome 1 is the single most involved chromosome in structural alterations in solid tumours (Trent, 1985), and the S-100 gene cluster locus is involved in a variety of tumours such as breast (Devilee *et al.*, 1991a; Wolman *et al.*, 1992) and gastric carcinomas (Sano *et al.*, 1991) and B-cell leukaemic clones (Ghose *et al.*, 1990). There are several reports that human malignant melanomas contain abnormalities (rearrangements) associated with chromosome 1, among others (Fountain *et al.*, 1990). Extra copies and rearrangements of chromosome 1 and chromosome 7 have been reported also in several other human tumour types (Heim and Mitelman, 1987; Presti *et al.*, 1991; Jhanwar *et al.*, 1992). As stated before, Lakshmi *et al.* (1991) provisionally mapped the *b-mts1* gene to chromosome 7q22 and detected no hybridisation to chromosome 1. There is also considerable evidence of abnormalities of chromosome 7 in a variety of human tumour types (Collard *et al.*, 1987b; Priest *et al.*, 1988; Fountain *et al.*, 1990; Bertrand *et al.*, 1991). Admittedly, the probe used by Lakshmi *et al.* (1991) is a murine probe; nevertheless, the hybridisation results may not be affected by this on account of the extensive sequence homology between the murine and the human clones. Engelkamp *et al.* (1993) have made a good case for chromosome 1 as the locus of the human *18A2/mts1* gene; unfortunately they have provided no *in situ* hybridisation evidence for this, but only for S-100α and D. Therefore, it would not be unreasonable to suggest that the assignment of these genes to chromosome 1q21 may be deemed as provisional. One may recall that S-100β is located on chromosome 21q22 and not in the gene cluster on chromosome 1q22 described by Engelkamp *et al.* (1993).

Apart from the apparent association with malignant processes, S-100 proteins are known to be expressed in a cell cycle-related fashion. This has been reviewed by Kligman and Hilt (1988). S-100β appears to be differentially expressed in the cell cycle, with enhanced expression in the G_1 phase. Marks *et al.* (1990) examined S-100β expression in cell lines derived from two melanomas and the C6 rat glioma. They found that whereas 80–95% of cells in the $S + G_2 + M$ phases expressed S-100β, only 50–70% of cells in the G_0G_1 expressed the protein.

S-100β is also known to inhibit microtubule polymerisation (Baudier *et al.*, 1982; Baudier and Cole, 1988). Its involvement in microtubule assembly is further supported by the down-regulation of the S-100β gene when microtubule assembly is disrupted by chemical treatments (Dunn *et al.*, 1987); this again may be a reflection of the involvement of S-100β in the cell division cycle. Lakshmi *et al.* (1993) and Parker *et al.* (1994b) have shown that enhanced expression of the *18A2/mts1* gene promotes microtubule depolymerisation in B16 murine melanoma cell lines. These studies clearly indicate that the expression of both S-100β and the *18A2/mts1* protein could be a prerequisite for the progression of cells into the synthetic phase of the cell cycle.

S-100β and 2A9 (also known as calcyclin) show high levels of expression in the G_1 phase of the cell cycle. In LAN-5 cells calcyclin gene expression is detectable upon treatment with retinoic acid together with an accumulation of cells in the G_1-phase and cell growth arrest (Tonini *et al.*, 1991). Recent work shows that the regulation of proliferation by calcyclin may be mediated by binding to CAP-50 which is a calcyclin-specific annexin (Minami *et al.*, 1992; Hidaka and Mizutani, 1993).

The expression of murine *18A2* and the human *h-mts1* genes can be modulated by mitogens such as lipopolysaccharides, IFN-γ and concanavalin A (Grigorian *et al.*, 1994). It is expressed abundantly in the S-phase, although its homologue 42A shows markedly increased expression following mitosis in certain species. The demonstration that there might be some discernible pattern of expression of S-100 family of genes in relation to the stage of the cell cycle, however, does little to illuminate whether they actually control the cell cycle traverse. Empirically, human carcinoma cells which constitutively express the *18A2/mts1* homologous gene have been reported to have large S-phase fractions compared with cell lines with low expression levels (Sherbet *et al.*, 1995). The first experimental demonstration that it might induce G_1-S transition has been reported by Parker *et al.* (1994b). They constructed a vector inserting the *18A2/mts1* under the control of the dexamethasone-inducible mammary tumour virus promoter. This vector was transfected into B16 melanoma F10 variant cells. Upon switching on expression of the transfected gene there was a 2.5-fold increase in the number of

in the S phase, whereas no such changes in cell cycle distribution were noted in control
that had been transfected with plasmid not carrying the insert and in untransfected
lines. This indicates that the gene product is driving the cells into the S-phase. This
has been suggested to be due to the promotion of microtubule depolymerisation by the *18A2/
mts*, which might serve as a signal for G_1-S transition of cells (Lakshmi *et al.*, 1993; Parker *et
al.*, 1994b). A second possibility is that this protein may form a complex with the p53
phosphoprotein and sequester the latter, effectively removing the control exerted by the
phosphoprotein on G_1-S transition. Both of these postulated modes of cell cycle control are
discussed in detail in an earlier section (see page 48). The possibility that the *18A2/mts1* may
be involved in the deregulation of cell cycle progression and as a late or a distal event in the
metastatic progression of cancer has to be taken seriously. These observations have prompted
an in-depth investigation of the relationship between metastatic potential and the expression
of the *18A2/mts1* gene in several laboratories.

Cell differentiation and *18A2/mts1* gene expression

It has been postulated that metastatic potential is possibly related to defective differentiation of
the tumour cell and the induction of melanogenesis has often been cited as an indicator of the
differentiated phenotype of melanomas. The process of melanogenesis is regulated by
melanocyte-stimulating hormone (MSH), together with changes in melanocyte morphology
(Lerner and McGuire, 1961; Dexter and Bennett, 1987; Preston *et al.*, 1987; Jimenez *et al.*,
1988). The inter-relationships between induction of differentiation, i.e. melanogenesis and
malignancy are not well understood. Riley PA (personal communication, 1987) argued that the
level of pigmentation in melanocytes is controlled by its dilution during cell division and that the
average degree of pigmentation, i.e. the degree of differentiation as indicated by the degree of
melanisation, is inversely related to the rate of proliferation of melanocytes. Aubert *et al.* (1980)
found no relationship between phenotypic features expressed *in vitro* and tumorgenicity and
metastatic ability *in vivo*. They suggest that melanogenesis is not related to malignancy. In
contrast, Silagi and Bruce (1970) reported that the malignancy and pigmentation can be
modified simultaneously and have suggested, therefore, that the two processes are regulated
by similar mechanisms. A direct correlation between melanogenesis and metastatic ability was
also noted by Kameyama *et al.* (1990).

It has been demonstrated, however, that while MSH treatment of the B16 cells enhances
metastasis (Bennett *et al.*, 1986; Parker *et al.*, 1991) it also enhances melanogenesis (Bennett *et
al.*, 1986). Furthermore, MSH immunoreactivity appears to be associated with peripheral
invading zones of the B16 murine melanoma (Zubair *et al.*, 1992). This contradicts the view
that metastasis and cell differentiation are mutually incompatible features. MSH treatment of the
B16 cell variants has been shown to enhance both lung colonisation and melanogenesis
(Sheppard *et al.*, 1984; Bennett *et al.*, 1986; Parker *et al.*, 1991). However, the Ca^{2+} channel

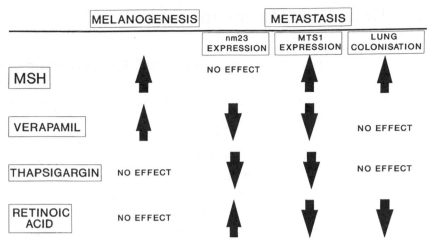

Figure 20. This figure summarises the effects of MSH and retinoic acid on *18A2/mts1* expression and lung colonisation by B16 melanoma cells. MSH enhances *18A2/mts1* expression and also lung colonisation. In contrast, retinoic acid has opposite effects on both. MSH not only enhances metastatic ability but also induces melanogenesis. The effect of verapamil, which is a Ca^{2+} blocker, is included here because it has been found to have no effect on the formation of metastatic deposits in the lung, but markedly increases melanogenesis. These data suggest a possible uncoupling of melanogenesis and metastatic potential. Based on data from Parker *et al.* (1991) and Parker and Sherbet (1993). Figure constructed in consultation with Dr C. Parker.

blocker verapamil was found to have no effect on lung colonisation but markedly enhanced melanogenesis in the B16 cell variants (Parker and Sherbet, 1993). In addition to this, it has been demonstrated that MSH up-regulates the expression of the dominant metastasis-associated gene *18A2/mts1* whereas verapamil down-regulates it (Parker *et al.*, 1991; Parker and Sherbet, 1992b) (Figure 20). Therefore it can be said that the processes of melanogenesis and metastasis can be uncoupled both at the genetic and phenotypic levels.

Retinoids have been known to produce a wide range of differentiation-related phenotypic changes in a variety of cell types (Jetten, 1985). Retinoic acid (RA) suppresses the invasive ability of A549 human lung carcinoma cells (Fazely and Ledinko, 1990) and melanoma cells (Wood *et al.*, 1990). RA is known to induce differentiation in a variety of cell types and several genomic targets have been indentified in the induction of differentiation (Parker and Sherbet, 1992a). We have shown that lung colonisation by B16-ML8 murine melanoma cells injected into the tail vein of mice is significantly reduced if the cells are exposed *in vitro* to RA before injection (Parker *et al.*, 1991). We have argued that if RA is capable of inhibiting both invasion and metastatic dissemination, it is possible that exposure to RA would modulate the effects of the putative metastasis-suppressor *nm23* and the dominant *18A2/mts1* genes.

Are *18A2/mts1* and *nm23* genes functionally related?

We have recently probed three B16 murine melanoma cell lines possessing demonstrably different metastatic ability for *nm23* and *18A2/mts1* expression. The expression of *nm23* did not show the expected inverse relationship with metastatic ability, whereas *18A2/mts1* expression was directly related. Treatment of highly metastatic cells with RA, a differentiation-inducing agent, down-regulated *18A2/mts1* expression. RA up-regulated *nm23* expression, albeit not in a consistent fashion. An examination of the relative expression of these genes (i.e. the ratio of *nm23* : *18A2/mts1*) has shown that in low metastatic variants, the ratio remained virtually constant over the 48-h RA treatment period, but it showed a steady increase in highly metastatic variants, suggesting that the two genes may be coordinately regulated in low metastatic tumours, but their regulation may be uncoupled in the highly metastatic tumour variants (Parker *et al.*, 1991). The possibility that the two genes may be uncoupled is supported by another line of experimental evidence. We isolated a heat-resistant cell line, HTG, from the BL6 murine melanoma and another cell line, the HUT, from a human hepatic tumour. In both cases, the parental cells expressed *18A2/mts1* or *h-mts1* (the homologous human gene), respectively, at a high level, but *nm23* at a lower level. In contrast, both the heat-resistant cell lines HTG and HUT, showed low murine or human *mts1* with unaltered *nm23* expression.

The apparent uncoupling of *18A2/mts1* and *nm23* expression in potentially malignant tumours has been confirmed by further work carried out by our research group using the B16 murine melanoma line F10-192/10 which is a transfectant cell line that carries the *18A2/mts1* placed under the control of dexamethasone-inducible mammary tumour virus promoter. When the cells were exposed to the steroid, *18A2/mts1* expression increased, together with several-fold enhancement of lung colonisation, but the expression of *nm23* appeared to be unaffected (Parker *et al.*, 1994b). We have reported recently that Ca^{2+} signalling is a common regulation pathway of these genes (Parker and Sherbet, 1992b) and there may be an uncoupling of this co-regulation in highly metastatic variants. At the mechanistic level, their co-regulation may be reflected in the physiologically opposite functions attributable to the proteins encoded by these genes. We know that the 18A2/mts1 promotes depolymerisation of microtubules but, in sharp contrast, nm23/NDP kinase is closely implicated in promoting polymerisation of these cytoskeletal structures.

18A2/mts1 and *nm23* genes and cytoskeletal integrity

The *18A2/mts1* gene codes for a protein which has sequence homology with S-100β protein, which is a member of the Ca^{2+}-binding protein family (Ebralidze *et al.*, 1990). S-100β is known to form a complex with the microtubule-associated *tau* protein and this complex inhibits microtubule polymerisation (Baudier *et al.*, 1982; Baudier and Cole, 1988). S-100 proteins bind to annexin II and p11 proteins which are the heavy and light chains of calpactin I (Bianchi *et al.*, 1992). S-100 proteins also bind to glial fibrillary acidic protein (GFAP) and inhibit its polymerisation in a Ca^{2+}-dependent manner into glial filaments, which constitute the major cytoskeletal component of glial cells (Bianchi *et al.*, 1993). Whether the inhibition of polymerisation always involves an intermediate target protein is uncertain. Bianchi *et al.* (1993) suggest that S-100 protein dimers may cross-link GFAP units and suggest that S-100 could bind to tubulin in a similar fashion with a tubulin dimer : S-100 dimer linkage. The *18A2/mts1* protein could be directly binding to tubulin in promoting the depolymerisation of tubulin reported to be a consequence of over-expression of the gene (Lakshmi *et al.*, 1993). In fact, the protein encoded by the *p9Ka*, the rat homologue of murine *18A2/mts1*, also shows association with cytoskeletal elements (Davies BR *et al.*, 1993; Gibbs *et al.*, 1994). The association of *pEL98* (the *18A2/mts1* from Balbc/3T3 cells) protein with cytoskeletal proteins has also been demonstrated (Takenaga *et al.*, 1994a). Watanabe *et al.* (1993) found that the disorganisation of microfilaments in rat fibroblasts transfected with the *src* oncogene corresponded with increases in the levels of the protein encoded by *18A2/mts1*.

Amino acid sequence homology has been demonstrated between *nm23* and the *awd* gene in *Drosophila* (Rosengard *et al.*, 1989) and also a nucleoside diphosphate kinase found in the slime mould *Dictyostelium discoideum* (Lacombe *et al.*, 1990; Wallet *et al.*, 1990). There is considerable evidence, therefore, that *nm23* and the *awd* genes code for a nucleoside diphosphate kinase (Biggs *et al.*, 1990; Wallet *et al.*, 1990). The nm23/NDP kinase is also involved with the polymerisation of spindle microtubules which requires transphosphorylation of GDP to GTP (Nickerson and Wells, 1988). This is consistent with the demonstration that the nm23 proteins also form complexes with tubulin (Lombardi *et al.*, 1995). There are also suggestions that *nm23* expression may be related to cell proliferation. It has been reported that the level of *nm23*-H1 expression declines in serum-deprived cells in culture and increases rapidly upon serum supplementation (Igawa *et al.*, 1994). There does not appear to be any pattern to H1 expression during the cell cycle, hence the details of the involvement of the gene in cell proliferation need to be studied further. However, microtubule polymerisation might be the point of expression where *nm23* and *18A2/mts1* genes exert their specific suppressor or dominant effects on the biological behaviour of tumour cells. A new possibility that has emerged from the work of Postel *et al.* (1993) is that the *nm23* protein might function as a transcriptional regulator of the *myc* oncogene. These authors have found that the c-*myc* transcription factor PuF shows sequence identity to the human *nm23*-H2 protein.

We have recently reported that modulation of the expression of the *18A2/mts1* and *nm23* genes alters the state of polymerisation of tubulin and that treatment with MSH, which up-regulates the *18A2/mts1* gene, increases the proportion of the depolymerised form of tubulin, whereas RA, which down-regulates *18A2/mts1* (and up-regulates *nm23*), decreases the depolymerisation of tubulin (Lakshmi *et al.*, 1993) thereby providing a link between the expression of *18A2/mts1* and the invasive behaviour of tumour cells. Further support for this cell motility function of the *18A2/mts1* protein has recently come from two sources: Takenaga *et al.* (1994b) found high expression of the gene in HL-60 cells differentiating into macrophages, but the levels were low in cells induced to differentiate in the granulocytic direction by all-*trans* RA; Merzak *et al.* (1994b) found that *b-mts1* was over-expressed in cell lines derived from invasive human gliomas compared with cell lines derived from non-invasive tumours. Finally, Takenaga *et al.* (1994c) transfected the *pEL98 (18A2/mts1)* cDNA into 3Y1-H (src transfected) cells with low cell motility and found their motility was significantly enhanced. They also reported that in cell clones derived from the Lewis lung carcinoma, gene expression correlated with cell motility.

The role of cytoskeletal elements in cancer invasion

Cytoskeletal structures play a leading role in cell motility and invasion, proliferation, differentiation and in the transduction of extracellular signals. In the light of this, there have been several studies on the changes in cytoskeletal elements consequent upon cell transformation or induction of differentiation. Changes in cytoskeleton-associated proteins and vimentin were described in both granulocytic and monocytic leukaemia cells some years ago by Bernal and Chen (1982) and Bernal and Stahel (1985). For example, alterations in microtubules, microtubule-associated proteins (MAPs) and intermediate filaments (IF) have been demonstrated in HL-60 leukaemia cells. Treatment of the leukaemic cells with RA, which induces terminal differentiation of these cells, has been found to increase the amount of microtubule protein and vimentin (an intermediate filament glycoprotein). Changes have also been reported in the microtubule-associated proteins MAP2 and tau (Leung *et al.*, 1992). It has been reported that breast cancer cell lines which express vimentin are more invasive than those which do not have vimentin (Thompson *et al.*, 1991).

There is some evidence that control of cell locomotion and invasion may be mediated by genes which control the dynamics of microtubule assembly. A striking example of this is the expression of MSH and its association with the invasive and metastatic behaviour of melanomas. Zubair *et al.* (1992) demonstrated that MSH immunoreactivity occurs predominantly in the peripheral invading zones of a B16-BL6 melanoma. It has recently been reported that treatment of B16 melanoma cells with MSH enhances metastatic ability of B16 melanoma cells and up-regulates *18A2/mts1* expression (Parker *et al.*, 1991). These effects are accompanied, in parallel, by an increase in depolymerisation of tubulin (Lakshmi *et al.*, 1993). Merzak *et al.* (1994b) have recently demonstrated that the *18A2/mts1* gene is expressed in invasive gliomas but not in non-invasive brain tumours or in fetal brain cells. It appears, therefore, that there is a clear physical link in the form of cytoskeletal dynamics between expression of *18A2/mts1* gene and tumour cell invasion.

Invasion by cancer cells is also regulated by hormones and growth factors. For instance, in oestrogen receptor (ER)-positive breast cancer cells lines such as MCF-7 and T47D, oestradiol stimulation increases their invasive ability but this does not occur in the ER-negative cell line

MDA-MB-231 (Albini *et al.*, 1987; Thompson *et al.*, 1988, 1989). Most interesting is the observation by Thompson *et al.* (1991) that oestradiol-regulated alterations are associated with the occurrence of vimentin. They found that vimentin-positive breast cancer cells showed far greater increases in invasion in response to oestradiol than cells which were vimentin-negative. Epidermal growth factor (EGF) not only produces changes in cellular morphology but also promotes cell invasion *in vitro* (Shiozaki *et al.*, 1995).

Recently, it has been demonstrated that the proliferative response of cancer cells to stimulation by growth factors is also associated with the cytoskeletal elements. In the A431 epidermoid carcinoma cell line, EGF-stimulated high-affinity EGF receptors are invariably associated with cytoskeletal structures (Roy *et al.*, 1989, 1991; van Bergen en Henegouwen *et al.*, 1989). This suggests that cytoskeletal elements play an important role in the transduction of the proliferative signal imparted by the binding of EGF to its receptor.

Growth factor receptors are associated with cytoskeletal elements

As discussed in a previous chapter, high EGF receptor (EGFr) expression has been correlated with axillary node involvement and higher levels of EGFr have been reported in metastatic tumour than in the primary lesion. Furthermore, high EGFr status correlates with poor differentiation and high tumour grade. It ought to be stated, however, that there are also studies which do not subscribe to these views. Nevertheless, for breast cancer an overall picture has emerged which suggests EGFr status as a strong marker of clinical aggressiveness and metastatic potential (see page 153).

Recently, we investigated whether the expression of *18A2/mts1* and *nm23* genes was related to EGFr expression (Parker *et al.*, 1992; Sherbet *et al.*, 1995). We found a constitutively high expression of *h-mts1* in the breast cancer cell line MDA-MB-231 and A431 (vulval epidermoid carcinoma) which are both also high expressors of EGFr. In contrast there was no detectable expression of this gene in the MCF7 cell line which is a low expressor of EGFr. The ZR-75-1 breast cancer cells in which *h-mts1* expression is low (Pedrocchi *et al.*, 1994) have also been described as containing low levels of high-affinity EGF receptors (Valverius *et al.*, 1990). Furthermore, the expression of *h-mts1* correlated with the degree of depolymerisation of tubulin. These data suggest that EGFr positivity and *h-mts1* (possibly also *nm23*) expression are related. Furthermore, the relative state of microtubule polymerisation strongly correlated with the expression of these two genes. Thus, MCF7 cells which showed the strongest expression of *nm23* showed the highest expression of polymerised tubulin compared with A431 and MDA cells in which *h-mts1* gene was highly expressed (Sherbet *et al.*, 1995).

There is currently considerable evidence suggesting that ligand-induced high-affinity EGF receptors are associated with cytoskeletal elements (Roy *et al.*, 1989, 1991; van Bergen en

Henegouwen *et al.*, 1989). As pointed out above, both *18A2-mts1/h-mts1* and *nm23* genes may be involved in, and possibly interfere with, the process of tubulin polymerisation and therefore these are reasonable grounds for undertaking a prospective study of the correlation between EGFr status and the expression of the metastasis-associated genes in breast cancer with a long-term view of assessing the potential of *mts1/nm23* expression as a marker for tumour progression and predicting prognosis. Preliminary data do indeed show that *h-mts1* expression in human breast cancer correlates directly with the potential for nodal metastasis and inversely with oestrogen receptor status, thus strongly suggesting that the expression of this gene indicates highly aggressive disease (Albertazzi *et al.*, 1996).

As discussed previously, the proposed mechanism of the up-regulation of *18A2/mts1* by MSH in the B16 murine melanoma is via activation of cAMP-PKA signal transduction, producing a transient increase in the early response genes and since *18A2/mts1* contains an AP1-like enhancer element in the 3' region of the gene this may induce its expression. EGF receptor when activated is believed to transduce its signal via subsequent activation of PKC. Conceivably, a result of this activation will be a transient increase in the expression of the early response genes which may, in turn, up-regulate the *18A2/mts1* gene. Therefore, this may suggest that *18A2/mts1* expression may be regulated by means of activation of PKC signal transduction by interaction of EGF with its receptor EGFr. There is now considerable experimental evidence linking *18A2/mts1* expression with metastasis; therefore, one may conclude that the correlation demonstrated between *18A2/mts1* expression with EGF receptor status may be significant and relevant to the process of progression of tumours to the metastatic state.

The p21^{ras} protein and the transduction of *18A2-mts1/h-mts1* proliferative signals

The ras proteins are a family of highly conserved proteins and have, in recent years, been shown to regulate transduction of signals associated with control of proliferation and growth. Since *ras* oncogene expression appears to bring in its wake the expression of S-100 related proteins, we shall only briefly discuss how one might envisage the role of 18A2/mts1 and homologous proteins and the *nm23*/NDP kinase in growth signal transduction.

The ras proteins bind to and hydrolyse GTP in a manner analogous to guanine nucleotide-binding regulatory proteins, viz. the heterotrimeric G proteins. Point mutations in p21^{ras} can, in addition to over-expression of the native protein, lead to a loss of growth control and can transform cells to a malignant phenotype. The mutant ras protein shows impaired GTPase activity. Conversely, the GTPase activity of the native ras protein is increased over 100-fold by interaction with a 120 kDa protein called the GTPase activating protein (GAP). Transforming p21^{ras} are not activated by GAP. Therefore, the constitutive presence of the active form of a (p21^{ras}/GTP) complex provides a continuous signal for cell proliferation and oncogenic transformation.

Recent work has shown that the GAP and two GAP-associated proteins, p62 and p190 are phosphorylated on tyrosine and serine residues by PDGF and EGF (Molloy *et al.*, 1989; Ellis *et al.*, 1990; Kaplan *et al.*, 1990). The *N*-terminal half of GAP contains two *src* homology SH2 domains which are the site of interaction of PDGF and EGF receptors with GAP or its associated protein p62 (Anderson *et al.*, 1990; Moran *et al.*, 1990). As we have discussed previously, the transduction of the growth factor signals also involve the cytoskeletal elements, especially in the depolymerised state, conceivably because this allows the EGF receptors to dimerise and autophosphorylate. It is therefore of more than coincidental interest that the two SH2 domains are separated by a sequence resembling the SH3 domain which Lehto *et al.* (1988) identified in a number of cytoskeletal proteins, and this SH3-like sequence could conceivably control the flow of information by regulating the association of EGF and GAP/GAP-associated proteins with the cytoskeletal elements.

Oncogenes such as *src* and *ras* have previously been shown to affect the regulation of F-actin which is a major component of the cytoskeleton (Holme *et al.*, 1986; Marchisio *et al.*, 1987; Sistonen *et al.*, 1987). Sistonen *et al.* (1987) demonstrated that microinjection of $p21^{ras}$ modified both the amount and pattern of F-actin expression in NIH 3T3 cells. More pertinent to the subject of this discussion are the findings of De Vouge and Mukherjee (1992) that the transformation of rat kidney cells with v-K-*ras* resulted in enhanced expression of the S-100 family protein p9Ka, which is a rat homologue of the 18A2/mts1 protein (Barraclough *et al.*, 1984, 1990). This is compatible with the work from our research group described in the various preceding sections, which brings together the relationships between *18A2/hmts1* gene expression, EGF receptor status, and tubulin depolymerisation in the context of the invasive and metastatic behaviour of cancer cells.

We have argued that *18A2-mts1/h-mts1* and *nm23* genes are expressed in a coordinated fashion and have provided evidence that their pathways might converge and have also pointed out how the state of tubulin polymerisation might be affected in opposite directions by the two genes. The function of $p21^{ras}$ in signal transduction provides another site of action. As discussed above, *18A2-mts1/h-mts1* protein expression is enhanced by the *ras* oncogene, whereas *nm23/* NDP kinase has been postulated to phosphorylate GDP to GTP, which is involved in both microtubule polymerisation as well as in signal transduction.

Molecular mechanisms of regulation of metastasis by *18A2/mts1* gene and its homologues

An initial step in uncovering the molecular mechanisms of regulation of metastasis-related genes and differentiation inducing agents is to identify molecular targets downstream. The immediate–early response genes *fos/jun* are involved in the transduction of growth factor signals to the genetic material, and these may therefore be regarded as the most likely targets. Changes in the expression of these genes consequent upon exposure of cells to agents that enhance invasion and metastasis and to growth factors has been studied. C-*fos* expression is induced in response to a variety of growth factors and differentiation-inducing agents (Curran, 1988). The *fos* protein interacts with the protein encoded by c-*jun*, which is also an immediate–early response gene, to form the heterodimeric transcription factor AP1 (Angel *et al.*, 1988; Lamph *et al.*, 1988; Quantin and Breathnach, 1988; Rauscher *et al.*, 1988; Ryseck *et al.*, 1988).

It is now known that deregulation of signal transduction contributes significantly to the development and progression of tumours (Weinberg, 1985; Kahn and Graf, 1986; Reddy *et al.*, 1988). Since metastasis manifests itself in the later stages of tumour development, deregulation of certain elements of signal transduction systems involved in the regulation of metastasis-associated genes may play a crucial role in determining metastatic behaviour.

We have previously proposed a mechanism by which MSH and RA may control the regulation of the *18A2/mts1* and the *nm23* genes via activation or inactivation of the cAMP signal transduction pathway (Parker *et al.*, 1991). MSH is known to produce a rapid influx of Ca^{2+} ions across the cell membrane. Therefore, we have also investigated the effects of verapamil, which is a Ca^{2+} channel blocker (Atlas and Adler, 1981; Janis *et al.*, 1987), and thapsigargin, a sesquiterpene lactone, which increases intracellular Ca^{2+} levels (Takemura *et al.*, 1989; Thastrup *et al.*, 1989), on the expression of the metastasis-associated genes *18A2/mts1* and *nm23* in metastatic variants of the B16 murine melanoma. Since many components of the various signal transduction pathways may involve Ca^{2+}/calmodulin-dependent activation we have also investigated the effect of the calmodulin inhibitor W-7 on the expression of these genes (Parker and Sherbet, 1992b).

Work carried out by our research group has shown that treatment with MSH of the low metastatic F1 variant of the B16 murine melanoma increases expression of the 'dominant' metastasis-associated gene *18A2/mts1*. The proposed mechanism for this up-regulation is that MSH treatment increases cAMP levels inside the cell which, in turn, activate the protein kinase A (PKA) signal transduction pathway. This will produce a transient increase in the expression of the 'early response genes' c-*fos* (which contains a cAMP responsive element (CRE) in the promoter region of the gene) and *junB* (C Parker and GV Sherbet, personal communication), and since *18A2/mts1* is known to contain an AP1-like enhancer sequence in the 3′ region of the gene, this may result in its increased expression. Recent work carried out by our group has shown that treatment of the low metastatic F1 and highly metastatic ML8 variants of the B16 murine melanoma with the Ca^{2+} channel blocker verapamil and thapsigargin (which raises intracellular Ca^{2+} levels from intracellular stores), down-regulated both *18A2/mts1* and *nm23* expression (Parker and Sherbet, 1992b). From this it would appear that, while verapamil and thapsigargin have opposite effects on intracellular Ca^{2+} levels both agents reduce *18A2/mts1* and *nm23* expression. A possible explanation for these effects may be that verapamil and thapsigargin modulate the effects of Ca^{2+}/calmodulin-dependent protein kinases and phosphatases, which are involved in signal transduction. Furthermore, treatment of the F1 and ML8 cell variants with the calmodulin inhibitor W-7 was also found to down-regulate *18A2/mts1* and *nm23* expression implicating calmodulin in the Ca^{2+}-mediated signal transduction pathway and the subsequent regulation of these genes. The transcription-activating factor CREB (cAMP response element binding protein) has been shown to be phosphorylated by Ca^{2+}/calmodulin-dependent protein kinase (PKII) (Dash et al., 1991; Sheng et al., 1991). This will activate the early response gene fos which may in turn upregulate 18A2/mts1 expression. Contrary to this the phosphatases PP-2A and PP-2B, which are stimulated by Ca^{2+}/calmodulin, have been shown to dephosphorylate phosphatase inhibitor 1 (Klee and Cohen, 1988; Hubbard and Cohen 1989). Phosphatase inhibitor 1 has been shown to inhibit the activity of the phosphatase PP-1 (Huang and Glinsmann, 1976; Hemmings et al., 1984; Stralfors et al., 1985). The inactivation of phosphatase inhibitor 1 by PP-2A and PP-2B may allow phosphatase PP-1 to dephosphorylate CREB thereby rendering it inactive. Phosphatase inhibitor 1 is also a substrate for calcineurin, a Ca^{2+}/calmodulin-dependent phosphatase. Since calcineurin is reported to have 100–1000 times greater affinity for calmodulin than PKII it will be preferentially activated when the Ca^{2+} level is relatively low (e.g. those levels resulting from release of calcium from intracellular stores) (Klee, 1991).

There is ample evidence suggesting that Ca^{2+} influx and release from intracellular stores have independent roles (Haverstick et al., 1991). It has also been suggested that low levels of intracellular Ca^{2+} (in the low micromolar range) inhibit the activity of adenylate cyclase (AC) in contrast to calmodulin stimulation of AC, possibly mediated by Ca^{2+} influx (Cooper, 1991). Therefore, it may be postulated that the release of Ca^{2+} from intracellular stores may activate specific components of the signal transduction pathways involved in gene regulation, e.g. via the activation of Ca^{2+}/calmodulin-dependent phosphatases PP-2B and calcineurin, whereas altering Ca^{2+} influx into the cell may modulate Ca^{2+}/calmodulin-dependent phosphorylation of CREB. Thus, there may be two mechanisms by which alterations in the intracellular Ca^{2+} might down-regulate the expression of the 18A2/mts1 gene. With nm23 expression it may also be the case that Ca^{2+}/calmodulin-dependent protein phosphatases and kinases are involved in modulating the activity of specific transcription-activating factors (Figure 21, see page 208).

Interestingly, contrary to what might be expected, verapamil and thapsigargin reduced nm23 expression (nm23 has been described as a metastasis suppressor gene) in the low metastatic F1 variant, but there was no corresponding increase in lung colonisation. In addition, 18A2/mts1 expression (18A2/mts1 augments metastasis) was found to be reduced, along with nm23 expression in the highly metastatic ML8 cell variant but again there was no corresponding change in lung colonisation (Parker and Sherbet, 1992b) (Figure 20, page 199). As mentioned above, it is only after treatment of the ML8 cells with RA, which caused an increase in the ratio of nm23 : 18A2/mts1, that a corresponding reduction in lung colonisation was seen. These observations support the thesis that the metastatic phenotype may be determined by the relative expression of both nm23 and mts1 and not by either gene individually.

By general reckoning, murine 18A2/mts1, with its homologues, may be a candidate metastasis gene. The ubiquitous expression of the gene in normal proliferating tissues and its ability to drive the cell into the S-phase, together with its apparent involvement and participation in the

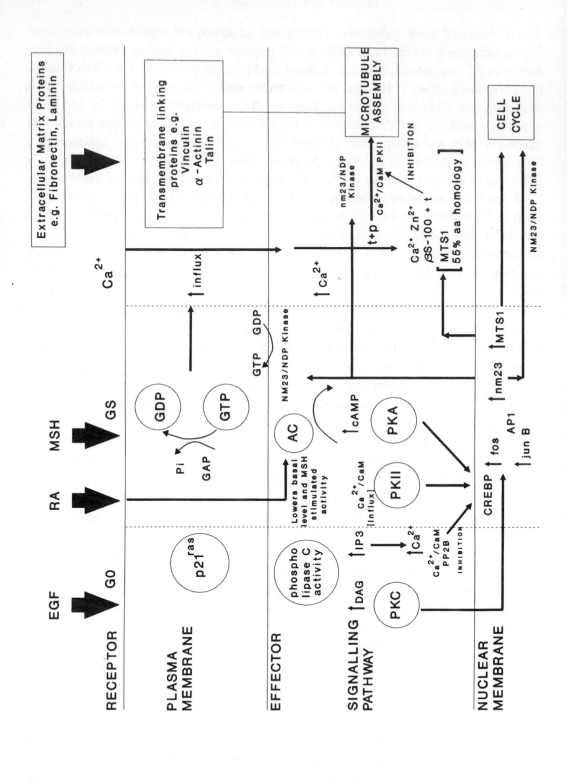

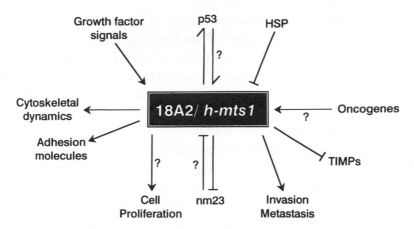

Figure 22.   This figure summarises the wide spectrum of biological functions in which the *18A2/h-mts1* gene appears to participate. The gene is strongly implicated in the progression of the cell cycle by sequestering p53. The promoter region of the murine *18A2/mts1* and its human homologue contain motifs with sequence similarity to the consensus p53-binding site derived by El-Deiry *et al.* (1992). The illustration also shows its possible involvement in a cell cycle indicated by its down-regulation by heat shock, together with the induction of HSP28 which is known to inhibit cell proliferation. The expression of *18A2/mts1* has profound effect on cytoskeletal dynamics and this may be the property which relates it closely with growth factor signal transduction as well as cell deformability and consequent acquisition of invasive potential. Invasive behaviour of cancer cells may be modified by the 18A2/mts1 protein and this is suggested by its apparent ability to down-regulate TIMPs. Invasive behaviour also may be affected by the changes in the lateral mobility of membrane receptors brought about by the alterations in the cytoskeletal organisation.

transduction of growth factor signals, clearly suggests that the *mts1* gene product subserves several physiological functions. However, the most exciting feature of the function of the *18A2-mts1/h-mts1* gene product is its apparent versatility in participation in cell motility and therefrom it derives a function in metastatic progression of cancer. It seems to participate in cell cycle regulation and cellular responses to growth factors (Figure 22). Whether the *18A2-mts1/h-mts1* gene is a metastasis-associated gene or a candidate metastasis gene is unimportant *per se*. Possibly, the multifarious functions of the protein confer the invasive and metastatic

Figure 21. (On facing page)   Postulated pathways of regulation of expression of *18A2/mts1* gene by growth factor and differentiation signals and how expression of *18A2/mt1* and *nm23* genes might inter-relate in altering the cytoskeletal dynamics and progression of the cell cycle. Figure constructed in consultation with Dr C. Parker.

properties on cells which have undergone the early stages of transformation, or there may be enhanced expression of the gene following cell transformation. Retroviral long terminal repeats (LTRs) have been shown to activate its transcription *in vitro* (Tarabykina *et al.*, 1996). LTR-mediated transcription of the gene has not been demonstrated *in vivo* but, in the light of the viral aetiology of some forms of cancer, this cannot be ruled out. Together with its ability to influence the cell cycle, albeit indirectly, and to modify the ability of the tumour cell to respond to extracellular proliferative signals, the 18A2/mts1 protein could be aiding the process of cancer progression. By the definition by Zachary and Rozengurt (1992) that 'exciting develop-ments in biology often occur as a result of the discovery that a given protein plays a fundamental role in diverse aspects of cell function', the *18A2/mts1* and related proteins may indeed provide an exciting prospect for the understanding of some basic features of cell invasion and cell cycle control in metastatic progression of cancer and enhance also the prospect of successful cancer therapy.

Epilogue

The basic features that characterise tumour development and its secondary spread were recognised many years ago and this is amply testified by the definitions of a tumour as 'an abnormal mass of tissue, the growth of which exceeds and is unco-ordinated with that of normal tissue, and persists in the same excessive manner after the cessation of the stimuli which evoked the change' (Willis, 1967). Quite transparently, this definition subsumes a heritable change, and over the years the question has been consistently posed whether there are identifiable genetic determinants involved in tumour development and progression. Willis (1934) had earlier provided a succinct and accurate description of metastatic tumour by stating that 'only those growths which are not continuous with the primary growth but have arisen from detached transported fragments of that tumour are entitled to be called metastases'. Here we have focused on genetic mechanisms involved in the invasive and metastatic behaviour of cancers, at the various levels in the cascade of metastatic spread, with special reference to a panoply of genes which are differentially expressed in normal tissues and their corresponding neoplastic counterparts and which markedly influence tumour growth and progression. A wide spectrum of biological processes are implicated in the pathogenesis, progression and prognosis of cancer. This book represents an attempt to gain insights into the deregulation of the cell cycle in tumour development and the functions of tumour suppressor genes, oncogenes and metastasis-associated genes in the clonal evolution of the invasive and metastatic phenotype, leading to the pathogenesis and progression of cancer.

Tumour evolution may be associated with increased genetic instability which could lead to the emergence of variant cell types which have more aggressive properties. Spontaneous mutation rates are known to be higher in cancer cells as compared with their non-malignant counterparts. A faster growth rate coupled with high rates of production of malignant cells may be expected to lead to the pathogenesis of highly aggressive primary cancer. This crucial relationship between tumour cell proliferation and secondary spread, not highlighted hitherto, concerns genes which are implicated both in cell proliferation and metastasis. Cancer has aptly been described as a disease of cell proliferation, and the deregulation of cell proliferation in tumour development, invasion and progression to the metastatic state, is given due cognisance, the major themes being the cell cycle control genes, e.g. *p53* and *rb*, and appropriately also, their downstream target genes. The proteins encoded by these suppressor genes can form complexes with other gene products and the concept has therefore arisen that there may be regulatory loops of gene function. Possibly sequestration of some of these suppresssor proteins and consequent abrogation of their functions, could lead to a loss of control over cell proliferation and apoptosis.

A pre-requisite of tumour dissemination is its neovascularisation. This process is extensively reviewed, both from the point of view of its induction and as a predictor of prognosis of cancer. There are several *dramatis personae* on the invasion stage, viz. genes coding for cell adhesion molecules and those encoding a range of proteases and their inhibitors. These contribute significantly to the invasive propensity of cancer cell and are powerful modulators of metastatic behaviour. A part of this book deals with the transduction of signals imparted by extraneous growth factors, the role of *ras* oncogene in this process, the involvement of cytoskeletal elements in signal transduction, and how signal transduction is modulated by genes such as *18A2/mts1* and *nm23* which affect the polymerisation of cytoskeletal elements, and have the potential to confer invasive properties.

Finally, there are several oncogenes and metastasis-associated genes which are differentially expressed between non-malignant tumours and their aggressive counterparts. Several genes which seriously affect the outcome of the disease have been identified, e.g. the APC and MCC genes, breast carcinoma suppressor genes, as well as the putative metastasis-suppressor *nm23* and the dominant S-100 family genes. Their biological function and the possible relationship between their expression and the progression of the disease have been the focus of considerable attention. Surprisingly, both *nm23* and the S-100 family genes may be related to the cell cycle. As we have seen the murine *18A2/mts1* and its human homologue *h-mts1*, a member of this gene family, appear to be able to control cell cycle progression as well as cancer invasion and metastasis. The latter influences may be attributable to the apparent ability of this gene to modulate the expression of some genes encoding adhesion factors and tumour cell-associated enzymes and their inhibitors, which are actively involved downstream in the metastatic cascade. These observations lead one often to ask whether there are also specific determinants for metastasis, i.e. are there candidate metastasis genes? The answer to this at the present is probably no. Admittedly there are several genes which can up-regulate both invasive and metastatic processes. But this may occur only in cells which have passed into the transformed state. Therefore these genes may not be metastasis genes *per se*, but only normal genes whose inappropriate expression can influence cell behaviour. Several features of invasive and metastasis-like behaviour may be encountered in normal embryonic development. It would be rewarding in various ways, not least to reinforce the preceding arguments, to see how the expression of these metastasis-associated genes relates to the cell behaviour in embryonal systems.

Continuing with the theme of cell proliferation in cancer: the initiation of DNA synthesis and mitosis are controlled by cyclin-dependent kinases and their inhibitors. Genes coding for cyclins have been named as proto-oncogenes and treatment of this topic forms an important part of the book. Many of their functions are intricately related to the functioning of the tumour suppressor gene *p53*. The latter is able to induce a powerful cyclin-dependent kinase inhibitor. The so-called multiple tumour suppressor gene $p16^{ink4}$ has been an important component of this discussion, since its product is also a cyclin-dependent kinase inhibitor. The retinoblastoma-susceptibility gene *rb* is another gene involved with cell cycle progression. All these genes show a range of abnormalities in a variety of human cancers. Thus we have attempted, and hopefully achieved here, a conceptual as well as a factual synthesis of the biological processes of invasion, proliferation, and metastasis, by linking the biological processes of cancer invasion and secondary spread with cell proliferation and its deregulation.

References

Aaltonen LA, Peltomaki P, Leach FS, Sistonen P, Pylkkanen L, Mecklin JP, Jarvinen H, Powell SM, Jen J, Hamilton SR, Peterson GM, Kinzler KW, Vogelstein B, De la Chapelle A (1993). Clues to the pathogenesis of familial colorectal cancer. *Science* **260**, 812-816.

Abbinantenissen JM, Simpson LG, Leikauf GD (1995). Corticosteroids increase secretory leukocyte protease inhibitor transcript levels in airway epithelial cells. *Amer J Physiol* **12**, L601-L606.

Abe T, Kobayashi N, Yoshimura K, Trapnell BC, Kim H, Hubbard RC, Brewer MT, Thompson RC, Crystal RG (1991). Expression of the secretory leukoprotease inhibitor gene in epithelial cells. *J Clin Invest* **87**, 2207-2215.

Abraham JA, Whang JL, Tumolo A, Mergia A, Fiddes JC (1986). Human basic fibroblast growth factor. Nucleotide sequence, genomic organisation and expression in mammalian cells. *Cold Spring Harb Symp Quant Biol* **51**, 657-668.

Abrahamson M, Barrett AJ, Salvesen G, Grubb A (1986). Isolation of six cysteine proteinase inhibitors from human urine. Their physico-chemical and enzyme kinetic properties and concentrations. *J Biol Chem* **261**, 11282-11289.

Adachi J, Shiseki M, Okazaki T, Ishimaru G, Noguchi M, Hirohashi S, Yokota J (1995). Microsatellite instability in primary and metastatic lung carcinomas. *Genes Chrom Cancer* **14**, 301-306.

Adamson MC, Dennis C, Delaney S, Christiansen J, Monkley S, Kozak CA, Wainwright B (1994). Isolation and genetic mapping of two novel members of the murine wnt gene family, wnt-11 and wnt-12, and the mapping of wnt-5a and wnt-7a. *Genomics* **24**, 9-13.

Addison C, Jenkins JR, Sturzbecher HW (1990). The p53 nuclear localisation signal is structurally linked to a p34 cdc2 kinase motif. *Oncogene* **5**, 423-426.

Adenis A, Huet G, Zerimech F, Hecquet B, Balduyck M, Peyrat JP (1995). Cathepsin B, cathepsin L, and cathepsin D activities in colorectal carcinomas. Relationship with clinicopathological parameters. *Cancer Lett* **96**, 267-275.

Adler RR, Brenner CA, Werb Z (1990). Expression of extracellular matrix degrading metalloproteinases and metalloproteinase inhibitors is developmentally regulated during endoderm differentiation of embryonal carcinoma cells. *Development* **110**, 211-220.

Adnane J, Gaudray P, Simon MP, Simony-Lafontaine J, Jeanteur P, Theillet C (1989). Proto-oncogene amplification and human breast tumour phenotype. *Oncogene* **4**, 1389-1395.

Agoff SN, Hou J, Linzer DIH, Wu B (1993). Regulation of the human HSP70 promoter. *Science* **259**, 84-87.

Aguilar-Santelises M, Rottenberg ME, Lewin N, Mellstedt H, Jondal M (1996). Bcl-2, bax and p53 expression in B-CLL in relation to *in vitro* survival and clinical progression. *Int J Cancer* **69**, 114-119.

Ahuja H, Bar-Eli M, Advani SH, Benchimol S, Cline MJ (1989). Alterations in the p53 gene and the clonal evolution of the blast crisis of chronic myelogenous leukaemia. *Proc Natl Acad Sci USA* **86**, 6783-6787.

Aihara M, Scardino PT, Truong LD, Wheeler TM, Goad JR, Yang G, Thompson TC (1995). The frequency of apoptosis correlates with the prognosis of Gleason grade 3 adenocarcinoma of the prostate. *Cancer* **75**, 522-529.

Akagi T, Kondo E, Yoshino T (1994). Expression of bcl-2 protein and bcl-2 mRNA in normal and neoplastic lymphoid tissues. *Leuk Lymph* **13**, 81-87.

Albertazzi E, Cajone F, Leone BE, Lakshmi MS, Sherbet GV (1996). Expression of metastasis associated *18A2/mts1* and *nm23* genes in human breast cancer: Relationship to nodal spread, oestrogen/progesterone receptor status and differentiation. *Proc 9th Int Conf Develop Diff Cancer*, Pisa, Italy, p. 153.

Alberts B, Bray D, Lewis J, Raff M, Roberts K, Watson JD (1983). *Molecular Biology of the Cell*. Garland Publ Co, New York, pp. 471-472.

Albini A, Iwamoto Y, Kleinman HK, Martin GR, Aaronson SA, Kozlowski JM, McEwan RN, Veilette A, Lippman ME (1987). A rapid *in vitro* assay for quantitating the invasive potential of tumour cells. *Cancer Res* **47**, 3239-3245.

Albini A, Melchiori A, Santi L, Liotta LA, Brown PD, Stetler-Stevenson WG (1991). Tumour cell invasion inhibited by TIMP-2. *J Natl Cancer Inst* **83**, 775-779.

Albino AP, Nanus DM, Mentle IR, Cordon-Cardo C, McNutt NS, Bressler J, Andreeff M (1989). Analysis of *ras* oncogenes in malignant melanoma and precursor lesions: correlation of point mutations with differentiation phenotype. *Oncogene* **4**, 1363-1374.

Albino AP, Sozzi G, Nanus D, Jhanwar SC, Houghton AN (1992). Malignant transformation of human melanocytes: induction of a complete melanoma phenotype and genotype. *Oncogene* **7**, 2315-2321.

Aldaz CM, Chen TP, Sahin A, Cunningham J, Bondy M (1995). Comparative allelotype of in situ and invasive human breast cancer. High frequency of microsatellite instability in lobular breast carcinomas. *Cancer Res* **55**, 3976-3981.

Alexander CM, Werb Z (1989). Proteinases and extracellular matrix remodelling. *Curr Opin Cell Biol* **1**, 974-982.

Alexander P (1984). The biology of metastases. *Cancer Topics* **4**, 116-117.

Algar EM, Kenney MT, Simms LA, Smith SI, Kida Y, Smith PJ (1995). Homozygous intragenic deletion in the wt1 gene in a sporadic Wilms' tumour associated with high levels of expression of a truncated transcript. *Human Mutation* **5**, 221-227.

Ali IU, Campbell G, Liberau R, Callahan R (1988). Amplification of c-erbB2 and aggressive breast tumours. *Science* **240**, 1795-1796.

Allen JI (1995). Molecular biology of colon polyps and colon cancer (1995). *Semin Surg Oncol* **11**, 399-405.

Allore R, O'Hanlon D, Proce R, Neilson K, Willord HF, Cox DR, Marks A, Dunn RJ (1988). Gene encoding the β subunit of S100 protein is on chromosome 21: Implications for Down's syndrome. *Science* **239**, 1311-1313.

Allore RJ, Friend WC, O'Hanlon D, Neilson KM, Baumal R, Dunn RJ, Marks A (1990). Cloning and expression of the human S100 beta gene. *J Biol Chem* **265**, 15537-15543.

Almasan A, Yin YX, Kelly RE, Lee EYHP, Bradley A, Li WW, Bertino JR, Wahl GM (1995). Deficiency of retinoblastoma protein leads to inappropriate S-phase entry, activation of E2F-responsive genes, and apoptosis. *Proc Natl Acad Sci USA* **92**, 5436-5440.

Alnemri ES, Fernandes TF, Haldar S, Croce CM, Litwack G (1992a). Involvement of bcl-2 in glucocorticoid-induced apoptosis of human pre-B-leukaemias. *Cancer Res* **52**, 491-495.

Alnemri ES, Robertson NM, Fernandes TF, Croce CM, Litwack G (1992b). Over-expressed full-length human Bcl-2 extends the survival of Baculovirus-infected SF9 insect cells. *Proc Natl Acad Sci USA* **89**, 7295-7299.

Ambartsumian N, Tarabykina S, Grigorian M, Tulchinsky E, Hulgaard E, Georgiev G, Lukanidin E (1995). Characterisation of two splice variants of metastasis-associated human *mts1* gene. *Gene* **159**, 125-130.

Ambros RA, Vigna PA, Figge J, Kallakury BVS, Mastrangelo, Eastman AY, Malfetano J, Figge HL, Ross JS (1994). Observations on tumour and metastatic suppressor gene status in endometrial carcinoma with particular emphasis on p53. *Cancer* **73**, 1686-1692.

Amin J, Ananthan J, Voellmy R (1988). Key features of the heat shock regulatory elements. *Mol Cell Biol* **8**, 3761-3769.

Amin KM, Litzky LA, Smythe WR, Mooney AM, Morris JM, Mews DJY, Pass HI, Kari C, Rodeck U, Rauscher FJ, Kaiser LR, Abdelda SM (1995). Wilms tumour 1 susceptibility (wt1) gene products are selectively expressed in malignant mesotheliomas. *Amer J Pathol* **146**, 344-356.

Anderson D, Koch CA, Grey L, Ellis C, Moran MF, Pawson T (1990). Binding of SH2 domains of phospholipase C$_\gamma$1, GAP and src to activated growth factor receptors. *Science* **250**, 979-982.

Andreassen A, Oyjord T, Hovig E, Florenes VA, Nesland JM, Myklebost O, Hoie J, Bruland OS, Borresen AL (1993). p53 abnormalities in different subtypes of human sarcomas. *Cancer Res* **53**, 468-471.

Angel P, Baumann I, Stein B, Delius H, Rahmsdorf HJ, Herrlich P (1987a). 12-O-tetradecanoly-phorbol-13-acetate induction of the human collagenase gene is mediated by an inducible enhancer element located in the 5' flanking region. *Mol Cell Biol* **7**, 2256-2266.

Angel P, Imagawa M, Chiu R, Stein B, Imbra R, Rahmsdorf HJ, Jonat C, Herrlich P, Karin M (1987b). Phorbol ester-inducible genes contain a common *cis* element recognised by a TPA-modulated *trans*-acting factor. *Cell* **49**, 729-739.

Angel P, Allegretto EA, Okino ST, Hattori K, Boyle WJ, Hunter T, Karim M (1988). Oncogene jun encodes a sequence-specific trans activator similar to AP1. *Nature* **332**, 166-171.

Anthoney DA, McIlwrath AJ, Gallagher WM, Edlin ARM, Brown R (1996). Microsatellite instability, apoptosis and loss of p53 function in drug-resistant tumour cells. *Cancer Res* **56**, 1374-1381.

Aprikian AG, Sarkis AS, Fair WR, Zhang ZF, Fuks Z, Cordon-Cardo C (1994). Immunohistochemical determination of p53 protein nuclear accumulation in prostatic adenocarcinoma. *J Urol* **151**, 1276-1280.

Armstrong JF, Pritchard-Jones K, Bickmore WA, Hastie ND, Bard JBL (1993). The expression of the Wilms tumour gene, *wt1*, in the developing mammalian embryo. *Mech Develop* **40**, 85-97.

Arnerlov C, Emdin SO, Lundgren B, Roos G, Soderstrom J, Bjersing L, Norgerg C, Angquist KA (1992). Mammographic growth rate, DNA ploidy, and S-phase fraction analysis in breast carcinoma. *Cancer* **70**, 1935-1942.

Arnold A, Kim HG, Gaz RD, Eddy RL, Fukushima Y, Byers MG, Shows TB, Kronenberg HM (1989). Molecular cloning and chromosomal mapping of DNA rearranged with the parathyroid hormone gene in a parathyroid adenoma. *J Clin Invest* **83**, 2034-2040.

Arnold A, Motokura T, Bloom T, Rosengerg C, Bale A, Kronenberg H, Ruderman J, Brown M, Kim HG (1992). PRAD1 (cyclin D1); A parathyroid neoplasia gene on 11q13. *Henry Ford Hosp Med J* **40**, 177-180.

Arregui CO, Carbonetto S, McKerracher L (1994). Characterisation of neural cell-adhesion sites. Point contacts are the sites of interaction between integrins and the cytoskeleton in PC12 cells. *J Neurosci* **14**, 6967-6977.

Arteaga CL, Hanauske AR, Clark GM, Osborne CK, Hazarika P, Pardue RL, Tio F, von Hoff DD (1988). Immunoreactive α-transforming growth factor activity in effusions from cancer patients as a marker of tumour burden and patient prognosis. *Cancer Res* **48**, 5203-5208.

Artuso M, Esteve A, Bresil H, Vuillaume M, Hall IJ (1995). The role of the ataxia telangiectasia gene in the p53, waf1/cip1 (p21)- and GADD45-mediated response to DNA damage produced by ionising radiation. *Oncogene* **11**, 1427-1435.

Aruffo A, Stamenkovic I, Melnick M, Underhill CB, Seed B (1990). CD44 is the principal cell surface receptor for hyaluronate. *Cell* **61**, 1303-1313.

Atkin NB, Baker MC (1986). Chromosome abnormalities as primary event in human malignant disease: Evidence from marker chromosomes. *J Natl Cancer Inst* **36**, 539-557.

Atlas D, Adler M (1981). α-Adrenergic antagonists as possible calcium channel inhibitors. *Proc Natl Acad Sci USA* **78**, 1237-1241.

Aubert C, Rouge F, Galindo JR (1980). Tumorigenicity of human malignant melanocytes in nude mice in relation to the differentiation in vitro. *J Natl Cancer Inst* **64**, 1029-1040.

Ausprunk DH, Folkman J (1977). Migration and proliferation of endothelial cells in preformed and newly formed blood vessels during tumour angiogenesis. *Microvas Res* **14**, 53065.

Ayhan A, Yasui W, Yukozaki H, Kitadai Y, Tahara E (1993). Reduced expression of nm23 protein is associated with advanced tumour stage and distant metastasis in human colorectal carcinomas. *Virchows Arch B* **63**, 213-218.

Baguley BC (1991). Cell cycling, cdc2, and cancer. *J Natl Cancer Inst* **83**, 896-898.

Bailly M, Bertrand S, Dore JF (1993). Increased spontaneous mutation rates and prevalence of karyotype abnormalities in highly metastatic human melanoma cell lines. *Melanoma Res* **3**, 51-61.

Baird P, Wadey R, Cowell J (1991). Loss of heterozygosity for chromosome 11p15 in Wilms tumours is not related to H-ras gene transforming mutations. *Oncogene* **6**, 1147-1149.

Baker RM, Brunette DM, Mankovitz R, Thompson LH, Whitmore GF, Siminovich L, Till JE (1974). Ouabain resistant mutants of mouse and hamster cells in culture. *Cell* **1**, 9-21.

Baker SJ, Fearon ER, Nigro JM, Hamilton SR, Preisinger AC, Jessup JM, Vantuinen P, Ledbetter DH, Barker DF, Nakamura Y, White R, Vogelstein B (1989). Chromosome 17 deletions and p53 gene mutations in colorectal carcinomas. *Science* **244**, 217-221.

Baker SJ, Preisinger AC, Jessup JM, Paraskeva C, Markowitz S, Wilson JKV, Hamilton S, Vogelstein B (1990a). p53 gene mutations occur in combination with 17p allelic deletions as late events in colorectal tumorigenesis. *Cancer Res* **50**, 7717-7722.

Baker SJ, Markowitz K, Fearon ER, Wilson JKV, Vogelstein B (1990b). Suppression of human colorectal carcinoma cell growth by wild type p53. *Science* **249**, 1912-1915.

Bakhshi A, Jensen JP, Goldman P, Wright JJ, McBride OW, Epstein AL, Korsmeyer SJ (1985). Cloning the chromosomal break point of t(14;18) human lymphomas. Clustering around J$_H$ on chromosome 14 and near a transcriptional unit of chromosome 18. *Cell* **41**, 899-906.

Balslev I, Christensen IJ, Rasmussen BB, Larsen JK, Lykkesfeldt AE, Thorpe SM, Rose C, Briand P, Mouridsen HT (1994). Flow cytometric DNA ploidy defines patients with poor prognosis in node-negative breast cancer. *Int J Cancer* **56**, 16-25.

Band V, De Caprio JA, Delmolino L, Kuleska V, Sager R (1991). Loss of p53 protein in human papillomavirus type 16 E6-immortalised human mammary epithelial cells. *J Virol* **65**, 6671-6676.

Bandara LR, Buck VM, Zamanian M, Johnston LH, La Thangue NB (1993). Functional synergy between DP-1 and E2F-1 in the cell cycle regulating transcription factor DRTF1/E2F. *EMBO J* **12**, 4317-4324.

Bandara LR, Lam EWF, Sorensen TS, Zamanian M, Girling R, La Thangue NB (1994). DP-1a: a cell cycle regulated and phosphorylated component of transcription factor DRTF1/E2F which is functionally important for recognition by pRb and the adenovirus E4 orf 6/7 protein. *EMBO J* **13**, 3104-3114.

Banerji SS, Theodorakis NG, Morimoto R (1984). Heat shock induced translational control of HSP70 and globin synthesis in chicken reticulocytes. *Mol Cell Biol* **4**, 2437-2448.

Banks RE, Gearing AJH, Hemingway IK, Norfolk DR, Perren TJ, Selby PJ (1993). Circulating intercellular adhesion molecule-1 (ICAM-1), E-selectin and vascular cell adhesion molecule (VCAM-1) in human malignancies. *Br J Cancer* **68**, 122-124.

Barak Y, Juven T, Haffner R, Oren M (1993). mdm2 expression is induced by wild type p53 activity. *EMBO J* **12**, 461-468.

Barak Y, Gottlieb E, Juven-Gershon T, Oren M (1994). Regulation of mdm2 expression by p53: Alternative promoters produce transcripts with nonidentical translation potential. *Genes Develop* **8**, 1739-1749.

Barboule N, Mazars P, Baldin V, Vidal S, Jozan S, Martel P, Valette A (1995). Expression of p21 (waf1/cip1) is heterogeneous and unrelated to proliferation index in human ovarian carcinoma. *Int J Cancer* **63**, 611-615.

Bardeesy N, Falkoff D, Petruzzi MJ, Nowak N, Zabel B, Adam M, Aguiar MC, Grundy P, Shows T, Pelletier J (1994). Anaplastic Wilms' tumour, a subtype displaying poor prognosis, harbours p53 gene mutations. *Nature Genet* **7**, 91-97.

Bargmann CI, Weinberg RA (1988). Increased tyrosine kinase activity associated with the protein encoded by the activated neu oncogene. *Proc Natl Acad Sci USA* **85**, 5394-5398.

Bargmann CI, Hung MC, Weinberg RA (1986a). The neu oncogene encodes an epidermal growth factor receptor-related protein. *Nature* **319**, 226-230.

Bargmann CI, Hung MC, Weinberg RA (1986b). Multiple independent activations of neu oncogene by a point mutation altering the transmembrane domain of p185. *Cell* **45**, 649-657.

Bargonetti J, Friedman PN, Kern SE, Vogelstein B, Prives C (1991). Wild-type but not mutant p53 immunopurified proteins bind to sequences adjacent to the SV40 origin of replication. *Cell* **65**, 1083-1091.

Bargonetti J, Reynisdottir I, Friedman PN, Prives C (1992). Site-specific binding of wild-type p53 to cellular DNA is inhibited by SV40 T antigen and mutant p53. *Genes Develop* **6**, 1886-1898.

Bargonetti J, Manfredi JJ, Chen XB, Marshak DR, Prives C (1993). A proteolytic fragment from the central region of p53 has marked sequence-specific DNA binding activity when generated from wild-type but not from oncogenic mutant p53 protein. *Genes Develop* **7**, 2565-2574.

Bargou RC, Daniel PT, Mapara MY, Bommert K, Wagener C, Kallinich B, Royer HD, Dorken B (1995). Expression of the blc-2 gene family in normal and malignant breast tissue. Low bax-α expression in tumour cells correlates with resistance to apoptosis. *Int J Cancer* **60**, 854-859.

Barletta C, Scillato F, Sega FM, Mannella E (1993). Genetic alteration in gastrointestinal cancer. A molecular and cytogenetic study. *Anticancer Res* **13**, 2325-2329.

Barnes R, Masood S, Barker E, Rosengard AM, Coggin DL, Crowell T, King CR, Porter-Jordan K, Wargotz ES, Liotta LA, Steeg PS (1991). Low nm23 protein expression in infiltrating ductal breast carcinomas correlates with reduced patient survival. *Amer J Path* **139** 245-250.

Barraclough R, Kimbell R, Rudland PS (1984). Increased abundance of a normal mRNA sequence accompanying conversion of mammary cuboidal epithelial cells to elongated myoepithelial-like cells in culture. *Nucl Acids Res* **21**, 8097-8114.

Barraclough R, Gibbs F, Smith JA, Haynes GA, Rudland PS (1990). Calcium ion binding by the potential calcium binding protein, p9Ka. *Biochem Biophys Res Commun* **169**, 660-666.

Barras LW, McMahon AP (1995). Biochemical analysis of murine wnt proteins reveals both shared and distinct properties. *Exp Cell Res* **220**, 363-373.

Barrett AJ (1984). Proteolytic and other metabolic pathways in lysosomes. *Biochem Soc Trans* **12**, 899-904.

Barrett AJ (1987). The cystatins: a new class of peptidase inhibitors. *Trends Biochem Sci* **12**, 193-196.

Barrett AJ, Kirschke H (1981). Cathepsin B, cathepsin H, cathepsin L. *Methods Enzymol* **80**, 535-561.

Barrett AJ, Fritz H, Grubb A, Isemura S, Jarvinen M, Katunuma N, Machleidt W, Muller-Esterl W, Sasaki M, Turk V (1986a). Nomenclature and classification of the proteins homologous with the cysteine proteinase inhibitor chicken cystatin. *Biochem J* **236**, 312.

Barrett AJ, Rawlings, ND, Davies ME, Machleidt W, Salvesen G, Turk V (1986b). Cysteine proteinase inhibitors of the cystatin superfamily. In: *Proteinase Inhibitors*, Barrett AJ, Salvesen G (eds). Elsevier, Amsterdam, pp. 489-513.

Bartek J, Bartkova J, Vojtesek B, Staskova Z, Rejthar A, Kdovarik J, Midgley CA, Gannon JV, Lane DP (1991). Aberrant expression of the p53 oncoprotein is a common feature of a wide spectrum of human malignancies. *Oncogene* **6**, 1699-1703.

Bartkova J, Bartek J, Lukas J, Vojtesek B, Staskova Z, Rejthar A, Kovarik J, Midgley CA, Lane DP (1991). p53 protein alterations in human testicular cancer including preinvasive intratubular germ cell neoplasia. *Int J Cancer* **49**, 196-202.

Bartkova J, Lukas J, Strauss M, Bartek J (1994a). The PRAD-1 cyclin D1 oncogene product accumulates aberrantly in a subset of colorectal carcinomas. *Int J Cancer* **4**, 568-573.

Bartkova J, Lukas J, Muller H, Lutzhoft D, Strauss M, Bartek J (1994b). Cyclin D1 protein expression and function in human breast cancer. *Int J Cancer* **57**, 353-361.

Barton CM, McKie AB, Hogg A, Bia B, Elia G, Phillips SMA, Ding SF, Lemoine NR (1995). Abnormalities of the RB1 and DCC tumour suppressor genes. Uncommon in human pancreatic adenocarcinoma. *Mol Carcinogen* **13**, 61-69.

Bashkin P, Doctrow S, Klagsbrun M, Svahn CM, Folkman J, Vlodavsky I (1989). Basic fibroblast growth factor binds to subendothelial extracellular matrix and is released by heparinase and heparin-like molecules. *Biochemistry* **28**, 1737-1743.

Basset P, Bellocq JP, Wolf C, Stoll I, Hutin P, Limacher JM, Podhajeer OL, Chenard MP, Rio MC, Chambon P (1990). A novel metalloproteinase gene specifically expressed in stromal cells of breast carcinomas. *Nature* **348**, 699-704.

Basset P, Wolf C, Chambon P (1993). Expression of the stromelysin-3 gene in fibroblastic cells of invasive carcinomas of the breast and other tissues. *Breast Cancer Res Treat* **24**, 185-193.

Battaglia F, Scambia G, Rossi S, Panici PB, Ballantrone R, Polizzi G, Querzoli P, Negrini R, Iacobelli S, Crucitti F, Mancuso S (1988). Epidermal growth factor receptor in human breast cancer: correlation with steroid hormone receptors and axillary lymph node involvement. *Eur J Cancer Clin Oncol* **24**, 1685-1690.

Baudier J, Cole RD (1988). Interaction between microtubule associated proteins and S100b regulate phosphorylation by Ca^{2+}/calmodulin dependent protein kinase II. *J Biol Chem* **263**, 5876-5883.

Baudier J, Briving C, Deinum J, Haglid K, Sorskog L, Wallin M (1982). Effects of S100 protein and calmodulin on Ca^{2+} induced disassembly of brain microtubule proteins *in vitro*. *FEBS Lett* **147**, 165-167.

Baudier J, Delphin C, Grunwald D, Khochbin S, Lawrence JJ (1992). Characterisation of the tumour suppressor protein p53 as a protein kinase C substrate and S100b binding protein. *Proc Natl Acad Sci USA* **89**, 11627-11631.

Bauer EA, Cooper TW, Huang JS, Altman J, Deuel TF (1985). Stimulation of *in vitro* human skin collagenase expression by platelet derived growth factor. *Proc Natl Acad Sci USA* **82**, 4132-4136.

Bauer J, Margolis M, Schreiner C, Edgell CJ, Azizkhan J, Lazarowski E, Juliano RL (1992). *In vitro* model of angiogenesis using a human endothelium-derived permanent cell line: contributions of induced gene expression, G-proteins, and integrins. *J Cell Physiol* **153**, 437-449.

Bauknecht T, Runge M, Schwall M, Pfleiderer A (1988). Occurrence of epidermal growth factor receptors in human adnexal tumours and their prognostic value in advanced ovarian carcinomas. *Gynecol Oncol* **29**, 147-157.

Bayle LH, Elenbaas B, Levine AJ (1995). The carboxyl-terminal domain of the p53 protein regulates sequence-specific DNA binding through its non-specific nucleic acid-binding activity. *Proc Natl Acad Sci USA* **92**, 5729-5733.

Becker KF, Atkinson MJ, Reich U, Becker I, Nekarda H, Siewert JR, Hofler H (1994). E-cadherin gene mutations provide clues to diffuse type gastric carcinomas. *Cancer Res* **54**, 3845-3852.

Behrendt T, Ronne E, Dano K (1995). The structure and function of the urokinase receptor, a membrane protein governing plasminogen activation on the cell surface. *Biol Chem Hoppe-Seyler* **376**, 269-279.

Behrens J, Mareel MM, Van RF, Birchmeier W (1989). Dissecting tumour cell invasion: epithelial cells acquire invasive properties after the loss of uvomorulin-mediated cell-cell adhesion. *J Cell Biol* **108**, 2435-2447.

Bell SM, Scott N, Cross D, Sagar P, Lewis FA, Blair GE, Taylor GR, Dixon MF, Quirke P (1993). Prognostic value of p53 over-expression and c-Ki-*ras* gene mutations in colorectal cancer. *Gastroenterol* **104**, 57-64.

Bello MJ, Decampos JM, Kusak ME, Vaquero L, Sarasa JL, Pestana A, Rey JA (1994). Molecular analysis of genomic abnormalities in human gliomas. *Cancer Genet Cytogenet* **73**, 122-129.

Belmont LD, Mitchison TJ (1996). Identification of a protein that interacts with tubulin dimers and increases the catastrophe rate of microtubules. *Cell* **84**, 623-631.

Benchimole S, Pim D, Crawford L (1982). Immunoassay of the cellular protein p53 in mouse and human cell lines. *EMBO J* **1**, 1055-1062.

Benchimole S, Lamb P, Crawford LV, Sheer D, Shows TB, Bruns GA, Peacock J (1985). Transformation associated p53 protein is encoded by a gene on human chromosome 17. *Somatic Cell Mol Genet* **11**, 505-509.

Benitez-Bribiesca L, Martinez G, Ruiz MT, Guttierez-Delgado F, Utrera D (1995). Proteinase activity in invasive cancer of the breast. Correlation with tumour progression. *Arch Med Res* **26**, S163-S168.

Bennett D, Dexter TJ, Ormerod EJ, Hart IR (1986). Increased experimental metastatic capacity of a murine melanoma following induction of differentiation. *Cancer Res* **46**, 3239-3244.

Bennett WP, Hollstein MC, Metcalf RA, Welsh JA, He A, Zhu SM, Kusters I, Resau JH, Trump BF, Lane DP, Harris CC (1992). P53 mutation and protein accumulation during multistage human esophageal carcinogenesis. *Cancer Res* **52**, 6092-6097.

Bensaude O, Morange M (1983). Spontaneous high expression of heat shock protein in mouse embryonal carcinoma cells and ectoderm from day 8 mouse embryo. *EMBO J* **2**, 173-177.

Bensaude O, Babinet C, Morange M, Jacob F (1983). Heat shock proteins, first major products of zygotic gene activity in mouse embryo. *Nature* **305**, 331-333.

Bepler G, Garciablanco MA (1994). Three tumour suppressor regions on chromosome 11p identified by high resolution deletion mapping in human non-small cell lung cancer. *Proc Natl Acad Sci USA* **91**, 5513-5517.

Berchuck A, Kamel A, Whitaker R, Kerns R, Olt G, Kinney R, Soper JT, Dodge R, Clarke-Pearson DL, Marks P, McKenzie S, Yin S, Bast RC, Jr (1990). Over-expression of HER-2/*neu* is associated with poor survival in advanced epithelial ovarian cancer. *Cancer Res* **50**, 4087–4091.

Berchuck A, Rodriguez G, Kinney RB, Soper JT, Dodge RK, Clarke-Pearson DL, Bast RC, Jr (1991a). Over-expression of HER-2/*neu* in endometrial cancer is associated with advanced stage disease. *Amer J Gynecol* **164**, 15–21.

Berchuck A, Rodriguez GC, Kamel A, Dodge RK, Soper JT, Clarke-Pearson DL, Bast RC, Jr (1991b). Epidermal growth factor receptor expression in normal ovarian epithelium and ovarian cancer. I. Correlation of receptor expression with prognostic factors in patients with ovarian cancer. *Amer J Obstet Gynecol* **164**, 669–674.

Berchuck A, Kohler MF, Marks JR, Wiseman R, Boyd J, Bast RC, Jr (1994). The p53 tumour suppressor gene frequently is altered in gynaecologic cancers. *Am J Obstet Gynecol* **170**, 246–252.

Beretta L, Dubois MF, Sobel A, Bensadue O (1995). Stathmin is a major substrate for mitogen-activated protein kinase during heat shock and chemical stress in HeLa cells. *Eur J Biochem* **227**, 388–395.

Berg EL, Goldstein LA, Jutila MA, Nakache M, Picker LJ, Streeter PR, Wu NW, Zhou D, Butcher EC (1989). Homing receptors and vascular addressins: cell adhesion molecules that direct lymphocyte traffic. *Immunol Rev* **108**, 5–18.

Berges RR, Furuya Y, Remington L, English HF, Jacks T, Isaacs JT (1993). Cell proliferation, DNA repair, and p53 function are not required for programmed death of prostatic glandular cells induced by androgen ablation. *Proc Natl Acad Sci USA* **90**, 8910–8914.

Bergthorsson JT, Egilsson V, Gudmundsson J, Arason A, Ingvarsson S (1995). Identification of a breast tumour with microsatellite instability in a potential carrier of the hereditary non-polyposis colon cancer trait. *Clin Genet* **47**, 305–310.

Berk AJ, Yew Pr (1992). Inhibition of p53 transactivation required for transformation by adenovirus early 1B protein. *Nature* **57**, 82–85.

Bernacki RJ, Bosmann BH (1972). Red cell hydrolase. II: Proteinase activities in human erythrocyte plasma membranes. *J Memb Biol* **7**, 1–14.

Bernal SD, Chen LB (1982). Induction of cytoskeleton-associated proteins during differentiation of human myeloid leukaemic cell lines. *Cancer Res* **42**, 5106–5116.

Bernal SD, Stahel RA (1985). Cytoskeleton associated proteins: their role as cellular integrators in the neoplastic process. *CRC Crit Rev Oncol Hematol* **3**, 191–204.

Bernhard EJ, Hagner B, Wong C, Lubenski I, Muschel RJ (1995). The effect of E1A transfection on MMP-9 expresssion and metastatic potential. *Int J Cancer* **60**, 718–724.

Bertrand S, Bailly M, Nguyen MJ, Dore JF (1991). Cytogenetic characterisation of human melanoma metastatic variants in immunosuppressed newborn rats: role of chromosome 7 and double minute (DM). *Clin Exp Metastasis* **8** (Suppl. 1), 35.

Berx G, Staes K, Van Hen Hengel J, Molemans F, Bussemakers MJG, van Bokhoven A, van Roy F (1995a). Cloning and characterisation of the human invasion suppressor gene E-cadherin (CDH-1). *Genomics* **26**, 281–289.

Berx G, Clenton-Janson AM, Nollet F, De Leeuw WJF, van de Vijver MJ, Cornelisse C, van Roy F (1995b). E-cadherin is a tumour invasion suppressor gene mutated in human lobular breast cancers. *EMBO J* **14**, 6107–6115.

Beutler E, Collins Z, Irwin LE (1967). Value of genetic variants of glucose-6-phosphate dehydrogenase in tracing the origin of malignant tumours. *N Engl J Med* **276**, 389–391.

Bevilacqua MP, Pober JS, Mendrick DL, Cotran RS, Gimbrone MA (1987). Identification of an inducible endothelial leukocyte adhesion molecule. *Proc Natl Acad Sci USA* **84**, 9238–9242.

Bevilacqua MP, Stengelin S, Gimbrone MA, Seed B (1989). Endothelial leukocyte adhesion molecule-1. An inducible receptor for neutrophils related to complement regulatory proteins and lectins. *Science* **243**, 1160-1165.

Bevilacqua G, Sobel ME, Liotta LA, Steeg PA (1989). Association of low nm23 RNA levels in human primary infiltrating ductal breast carcinoma with lymph node involvement and other histopathological indicators of high metastatic potential. *Cancer Res* **49**, 5185-5190.

Bianchi E, Cohen RL, Thor AT, Todd RF, Mizukami IF, Lawrence DA, Ljung BM, Shuman MA, Smith HS (1994). The urokinase receptor is expressed in invasive breast cancer but not in normal breast tissue. *Cancer Res* **54**, 861-866.

Bianchi R, Pula G, Ceccarelli P, Gianbanco L, Donato R (1992). S-100 protein binds to annexin II and p11, the heavy and light chains of calpactin I. *Biochim Biophys Acta* **1160**, 67-75.

Bianchi R, Gianbanco I, Donato R (1993). S-100 protein, but not calmodulin, binds to the glial fibrillary acidic protein and inhibits its polymerisation in a Ca^{2+} dependent manner. *J Biol Chem* **268**, 12669-12674.

Bienz M (1984). Developmental control of the heat shock response in *Xenopus*. *Proc Natl Acad Sci USA* **81**, 3138-3142.

Biggs J, Hersperger E, Steeg PS, Liotta LA, Shearn A (1990). *Drosophila* gene that is homologous to a mamalian gene associated with tumour metastasis codes for a nucleoside diphosphate kinase. *Cell* **63**, 933-940.

Bischoff JR, Friedman PN, Marshak DR, Prives C, Beach D (1990). Human p53 is phosphorylated by p60-cdc2 and cyclin B-cdc2. *Proc Natl Acad Sci USA* **87**, 4766-4770.

Blasband A, Schryver B, Papkoff J (1992). The biochemical properties and transforming potential of human wnt-2 are similiar to wnt-1. *Oncogene* **7**, 153-161.

Bodmer WF, Bailey CJ, Bodmer J, Bussey HJR, Ellis A, Gorman P, Lucibell FC, Murday VA, Rider SH, Scambler P, Sheer D, Solomon E, Spurr NK (1987). Localisation of the gene for familial adenomatous polyposis on chromosome 5. *Nature* **328**, 614-616.

Bohm M, Totzeck B, Birchmeier W, Wieland I (1994). Differences of E-cadherin expression levels and patterns in primary and metastatic human lung cancer. *Clin Exp Metastasis* **12**, 55-62.

Boise LH, Gonzalez-Garcia M, Postema CE, Ding Y, Lindsten T, Turka LA, Mao XH, Nunez G, Thompson CB (1993). Bcl-x, a bcl-2 related gene that functions as a dominant regulator of apoptotic cell death. *Cell* **74**, 597-608.

Boise LH, McShan CL, Thompson CB (1996). Introduction of the cell survival gene bcl-x(L) improves the viability of CTLL-2 cells without affecting their IL-2 proliferative response. Implications for the development of bioassays. *J Immunol Methods* **191**, 143-148.

Bolla M, Chedin M, Souvignet C, Marron J, Arnould C, Chambaz E (1990). Estimation of epidermal growth factor receptor in 177 breast cancers: correlation with prognostic factors. *Breast Cancer Res Treat* **16**, 97-102.

Bonay M, Soler P, Riquet M, Battesti JP, Hance AJ, Tazi A (1994). Expression of heat shock protein in human lung and lung cancers. *Amer J Resp Cell Mol Biol* **10**, 453-461.

Bond U, Schlesinger MJ (1985). Ubiquitin is a heat shock protein in chicken embryo fibroblasts. *Mol Cell Biol* **5**, 949-956.

Bond U, Schlesinger MJ (1986). The chicken ubiquitin gene contains a heat shock promoter and expresses an unstable mRNA in heat shocked cells. *Mol Cell Biol* **6**, 4601-4610.

Bondy, CP, Wilson S, Chambers AF (1985). Experimental metastatic ability of H-*ras* transformed NIH 3T3 cells. *Cancer Res* **45**, 6005-6009.

Bookstein R, Rio P, Madreperla SA, Hong F, Allred C, Grizzle WE, Lee WH (1990a). Promoter deletion and loss of retinoblastoma gene expression in human prostate carcinoma. *Proc Natl Acad Sci USA* **87**, 7762-7766.

Bookstein R, Shew JY, Chen PL, Scully P, Lee WH (1990b). Suppression of tumorigenicity of human prostate carcinoma cells by replacing a mutated *RB* gene. *Science* **247**, 712–715.

Borg, A, Tandon AK, Sigurdsson H, Clark GM, Ferno M, Fuqua AAW, Killander D, MacGuire WL (1990). HER-2/neu amplification predicts poor survival in node positive breast cancer. *Cancer Res* **50**, 4332–4337.

Borrensen AL (1992). Oncogenesis in ovarian cancer. *Acta Obstet Gynecol* **71** (Suppl. 155), 25–30.

Borzillo GV, Endo K, Tsujimoto Y (1992). Bcl-2 confers growth and survival advantage to interleukin 7-dependent early pre-B cells, which become factor independent by a multistep process in culture. *Oncogene* **7**, 869–876.

Bos JL (1985). The *ras* family and human carcinogenesis. *Mutagenesis Res* **195**, 255–271.

Bos JL, Fearon ER, Hamilton SR, Verlaan-de Vries M, van Boom JH, van der Eb AJ, Vogelstein B (1987). Prevalence of *ras* gene mutations in human colorectal cancers. *Nature* **327**, 293–297.

Bosch F, Jares P, Campo E, Lopezguillermo A, Piris MA, Villamor N, Tassies D, Faffe ES, Monteserrat E, Rozman C, Cardesa A (1994). PRAD-1 cyclin D1 gene over-expression in chronic lymphoproliferative disorders. A highly specific marker of mantle cell lymphoma. *Blood* **84**, 2726–2732.

Bottini F, Maxxocco K, Abbondi T, Tonini GP (1994). Identification of an AP-1-like sequence in the promoter region of calcyclin, an S-100-like gene. Enhancement of binding during retinoic acid-induced neuroblastoma cell differentiation. *Neurosci Lett* **181**, 35–38.

Bouck N (1990). Tumour angiogenesis: the role of oncogenes and tumour suppressor genes. *Cancer Cells* **2**, 179–185.

Bourguignon LYW, Lokeshwar VB, Chen X, Kerrick WGL (1993). Hyaluronic acid-induced lymphocyte signal-transduction and HA receptor (GP85/CD44)-cytoskeleton interaction. *J Immunol* **151**, 6634–6644.

Boyd D, Florent G, Kim P, Brattain M (1988). Determination of the levels of urokinase and its receptor in human colon carcinoma cell lines. *Cancer Res* **48**, 3112–3116.

Boyd J, Takahashi H, Waggoner SE, Jones LA, Hajek RA, Wharton JT, Liu FS, Fujino T, Barrett JC, McLachlan JA (1996). Molecular genetic analysis of clear cell adenocarcinomas of the vagina and cervix associated and unassociated with diethylstilboestrol exposure in utero. *Cancer* **77**, 507–513.

Boyd M, Harris F, McFarnale R, Davidson HR, Black DM (1995). A human BRCA1 gene knockout. *Nature* **375**, 541–542.

Boyer JC, Thomas DC, Maher VM, McCormick JJ, Kunkel TA (1993). Fidelity of DNA replication by extracts of normal and malignantly transformed human cells. *Cancer Res* **53**, 3270–3275.

Boynton RF, Huang Y, Blount PL, Reid BJ, Raskind WH, Haggitt RC, Newkirk C, Resau JH, Yin J, McDaniel T, Meltzer SJ (1991). Frequent loss of heterozygosity at the retinoblastoma locus in human oesophageal cancers. *Cancer Res* **51**, 5766–5769.

Brabant G, Hoang-Vu C, Cetin Y, Dralle H, Scheumann G, Molne J, Hansson G, Jansson S, Ericson LE, Nilsson M (1993). E-cadherin: A differentiation marker in thyroid malignancies. *Cancer Res* **53**, 4987–4993.

Bracke ME, Charlier C, Bruyneel EA, Labit C, Mareel MM, Castronovo V (1994). Tamoxifen restores the E-cadherin function in human breast cancer MCF-7/6 cells and suppresses their invasive phenotype. *Cancer Res* **54**, 4607–4609.

Braddock PS, Hu DE, Fan TPD, Stratford IJ, Harris AL, Bicknell R (1994). A structure-activity analysis of antagonism of the growth factor and angiogenic activity of basic fibroblast growth factor by suramin and related polyanions. *Br J Cancer* **69**, 890–898.

Bradley RS, Brown AMC (1995). A soluble form of wnt-1 protein with mitogenic activity on mammary epithelial cells. *Mol Cell Biol* **15**, 4616-4622.

Bradley RS, Cowin P, Brown AMC (1993). Expression of wnt-1 in PC12 cells results in modulation of plakoglobin and E-cadherin and increased cellular adhesion. *J Cell Biol* **123**, 1857-1865.

Brady HJM, Salomons GS, Bobedijk RC, Berns AJM (1996). T-cells from bax-α transgenic mice show accelerated apoptosis in response to stimuli but do not show restored DNA damage-induced cell death in the absence of p53 (1996). *EMBO J* **15**, 1221-1230.

Braithwaite A, Nelson C, Skulimowski A, McGovern J, Pigott D, Jenkins J (1990). Transactivation of the p53 oncogene by E1a gene products. *Virology* **177**, 595-605.

Brattsand G, Marklund U, Nylander K, Roos G, Gullberg M (1994). Cell cycle regulated phosphorylation of oncoprotein-18 on ser16, ser25 and ser38. *Eur J Biochem* **220**, 359-368.

Braunhut SJ, Moses MA (1994). Retinoids modulate endothelial cell production of matrix-degrading proteinases and tissue inhibitors of metalloproteinases (TIMP). *J Biol Chem* **269**, 13472-13479.

Bregman MD, Abdel-Malek ZA, Meyskens FL, Jr (1985). Anchorage-independent growth of murine melanoma in serumless media is dependent on insulin or melanocyte stimulating hormone. *Exp Cell Res* **157**, 419-428.

Brem SS, Gullino PM, Medina D (1977). Angiogenesis: A marker for neoplastic transformation of mammary papillary hyperplasia. *Science* **195**, 880-882.

Brem SS, Jensen HM, Gullino PM (1978). Angiogenesis as a marker of preneoplastic lesions of the human breast. *Cancer* **41**, 239-244.

Brenner CA, Adler RR, Rappolee DA, Pedersen R, Werb Z (1989). Genes for extracellular matrix degrading metalloproteinases and their inhibitors, TIMP, are expressed during early mammalian development. *Genes Develop* **3**, 848-859.

Brenner DA, O'Hara M, Angel P, Chojkier M, Karin M (1989). Prolonged activation of *jun* and collagenase genes by tumour necrosis factor-alpha. *Nature* **337**, 661-663.

Brewster SF, Browne S, Brown KW (1994a). Somatic allelic loss at the DCC, APC, NM23-H1 and p53 tumour suppressor gene loci in human prostatic carcinoma. *J Urol* **151**, 1073-1077.

Brewster SF, Gingell JC, Browne S, Brown KW (1994b). Loss of heterozygosity on chromosome 18q is associated with muscle invasive transitional cell carcinoma of the bladder. *Br J Cancer* **70**, 697-700.

Brezicka FT, Olling S, Bergman B, Berggren H, Engstrom CP, Hammarstrom S, Holmgren J, Larsson S, Lindholm L (1992). Co-expression of ganglioside antigen FUC-GM1, neural cell adhesion molecule, carcinoembryonic antigen, and carbohydrate tumour associated antigen CA-50 in lung cancer. *Tumour Biol* **13**, 308-315.

Brieger J, Weidmann E, Fenchel K, Mitrou PS, Hoelzer D, Bergmann L (1994). The expression of the Wilms tumour gene in acute myelocytic leukaemias as a possible marker for leukaemic blast cells. *Leukaemia* **8**, 2138-2143.

Brinckerhoff CE (1987). Regulation of collagenase gene expression in synovial cells. *J Rheumatol* **14**, 61-63.

Brinckerhoff CE, Plucinska IM, Sheldon LA, O'Connor GT (1986). Half-life of synovial collagen-ase mRNA is modulated by phorbol myristate acetate but not by all-*trans* retinoic acid or dexamethasone. *Biochemistry* **25**, 6378-6384.

Bringuier PP, Umbas R, Schaafsma HE, Karthaus HFM, De Bruyne FMJ, Schalken JA (1993). Decreased E-cadherin immunoreactivity correlates with poor survival in patients with bladder tumours. *Cancer Res* **53**, 3241-3245.

Brogi E, Schatteman G, Wu T, Kim EA, Varticovski L, Keyt B, Isner JM (1996). Hypoxia-induced paracrine regulation of vascular endothelial growth factor receptor expression. *J Clin Invest* **97**, 469-476.

Bromme D, Okamoto K (1995). Human cathepsin 02, a novel cysteine protease highly expressed in osteoclastomas and ovary. Molecular cloning, sequencing and tissue distribution. *Biol Chem Hoppe-Seyler* **376**, 379-384.

Bronner CE, Baker SM, Morrison PT, Warren G, Smith LG, Lescoe MK, Kane M, Earabino C, Lipford J, Lindblom A, Tannergard P, Bollag RJ, Godwin AR, Ward DC, Nordenskjold M, Fischel R, Kolodner R, Liskay RM (1994). Mutation in the mismatch repair gene homologue hMLH1 is associated with hereditary non-polyposis colon cancer. *Nature* **368**, 258-261.

Bronner-Fraser M (1988). Distribution and function of tenascin during cranial neural crest development in the chick. *J Neuro Sci* **21**, 135-147.

Brooks PC, Clark RAF, Cheresh DA (1994). Requirement of vascular integrin $\alpha_v\beta_3$ for angiogenesis. *Science* **264**, 569-571.

Brouillet JP, Spyratos F, Hacene K, Fauque J, Freiss G, Dupont F, Maudelonde T, Rochefort H (1993). Immunoradiometric assay of pro-cathepsin D in breast cancer cytosol. Relative prognostic value versus total cathepsin D. *Eur J Cancer* **29A**, 1248-1251.

Browder LW, Pollock M, Heikkila JJ, Wilkes J, Wang T, Krone P, Ovsenek N, Kloc M (1987). Decay of the oocyte type heat shock response in *Xenopus laevis*. *Develop Biol* **124**, 191-199.

Bruening W, Gros P, Sato T, Stanmir J, Nakamura Y, Housman D, Pelletier J (1993). Analysis of the 11p13 Wilms tumour suppressor gene (wt1) in ovarian tumours. *Cancer Invest* **11**, 393-399.

Bruner JM, Saya H, Moser RP (1991). Immunocytochemical detection of p53 in human gliomas. *Modern Pathol* **4**, 671-674.

Brzin J, Popovic T, Turk V, Borchart U, Machleidt W (1984). Human cystatin, a new protein inhibitor of cysteine proteinases. *Biochem Biophys Res Commun* **118**, 103-109.

Buchkovich K, Duffy LA, Harlow E (1989). The retinoblastoma protein is phosphorylated during specific phases of the cell cycle. *Cell* **58**, 1097-1105.

Buckbinder L, Talbott R, Velascomiguel S, Takenaka I, Faha B, Seizinger BR, Kley N (1995). Induction of the growth inhibitor IGF-binding protein-3 by p53. *Nature* **377**, 646-649.

Buckley MF, Sweeney KJE, Hamilton JA, Sini RL, Manning DL, Nicholson RI, De Fazio A, Watts CKW, Musgrove EA, Sutherland RL (1993). Expression and amplification of cyclin genes in breast cancer. *Oncogene* **8**, 2127-2133.

Budihna M, Strojan P, Smid L, Skrk J, Vrhovec I, Zupevc A, Rudolf Z, Zargi M, Krasovec M, Svetic B, Kopitarjerala N, Kos J (1996). Prognostic value of cathepsin B, cathepsin H, cathepsin L, cathepsin D and their endogenous inhibitors stefin A and stefin B in head and neck carcinoma. *Biol Chem Hoppe-Seyler* **377**, 385-390.

Budnik A, Grewe M, Gyufko K, Krutmann J (1996). Analysis of the production of soluble ICAM-1 molecules by human cells. *Exp Hematol* **24**, 352-359.

Buo L, Lyberg T, Jorgensen L, Johansen HT, Aasen AO (1993). Location of plasminogen activator (PA) and PA inhibitor in human colorectal adenocarcinomas. *APMIS* **101**, 235-241.

Burgeson RE, Chiquet M, Deutzmann R, Ekblom P, Engel J, Kleinman HK, Martin GR, Meneguzzi G, Paulsson M, Sanes J, Timpl R, Tryggvason K, Yamada Y, Yurchenco PD (1994). A new nomenclature for the laminin. *Matrix Biol* **14**, 209-211.

Burks RT, Kessis TD, Cho KR, Hendrick L (1994). Microsatellite instability in endometrial carcinoma. *Oncogene* **9**, 1163-1166.

Burno DK, Fabian DF, Lefor AT (1996). ICAM-1 increases *in vitro* adhesion and cytotoxicity in a murine fibrosarcoma. *J Surg Res* **60**, 398-402.

Bussolino F, Di Renzo MF, Ziche M, Bocchietto E, Olivero M, Naldini L, Gaudino G, Tamagnone L, Coffer A, Comoglio PM (1992). Hepatocyte growth factor is a potent angiogenic factor which stimulates endothelial cell motility and growth. *J Cell Biol* **119**, 629-641.

Cahilly-Snyder L, Yang-Feng T, Francke U, George DL (1987). Molecular analysis and chromosomal mapping of amplified genes isolated from a transformed mouse 3T3 cell lines. *Somat Cell Mol Genet* **13**, 235-244.

Cajone C, Debiasi S, Parker C, Lakshmi MS, Sherbet GV (1994). Metastasis associated MTS1 gene expression is down-regulated by heat shock in variant cell lines of the B16 murine melanoma. *Melanoma Res* **4**, 143-150.

Calabretta B, Battini R, Kaczmarck L, De Riel JK, Baserga R (1986). Molecular cloning of a cDNA for a growth factor inducible gene with strong homology to S100, a calcium binding protein. *J Biol Chem* **261**, 12628-12632.

Caldas C, Hahn SA, Dacosta LT, Redston MS, Schutte M, Seymour AB, Weinstein CL, Hruban RH, Yeo CJ, Kern SE (1994). Frequent somatic mutations and homozygous deletions of the p16 (MTS1) gene in pancreatic adenocarcinoma. *Nature Genet* **8**, 27-32.

Caligo MA, Cipollini G, Di Valromita AC, Buitocchi M, Bevilacqua G (1992). Decreasing expression of *nm23* gene in metastatic murine mammary tumours of viral etiology (MMTV). *Anticancer Res* **12**, 969-974.

Caligo MA, Grammatico P, Cipollini G, Varesco L, Delporto G, Bevilacqua G (1994). A low *nm23.H1* gene expression identifying high malignancy human melanomas. *Melanoma Res* **4**, 179-184.

Calin G (1994). Oncogenes and tumour suppressor genes. Two different looks of the same gene. *Oncol Rep* **1**, 987-991.

Calkins CC, Sloane BF (1995). Mammalian cysteine protease inhibitors. Biochemical properties and possible role in tumour progression. *Biol Chem Hoppe-Seyler* **376**, 71-80.

Call KM, Glaser T, Ito CY, Buckler AJ, Pelletier J, Haber DA, Rose EA, Kral A, Yeger H, Lewis WH, Jones C, Housman DE (1990). Isolation and characterisation of a zinc finger polypeptide gene at the human chromosome 11 Wilms tumour locus. *Cell* **60**, 509-520.

Callahan R (1996). MMTV-induced mutations in mouse mammary tumours. Their potential relevance to human breast cancer. *Breast Cancer Res Treat* **39**, 33-44.

Callender T, Elnaggar AK, Lee MS, Frankenthaler R, Luna HA, Batsakis JG (1994). PRAD-1 (CCND1) cyclin D1 oncogene amplification in primary head and neck squamous cell carcinoma. *Cancer* **74**, 152-158.

Camonis JH, Kalekine M, Gondre B, Gerreau H, Boy-Marcotta E, Jacquet M (1986). Characterisation, cloning and sequence analysis of the cdc25 gene which control the cyclic AMP level of *Saccharomyces cerevisiae*. *EMBO J* **5**, 375-381.

Campbell C, Quinn AG, Ro YS, Angus B, Rees JL (1993). p53 mutations are common and early events that precede tumour invasion in squamous cell neoplasia of the skin. *J Invest Dermatol* **100**, 746-748.

Campbell EJ, Cury JD, Shapiro SD, Goldberg GI, Welgus HG (1991). Neutral proteinases of human mononuclear phagocytes. Cellular differentiation markedly alters cell phenotype for serine proteinases, metalloproteinases, and tissue inhibitor of metalloproteinases. *J Immunol* **146**, 1286-1293.

Campbell IG, Foulkes WD, Senger G, Trowsdale J, Garinchesa P, Rettig WJ (1994). Molecular cloning of the B-CAM cell surface glycoprotein of epithelial cancers. A novel member of the immunoglobulin superfamily. *Cancer Res* **54**, 5761-5765.

Campo E, Miquel R, Jares P, Bosch F, Juan M, Leone A, Vives J, Cardesa A, Yague J (1994). Prognostic significance of the loss of heterozygosity of nm23-H1 and p53 genes in human colorectal carcinomas. *Cancer* **73**, 2913-2921.

Candidus S, Bischoff P, Becker KF, Hofler H (1996). No evidence for mutations in the α-catenin and β-catenin genes in human gastric and breast carcinomas. *Cancer Res* **56**, 49-52.

Canman CE, Wolfe AC, Chen CY, Fornace AJ, Kastan MB (1994). The p53-dependent G1 cell cycle checkpoint pathway and ataxia telangiectasia. *Cancer Res* **54**, 5054-5058.

Cannistra AA, Abujawdeh G, Niloff J, Strobel T, Swanson J, Andersen J, Ottensmeier C (1995). CD44 variant expression is a common feature of epithelial ovarian cancer. Lack of association with standard prognostic factors. *J Clin Oncol* **13**, 1912-1921.

Carduff RF, Johnston CM, Frank TS (1995). Mutations of the Ki-*ras* oncogene in carcinoma of the endometrium. *Am J Path* **146**, 182-188.

Carduff RF, Johnston CM, Svoboda-Newman SM, Poy EL, Merajver SD, Frank TS (1996). Clinical and pathological significance of microsatellite instability in sporadic endometrial carcinoma. *Amer J Path* **148**, 1671-1678.

Carmichael DF, Sommer A, Thompson RC, Anderson D, Smith CG, Welgus H, Stricklin GP (1986). Primary structure and cDNA cloning of human fibroblast collagenase inhibitor. *Proc Natl Acad Sci USA* **83**, 2407-2411.

Carmo-Fonseca M, Pepperkok R, Caravalho MT, Lamond AI (1992). Transcription-dependent colocalisation of the U1, U2, U4/U6 and I5 snRNPs in coiled bodies. *J Cell Biol* **117**, 1-14.

Caron de Fromentel C, Soussi T (1992). TP53 tumour suppressor gene: A model for investigating human mutagenesis. *Genes Chrom Cancer* **4**, 1-15.

Caron-Leslie LAM, Schwartzman RA, Gaido ML, Compton MM, Cidlowski JA (1991). Identification and characterisation of glucocorticoid-regulated nuclease(s) in lymphoid cells undergoing apoptosis. *J Steroid Biochem Mol Biol* **40**, 661-671.

Carrier F, Smith ML, Bae I, Kilpatrick KE, Lansing TJ, Chen CY, Engelstein M, Friend SH, Henner WD, Gilmer TM, Kastan MB, Fornace AJ (1994). Characterisation of human GADD45, a p53-regulated protein. *J Biol Chem* **269**, 32672-32677.

Casson AG, Mukhopathyaya T, Cleary KR, Ro JY, Levin B, Roth JA (1991). P53 gene mutations in Barretts epithelium and esophageal cancer. *Cancer Res* **51**, 4495-4499.

Cavailles V, Augereau P, Garcia M, Rochefort H (1988). Estrogens and growth factors induce the mRNA of the 52 K-procathepsin D secreted by breast cancer cells. *Nucl Acids Res* **16**, 1903-1919.

Cavailles V, Garcia M, Rochefort H (1989). Regulation of cathepsin D and pS2 gene expression by growth factors in MCF7 human breast cancer cells. *Mol Endocrinol* **3**, 552-558.

Cave H, Gerard B, Martin E, Guidal C, Devaux I, Weissenbach J, Elion J, Vilmer E, Grandchamp B (1995). Loss of heterozygosity in the chromosomal region 12p12-13 is very common in childhood acute lymphoblastic leukaemia and permits the precise localisation of a tumour suppressor gene distinct from p27 (kip1). *Blood* **86**, 3869-3875.

Cawkwell L, Lewis FA, Quirke P (1994). Frequency of allele loss of DCC, p53, wt1, NF1, nm23 and APC/MCC in colorectal cancer assayed by fluorescent multiplex polymerase chain reaction. *Br J Cancer* **70**, 813-818.

Chadeneau C, Hay K, Hirte HW, Gallinger S, Bacchetti S (1995). Telomerase activity associated with acquisition of malignancy in human colorectal cancer. *Cancer Res* **55**, 2533-2536.

Chambers AF, Ling V (1984). Selection for experimental metastatic ability of heterologous tumour cells in the chick embryo after DNA mediated transfer. *Cancer Res* **44**, 3970-3975.

Chambers AF, Wilson S (1985). Cells transformed with a *ts* viral *src* mutant are temperature sensitive for *in vitro* growth. *Mol Cell Biol* **5**, 728-733.

Chambers AF, Harris JF, Grundy JS (1988). Rates of generation of methotrexate-resistant variants in cells temperature-sensitive for malignant transformation. *Somatic Cell Mol Genet* **14**, 252-259.

Chambers AF, Denhardt GH, Wilson S (1990). Ras transformed NIH 3T3 cell lines, selected for metastatic ability in chick embryos, have increased proportion of p21-expressing cells and are metastatic in nude mice. *Invasion Metastasis* **10**, 225-240.

Chammas R, Brentani R (1991). Integrins and metastases: An overview. *Tumour Biol* **12**, 309-320.

Champeme MH, Bieche I, Lizard S, Lidereau R (1995). 11q13 amplification in local recurrence of human primary breast cancer. *Genes Chrom Cancer* **12**, 128-133.

Chant ID, Rose PE, Morris AG (1995). Analysis of heat shock protein expression in myeloid leukaemia cells by flow cytometry. *Br J Haematol* **90**, 163-168.

Charlieu JP, Larsson S, Miyagawa K, van Heyningen V, Hastie ND (1995). Does the Wilms tumour suppressor gene, wt1, play roles in both splicing and transcription. *J Cell Sci* **S19**, 95-99.

Charpin C, De Victor B, Bonnier P, Andrac L, Lavaut MN, Allasia C, Piana L (1993). Cathepsin D immunocytochemical assays on breast carcinomas. Image analysis and correlation to prognostic factors. *J Pathol* **170**, 463-470.

Chellappan SP, Hiebert S, Mydryj M, Horowitz JM, Nevins JR (1991). The E2F transcription factor is a cellular target for the RB protein. *Cell* **65**, 1053-1061.

Chen CY, Odliner JD, Zhan QM, Fornace AJ, Vogelstein B, Kastan MB (1994). Interactions between p53 and mdm2 in a mammalian cell cycle checkpoint pathway. *Proc Natl Acad Sci USA* **91**, 2684-2688.

Chen JD, Wu XW, Lin JY, Levine AJ (1996). Mdm-2 inhibits the G(1) arrest and apoptosis functions of the p53 tumour suppressor protein. *Mol Cell Biol* **16**, 2445-2452.

Chen PL, Scully P, Shew JY, Wang JYY, Lee WH (1989). Phosphorylation of the retinoblastoma gene product is modulated during the cell cycle and cellular differentiation. *Cell* **58**, 1193-1198.

Chen W, Obrink B (1991). Cell-cell contacts mediated by E-cadherin (uvomorulin) restrict invasive behaviour. *J Cell Biol* **114**, 319-327.

Chen WT (1992). Membrane proteases: roles in tissue remodelling and tumour invasion. *Curr Opin Cell Biol* **4**, 802-809.

Chen YH, Dong JP, Lu YD, McGee JOD (1995). Quantitative detection of amplification of proto-oncogenes in breast cancer. *Chinese Med J* **108**, 849-854.

Chen YM, Chen CF, Riley DJ, Allred DC, Chen PL, von Hoff D, Osborne CK, Lee WH (1995). Aberrant subcellular localisation of BRCA1 in breast cancer. *Science* **270**, 789-791.

Cheng J, Scully P, Shew JY, Lee WH, Vila V, Haas M (1990). Homozygous deletion of the retinoblastoma gene in an acute lymphoblastic leukaemia (T) cell line. *Blood* **75**, 730-735.

Chen-Levy Z, Nourse J, Clearly ML (1989). The bcl-2 candidate proto-oncogene product is a 24-kilodalton integral membrane protein highly expressed in lymphoid cell lines and lymphomas carrying the t(14;18) translocation. *Mol Cell Biol* **9**, 701-710.

Chilosi M, Doglioni C, Menestrina F, Montagna L, Rigo A, Lestani M, Barbareschi M, Scarpa A, Mariuzzi GM, Pizzolo G (1994). Abnormal expression of the p53 binding protein mdm2 in Hodgkin's disease. *Blood* **84**, 4295-4300.

Chin KV, Ueda K, Pastan I, Goettesman MM (1992). Modulation of activity of the promoter of the human *MDR1* gene by *ras* and *p53*. *Science* **255**, 459-462.

Chiquetehrismann R, Hagios C, Matsumoto K (1994). The tenascin gene family. *Persp Develop Neurobiol* **2**, 3-7.

Chirico WJ, Waters MG, Blobel G (1988). 70k Heat shock related proteins stimulate protein translocation into microsomes. *Nature* **332**, 805-810.

Chiviri RGS, Garofalo A, Padura IM, Mantovani A, Giavazzi R (1993). Interleukin-1 receptor antagonist inhibits the augmentation of metastasis induced by interleukin-1 or lipopolysaccharide in a human melanoma-nude mouse system. *Cancer Res* **53**, 5051-5054.

Cho KR, Fearon ER (1995). DCC - Linking tumour suppressor gene and altered cell surface interactions in cancer. *Eur J Cancer* **31A**, 1055-1060.

Cho KR, Oliner JD, Simons JW, Hedrick L, Fearon ER (1994). The DCC gene. Structural analysis and mutations in colorectal carcinoma. *Genomics* **19**, 525-531.

Cho YJ, Gorina S, Jeffrey PD, Pavletich NP (1994). Crystal structure of a p53 tumour suppressor DNA complex. Understanding tumorigenic mutations. *Science* **265**, 346-355.

Chong JM, Fukayama M, Hayashi Y, Takizawa T, Koike M, Konishi M, Kikuchiyanoshita R, Miyaki M (1994). Microsatellite instability in the progression of gastric carcinoma. *Cancer Res* **54**, 4595-4597.

Chou D, Miyashita T, Morenweiser HW, Ueki K, Kastury K, Druck T, von Deimling A, Huebner K, Reed JC, Louis DN (1996). The *bax* gene maps to the glioma candidate region at 19q13.3, but is not altered in human gliomas. *Cancer Genet Cytogenet* **88**, 136-140.

Chozick BS, Weicker ME, Pezzullo JC, Jackson CL, Finkelstein SD, Ambler MW, Epstein MH, Finch PW (1994). Pattern of mutant p53 expression in human astrocytomas suggests the existence of alternate pathways of tumorigenesis. *Cancer* **73**, 406-415.

Chua CC, Chua BHL (1990). Tumour necrosis factor-α induces messenger RNA for collagenase and TIMP in human skin fibroblasts. *Connect Tiss Res* **25**, 161-170.

Chung RY, Whaley J, Kley N, Anderson K, Louis D, Menon A, Hettlich C, Freiman R, Hedlewhyte ET, Martuza R, Henkins R, Yandell D, Seizinger BR (1991). Tp53 mutation and 17p deletion in human astrocytomas. *Genes Chrom Cancer* **3**, 323-331.

Ciechanover A, DiGiuseppe JA, Bercovich B, Orian A, Richter JD, Schwartz AL, Brodeur GM (1991). Degradation of nuclear oncoproteins by the ubiquitin system *in vitro*. *Proc Natl Acad Sci USA* **88**, 139-143.

Cifone MA, Fidler IJ (1981). Increasing metastatic potential is associated with increasing genetic instability of clones isolated from murine neoplasms. *Proc Natl Acad Sci USA* **78**, 6949-6952.

Cillo C, Dick JE, Ling V, Hill RP (1987). Generation of drug-resistant variants in metastatic B16 murine melanoma cell lines. *Cancer Res* **47**, 2604-2608.

Ciocca DR, Osterreich S, Chamness GC, McGuire WL, Fuqua SAW (1993). Biological and clinical implications of heat shock protein 27000 (HSP27). A review. *J Natl Cancer Inst* **85**, 1558-1570.

Cioce V, Castronovo V, Shmookler BM, Garbisa S, Grigioni WF, Liotta LA, Sobel M (1991). Increased expression of laminin receptor in human colon cancer. *J Natl Cancer Inst* **83**, 29-36.

Ciomei M, Pastori W, Mariani M, Sola F, Grandi M, Mongelli N (1994). New sulfonated distamycin-A derivatives with bFGF complexing activity. *Biochem Pharmcol* **47**, 295-302.

Clark CC, Cohen I, Eichstetter I, Cannizzaro LA, McPherson JD, Wasmuth JJ, Iozzo RV (1993). Molecular cloning of the human protooncogene wnt-5a and mapping of the gene (*wnt-5a*) to chromosome 3p14-p21. *Genomics* **18**, 249-260.

Clark GM, Dressler LG, Owens MA, Pounds G, Okdaker T, McGuire WM (1989). Prediction of relapse or survival in patients with node-negative breast cancer by DNA flow cytometery. *N Engl J Med* **320**, 627-633.

Clark SD, Wilhelm SM, Stricklin GP, Welgus HG (1985). Phorbol myristate acetate induces increased production of collagenase inhibitor in human skin fibroblasts. *J Invest Dermatol* **84**, 297.

Clark SD, Kobayashi DK, Welgus HG (1987). Regulation of the expression of tissue inhibitor of metalloproteinases and collagenase by retinoids and glucocorticoids in human fibroblasts. *J Clin Invest* **80**, 1280-1287.

Clarke AR, Purdie CA, Harrison DJ, Morris RG, Bird CC, Hooper MC, Wyllie AH (1993). Thymocyte apoptosis induced by p53-dependent and independent pathways. *Nature* **362**, 849-852.

Clarke AR, Gledhill S, Hooper ML, Bird CC, Wyllie AH (1994). P53 dependence on early apoptotic and proliferative responses within the mouse intestinal epithelium following gamma irradiation. *Oncogene* **9**, 1767-1773.

Clarke CF, Cheng K, Frey AB, Stein R, Hinds PW, Levine AJ (1988). Purification of complexes of nuclear oncogene p53 with rat and *Escherichia coli* heat shock proteins: *in vitro* dissociation of hsc70 and DnaK from murine p53 by ATP. *Mol Cell Biol* **8**, 1206-1215.

Clarke MR, Landreneau RJ, Resnick NM, Crowley R, Dougherty GJ, Cooper DL, Yousem SA (1995). Prognostic significance of CD44 expression in adenocarcinoma of the lung. *J Clin Pathol Mol Pathol* **48**, m200-m204.

Cleary ML, Sklar J (1985). Nucleotide sequence of a t(14;18) chromosomal breakpoint in follicular lymphoma and demonstration of a break point cluster region near a transcriptionally active locus on chromosome 18. *Proc Natl Acad Sci USA* **82**, 7439-7443.

Cleary ML, Smith SD, Sklar J (1986a). Cloning and structural analysis of cDNAs for bcl-2 and a hybrid bcl-2/immunoglobulin transcript resulting from the t(14;18) translocation. *Cell* **47**, 19-28.

Cleary ML, Galili N, Sklar J (1986b). Detection of a second t(14;18) breakpoint cluster region in human follicular lymphomas. *J Exp Med* **164**, 315-320.

Cliby W, Ritland S, Hartmann L, Dodson M, Halling KC, Keeney G, Podratz KC, Jenkins RB (1993). Human epithelial ovarian cancer allotype. *Cancer Res* **53**, 2392-2398.

Cohen JJ, Duke RC (1984). Glucocorticoid activation of a calcium-dependent endonuclease in thymocyte nuclei leads to cell death. *J Immunol* **132**, 38-42.

Cohen JJ, Duke RC, Fadok VA, Sellins KS (1992). Apoptosis and programmed cell death in immunity. *Annu Rev Immunol* **10**, 267-293.

Cohn KH, Wang F, Desoto La Paix F, Solomon WB, Patterson LG, Arnold MR, Weimer J, Feldman JG, Levy AT, Leone A, Steeg PS (1991). Association of nm23-H1 allelic deletions with distant metastasis in colorectal carcinoma. *Lancet* **338**, 722-724.

Collard JG, Schihven KF, Roos E (1987a). Invasive and metastatic potential induced by *ras* transfection into mouse BW 5147 T-lymphoma cells. *Cancer Res* **47**, 754-759.

Collard JG, van de Poll M, Scheffer A, Roos E, Hopman AHM, van Kessel AHMG, van Dongen JJM (1987b). Location of genes involved in invasion and metastasis on human chromosome 7. *Cancer Res* **47**, 6666-6670.

Collier IE, Wilhelm SM, Eisen AZ, Marmer BL, Grant GA, Seltzer JL, Kronberger A, He C, Bauer EA, Goldberg GI (1988). H-*ras* oncogene transformed human bronchial epithelial cells (TBE-1) secrete a single metalloprotease capable of degrading basement membrane antigen. *J Biol Chem* **263**, 6579-6587.

Collins K, Kobayashi R, Greider CW (1995). Purification of *Tetrahymena* telomerase and cloning of genes encoding the two protein components of the enzyme. *Cell* **81**, 677-686.

Combaret V, Lasset C, Bouvier R, Frappaz D, Thiesse P, Rebillard AC, Philip T, Favrot MC (1995). CD44, a new prognostic marker for neuroblastoma. *Bull Cancer*, **82**, 131-136.

Compton MM, Cidlowski JA (1992). Thymocyte apoptosis, a model of programmed cell death. *Trends Endocrinol Metab* 3, 17-23.

Cooper DMF (1991). Inhibition of adenylate cyclase by Ca^{2+} - A counterpart to stimulation by Ca^{2+}/calmodulin. *Biochem J* 278, 903-904.

Coppes MJ, Campbell CE, Williams BRG (1993). The role of wt1 in Wilms tumorigenesis. *FASEB J* 7, 886-895.

Coppock DL, Buffolino P, Kopman C, Nathanson L (1995). Inhibition of the melanoma cell cycle and regulation at the G1/S transition by 12-O-tetradecanoylphorbol-13-acetate (TPA) by modulation of cdk2 activity. *Exp Cell Res* 221, 92-102.

Cordon-Cardo C, Latres E, Drobnjak M, Oliva MR, Pollack D, Woodruff JM, Marechal V, Chen JD, Brennan MF, Levine AJ (1994). Molecular abnormalities of mdm2 and p53 genes in adult soft tissue sarcomas. *Cancer Res* 54, 794-799.

Coss RA, Dewey WC, Bamburg JR (1982). Effects of hyperthermia on dividing Chinese hamster ovary cells and on microtubules *in vitro*. *Cancer Res* 42, 1059-1071.

Costa M, Danesi R, Agen C, Di Paolo A, Basolo F, Delbianchi S, Deltacca M (1994). MCF-10A cells infected with *int-2* oncogene induce angiogenesis in chick embryo chorioallantoic membrane and in the rat mesentery. *Cancer Res* 54, 9-11.

Coulson PB, Thornthwaite JT, Woolley TW, Sugarbaker EV, Seckinger D (1984). Prognostic indicators including DNA histogram type, receptor content, and staging related to human breast cancer patient survival. *Cancer Res* 44, 4187-4196.

Counter CM, Avilion AA, LeFeuvre CE, Stewart NG, Greider CW, Harley CB, Bacchetti S (1992). Telomere shortening associated with chromosome instability is arrested in immortal cells which express telomerase activity. *EMBO J* 11, 1921-1929.

Counter CM, Kurte HW, Bacchetti S, Harley CB (1994a). Telomerase activity in human ovarian carcinoma. *Proc Natl Acad Sci USA* 91, 2900-2904.

Counter CM, Botelho FM, Wang P, Harley CB, Bacchetti S (1994b). Stabilisation of short telomeres and telomerase activity accompany immortalisation of Epstein–Barr virus transformed human B lymphocytes. *J Virol* 68, 3410-3414.

Cowell JK, Groves N, Baird P (1993), Loss of heterozygosity at 11p13 in Wilms tumours does not necessarily involve mutations in the *wt1* gene. *Br J Cancer* 67, 1259-1261.

Craft PS, Harris AL (1994). Clinical prognostic significance of tumour angiogenesis. *Ann Oncol* 5, 305-311.

Craig EA (1993). Chaperones: Helpers along the pathways to protein folding. *Science* 260, 1902-1903.

Craig RW (1995). The *bcl-2* gene family. *Sem Cancer Biol* 6, 35-43.

Cristofolini M, Boi S, Girlando S, Zumiani G, Cristofolini P, Palma PD, Doglioni C, Barbareschi M (1993). p53 protein expression in nevi and melanomas. *Arch Dermatol* 129, 739-743.

Croce CM (1997). Bcl-2 is the guardian of microtubule integrity. In: *Proc 9th Lorne Cancer Conference*, Lorne, Australia.

Crossin KL, Carney DH (1981a). Evidence that microtubule depolymerisation early in the cell cycle is sufficient to initiate DNA synthesis. *Cell* 23, 61-71.

Crossin KL, Carney DH (1981b). Microtubule stabilisation by taxol inhibits initiation of DNA synthesis by thrombin and by epidermal growth factor. *Cell* 27, 341-350.

Crossin KL, Hoffman S, Grumet M, Thiery JP, Edelman GM (1986). Site restricted expression of cytotactin during development of the chicken embryo. *J Cell Biol* 102, 1917-1930.

Cryns V, Thor A, Louis D, Benedict W, Arnold A (1993). Tumour suppressor gene abnormalities in human parathyroid carcinoma. *J Bone Mineral Res* 8, 5148.

Culty M, Shizari M, Thompson EW, Underhill CB (1994). Binding and degradation of hyaluronan

by human breast cancer cell lines expressing different forms of CD44. Correlation with
    invasive potential. *J Cell Physiol* **160**, 275-286.

Cunningham BA, Hemperly JJ, Murray BA, Prediger EA, Brackenbury R, Edelman GM (1987).
    Neural cell adhesion molecule: structure, immunoglobulin-like domains, cell surface modula-
    tion and alternative splicing. *Science* **236**, 799-806.

Curran T (1988). *The Oncogene Handbook*, Reddy EP (ed.). Elsevier, Amsterdam, p. 307.

Curtis L, Wyllie AH, Shaw JJ, Williams GT, Radulescu A, Demicco C, Haugen DRF, Varhaug JE,
    Lillehaug JR, Wynford-Thomas D (1994). Evidence against involvement of APC mutation in
    papillary thyroid carcinoma. *Eur J Cancer* **30A**, 984-987.

Czubayko F, Smith RV, Chung HC, Wellstein A (1994). A secreted binding protein can activate
    non-secreted FGF in tumours. *J Biol Chem* **269**, 28243-28248.

D'Agnano I, Bucci B, Mottolese M, Benevolo M, Conti L, Botti C, Vecchione A, Casillo S, Zupi G
    (1996). DNA ploidy, cell kinetics, and epidermal growth factor receptor and HER2/*neu*
    oncoprotein expression in primary operable breast cancer. *Ann NY Acad Sci* **784**, 472-481.

Dahse R, Fiedler W, Ernst G, Kosmehl H, Schlichter A, Schubert J, Calussen U (1996). Changes in
    telomere lengths in renal cell carcinomas. *Cell and Mol Biol* **42**, 477-485.

Daidone MG, Silvestrini R, D'Errico A, Di Fronzo G, Benini E, Mancini AM, Garbisa S, Liotta LA,
    Grigioni WF (1991). Laminin receptors, collagenase IV and prognosis in node negative breast
    cancers. *Int J Cancer* **48**, 529-532.

Dalet-Fumeron V, Guinec N, Pagano M (1993). *In vitro* activation of pro-cathepsin B by three
    serine proteinases: leukocyte elastase, cathepsin G, and the urokinase type plasminogen
    activator. *FEBS Lett* **332**, 251-254.

Dameron KM, Volpert OV, Tainsky MA, Bouck N (1994). Control of angiogenesis in fibroblasts
    by p53 regulation of thrombospondin-1. *Science* **265**, 1582-1584.

Danen EHJ, Tenberge PJM, Vanmuijen GNP, Vanthofgrootenboer AE, Brocker EB, Ruiter DJ
    (1994). Emergence of alpha-5-beta-1 fibronectin receptor and alpha-V-beta-3 vitronectin
    receptor expression in melanocytic tumour progression. *Histopathology* **24**, 249-256.

Dang CV, Lee WMF (1989). Nuclear and nucleolar targeting sequences of c-erbA, c-myb, N-myc,
    p53, HSP70 and HIV tat proteins. *J Biol Chem* **264**, 18019-18023.

Danks RA, Chopra G, Gonzales MF, Orian JM, Kaye AH (1995). Aberrant p53 expression does
    not correlate with prognosis in anaplastic astrocytoma. *Neurosurgery* **37**, 246-254.

Dash PK, Kark KA, Colocis MA, Prywes R, Kandel ER (1991). cAMP response element-binding
    protein is activated by Ca^{2+}/calmodulin, as well as cAMP protein kinase. *Proc Natl Acad Sci
    USA* **88**, 5061-5065.

Datto MB, Yu Y, Wang XF (1995a). Functional analysis of the transforming growth factor beta
    responsive elements in the waf1/cip1/p21 promoter. *J Biol Chem* **270**, 28623-28628.

Datto MB, Li Y, Panus JF, Howe DJ, Xiong Y, Wang XF (1995b). Transforming growth factor beta
    induces the cyclin dependent kinase inhibitor p21 through a p53-independent mechanism.
    Proc Natl Acad Sci USA **92**, 5545-5549.

Davidoff AM, Iglehart D, Marks JR (1992). Immune response to p53 is dependent upon p53/
    HSP70 complexes in breast cancer. *Proc Natl Acad Sci USA* **89**, 3439-3442.

Davies B, Waxman J, Wasan H, Abel P, Williams G, Krausz T, Neal D, Thomas D, Hanby A,
    Balkwill F (1993). Levels of matrix metalloproteases in bladder cancer correlate with tumour
    grade and invasion. *Cancer Res* **53**, 5365-5369.

Davies BR, Davies MPA, Gibbs FEM, Barraclough R, Rudland PS (1993). Induction of the
    metastatic phenotype by transfection of a benign mammary epithelial cell line with the gene
    for p9Ka, a rat calcium-binding protein, but not with the oncogene EJ-*ras*-1. *Oncogene* **8**,
    999-1008.

Davies ME, Barrett AJ (1984). Immunolocalisation of human cystatins in neutrophils and lymphocytes. *Histochemistry* **80**, 373-377.

Davis-Smyth T, Chen H, Park J, Presta LG, Ferrara N (1996). The 2nd immunoglobulin-like domain of the VEGF tyrosine kinase receptor flt-1 determines ligand binding and may initiate a signal transduction cascade. *EMBO J* **15**, 4919-4927.

Dealy CN, Roth A, Ferrari D, Brown AMC, Kosher RA (1993). Wnt-5a and wnt-7a are expressed in the developing chick limb bud in a manner suggesting roles in pattern formation along the proximodistal and dorsoventral axes. *Mech Develop* **43**, 175-186.

Dear TN, Kefford RF (1991). The WDNM1 gene product is a novel member of the 'four disulphide core' family of proteins. *Biochem Biophys Res Commun* **176**, 247-254.

Dear TN, Ramshaw IA, Kefford RF (1988). Differential expression of a novel gene WDNM1 in nonmetastatic rat mammary adenocarcinoma cells. *Cancer Res* **48**, 5203-5209.

Dear TN, McDonald DA, Kefford RF (1989). Transcriptional down regulation of a rat gene WDNM2 in metastatic DMBA-8 cells. *Cancer Res* **49**, 5323-5328.

Deb S, Jackson CT, Subler MA, Martin DW (1992). Modulation of cellular land viral promoters by mutant human p53 proteins found in tumour cells. *J Virol* **66**, 6164-6170.

Deb SP, Munoz RM, Brown DR, Subler MA, Deb S (1994). Wild type human p53 activates the human epidermal growth factor receptor promoter. *Oncogene* **9**, 1341-1349.

Debbas M, White E (1993). Wild type p53 mediates apoptosis by E1A, which is inhibited by E1B. *Genes Develop* **7**, 546-554.

De Benedetti L, Sciallero S, Gismondi V, James R, Bafico A, Biticchi, R, Masetti E, Bonelli L, Heouaine A, Picasso M, Groden J, Robertson M, Risio M, Caprilli R, Bruzzi P, White RL, Aste H, Santi L, Varesco L, Ferrara GB (1994). Association of APC gene mutations and histological characteristics of colorectal adenomas. *Cancer Res* **54**, 3553-3556.

DeClerck YA, Yean TD, Ratzkin BJ, Lu HS, Langley KE (1989). Purification and characterisation of two related but distinct metalloproteinase inhibitors secreted by bovine aortic endothelial cells. *J Biol Chem* **264**, 17445-17453.

DeClerck YA, Perez N, Shimada H, Boone TC, Langley KE, Taylor SM (1992). Inhibition of invasion and metastasis in cells transfected with an inhibitor of metalloproteinases. *Cancer Res* **52**, 701-708.

Dedhar S (1990). Integrins and tumour invasion. *BioEssays* **12**, 583-590.

Dedhar S and Saulnier R (1990). Alterations in integrin receptor expression on chemically transformed human cells: Specific enhancement of laminin and collagen receptor complexes. *J Cell Biol* **110**, 481-489.

Delahunt B, Farrant GJ, Bethwaite PB, Nacey JN, Lewis ME (1994). Assessment of proliferative activity in Wilms tumour. *Anal Cell Path* **7**, 127-138.

DeLarco A, Garcia J, Arribas C, Barrio R, Blazques MG, Izquierdo JM, Isquierdo M (1993). Timing of p53 mutations during astrocytoma tumorigenesis. *Human Mol Genet* **2**, 1687-1690.

Delia D, Aiello A, Formelli F, Fontanella E, Costa A, Miyashita T, Reed JC, Pierotti MA (1995). Regulation of apoptosis induced by the retinoid N-(4-hydroxyphenyl) retinamide and effect of deregulated *bcl-2*. *Blood* **85**, 359-367.

Demetrick DJ, Matsumoto S, Hannon GJ, Okamoto K, Xiong Y, Zhang H, Beach DH (1995). Chromosomal mapping of the genes for the human cell cycle proteins cyclin-C (CCNC), cyclin-E (CCNE), P21 (CDKN1) and KAP (CDKN3). *Cytogenet Cell Genet* **69**, 190-192.

D'Emilia J, Bulovas K, D'Ercole K, Wolf B, Steel G, Jr, Summerhayes IC (1989). Expression of the c-erb B2 gene product (p185) at different stages of neoplastic progression in the colon. *Oncogene* **4**, 1233-1239.

Denning SM, Le PT, Singer KH, Haynes BF (1990). Antibodies against the CD44 p80, lymphocyte homing receptor molecule augment human peripheral blood T cell activation. *J Immunol* **144**, 7-15,

Denton KJ, Stretch JR, Gatter KC, Harris AL (1992). A study of adhesion molecules as markers of progression in melanoma. *J Pathol* **167**, 187-191.

Deshaies RJ, Koch BD, Werner-Washburne M, Craig EA, Schekman R (1988). A subfamily of stress proteins facilitates translocation of secretory and mitochondrial precursor polypeptides. *Nature* **332**, 800-805.

Devilee P, van Vliet M, Bardoel A, Kievits T, Kuipers-Dijkshoorn N, Parson PL, Cornelisse CJ (1991a). Frequent somatic imbalance of marker alleles for chromosome 1 in human primary breast carcinoma. *Cancer Res* **51**, 1020-1025.

Devilee P, van Vliet M, van Sloun P, Kijkshoorn NK, Hermans J, Pearson PL, Cornelisse CJ (1991b). Allelotype of human breast carcinoma: a second major site for loss of heterozygosity. *Oncogene* **6**, 1705-1711.

De Vouge MW, Mukherjee BB (1992). Transformation of rat kidney cells by v-K-*ras* enhances expression of transin 2 and an S-100 related calcium binding protein. *Oncogene* **7**, 109-110.

Dexter TJ, Bennett DC (1987). Differentiation apparently repressed by the nucleus. Rapidly induced pigmentation of enucleated melanoma cells. *Exp Cell Res* **168**, 255-264.

Dey BR, Sukahtme VP, Roberts AB, Sporn MB, Rauscher III FJ, Kim SJ (1994). Repression of transforming growth factor-β gene by the Wilms tumour suppressor *wt1* gene product. *Mol Endocrinol* **8**, 592-602.

Diaz-Flores L, Gutierrez R, Varela H (1994). Angiogensis, an update. *Histol Histopathol* **9**, 807-843.

Dickinson AJ, Fox SB, Persad RA, Hollyer J, Sibley GNA, Harris AL (1994). Quantification of angiogenesis as an independent predictor of prognosis in invasive bladder carcinoma. *Br J Urol* **74**, 762-766.

Dickson CR, Smith R, Brookes S, Peters G (1984). Tumorigenesis by mouse mammary tumour virus: proviral activation of a cellular gene in the common integration region int-2. *Cell* **37**, 529-536.

Diller L, Kassel J, Nelson CE, Gryka MA, Litwack C, Gebhardt M, Bressac B, Ozturk M, Baker SJ, Vogelstein B, Friend SH (1990). p53 functions as a cell cycle control protein in osteosarcomas. *Mol Cell Biol* **10**, 5772-5781.

Diment S, Leech MS, Stahl PD (1988). Cathepsin D is membrane associated in macrophage endosome. *J Biol Chem* **263**, 6901-6907.

Dionne CA, Jaye M, Schlessinger J (1991). Structural diversity and binding of FGF receptors. *Ann NY Acad Sci* **638**, 161-166.

DiPaolo G, Pellier V, Catsicas M, Antosson B, Catsicas S, Grenningloh G (1996). The phosphoprotein stathmin is essential for nerve growth factor-stimulated differentiation. *J Cell Biol* **133**, 1383-1390.

DiPaolo JA, Woodworth CD, Popescu NC, Notario V, Doniger J (1989). Induction of human cervical squamous cell carcinoma by sequential transfection with human papillomavirus 16 DNA and viral Harvey *ras. Oncogene* **4**, 395-399.

Direnzo MF, Poulsom R, Olivero M, Comoglio PM, Lemoine NR (1995a). Expression of the met hepatocyte growth factor receptor in human pancreatic cancer. *Cancer Res* **55**, 1129-1138.

Direnzo MF, Olivero M, Giacomini A, Porte H, Chastre E, Mirossay L, Nordlinger B, Bretti S, Bottardi S, Giordano S, Plebani M, Gespach C, Comoglio PM (1995b). Over-expression and amplification of the met/HGF receptor gene during the progression of colorectal cancer. *Clin Cancer Res* **1**, 147-154.

Docherty AJP, Lyons A, Smith BJ, Wright EM, Stephens PE, Harris TJR, Murphy G, Reynods JJ

(1985). Sequence of human tissue inhibitor of metalloproteinases and its identity to erythroid-potentiating activity. *Nature* **318**, 66-69.

Dodson MK, Cliby WA, Xu HJ, De Lacey KA, HU SX, Keeney GL, Li J, Podratz KC, Henkins RB, Benedict WF (1994). Evidence of functional RB protein in epithelial ovarian carcinomas despite loss of heterozygosity at the *RB* locus. *Cancer Res* **54**, 610-613.

Doherty P, Barton CH, Dickson G, Seaton P, Rowett LH, Moore SE, Gower HJ, Walsh FS (1989). Neuronal process outgrowth of human sensory neurons on monolayers of cells transfected with cDNAs for five human NCAM isoforms. *J Cell Biol* **109**, 789-798.

Doherty P, Fruns M, Seaton P, Dickson G, Barton CH, Sears TA, Walsh FS (1990a). A threshold effect of the major isoforms of NCAM on neurite outgrowth. *Nature* **343**, 464-466.

Doherty P, Cohen J, Walsh FS (1990b). Neurite outgrowth in response to transfected NCAM changes during development and is modulated by polysialic acid. *Neuron* **6**, 209-219.

Donato R (1991). Perspectives in S-100 protein biology. *Cell Calcium* **12**, 713-726.

Donehower LA, Harvey M, Slagel BL, McArthur MJ, Montgomery CA, Jr, Butel JS, Bradley A (1992). Mice deficient for p53 are developmentally normal but susceptible to spontaneous tumours. *Nature* **356**, 215-221.

Donehower LA, Godley LA, Aldaz CM, Pyle R, Shi YP, Pinkel D, Gray J, Bradley A, Medina D, Varmus HE (1995). Deficiency of *p53* accelerates mammary tumorigenesis in *wnt-1* transgenic mice and promotes chromosomal instability. *Genes Develop* **9**, 882-895.

Dorin JR, Emslie E, van Heiningen V (1990). Related calcium binding proteins map to the same region of chromosome 1 and to an extended region of synteny on mouse chromosome 3. *Genomics* **8**, 420-426.

Dossantos NR, Seruca R, Constancia M, Seixas M, Sobrinosimoes M (1996). Microsatellite instability at multiple loci in gastric carcinoma. Clinocopathological implications and prognosis. *Gastroenterol* **110**, 38-44.

Dowdy SF, Hinds PW, Kenway L, Reed S, Arnold A, Weinberg RA (1993). Physical interaction of the retinoblastoma protein with human D cyclins. *Cell* **73**, 499-511.

Downward J, Yarden Y, Mayes E, Scrace G, Totty N, Stockwell P, Ullrich A, Schlessinger J, Waterfield MD (1984). Close similarity of epidermal growth factor receptor and v-erbB oncogene protein sequences. *Nature* **307**, 521-527.

Drake CJ, Davis LA, Little CD (1991). Antibodies to β1-integrins cause alterations of aortic vasculogenesis *in vivo. Develop Dynamics* **193**, 83-91.

Drummond IA, Madden SL, Rohwer-Nutter P, Bell GI, Sukhatme VP, Rauscher FJ, III (1992). Repression of the insulin-like growth factor II gene by the Wilms tumour suppressor wt1. *Science* **257**, 674-678.

D'Souza B, Taylor-Papadimitriou J (1994). Over-expression of erbB2 in human mammary epithelial cells signals inhibition of transcription of the E-cadherin gene. *Proc Natl Acad Sci USA* **91**, 7202-7206.

Duffy MJ, Reilly D, McDermott E, O'Higgins N, Fennelly JJ, Andreasen PA (1994). Urokinase plasminogen activator as a prognostic marker in different subgroups of patients with breast cancer. *Cancer* **74**, 2276-2280.

Duggan C, Maguire T, McDermott E, O'Higgins N, Fennelly JJ, Duffy MJ (1995). Urokinase plasminogen activator and urokinase plasminogen activator receptor in breast cancer. *Int J Cancer* **61**, 597-600.

Duncan A, Higgins J, Dunn RJ, Allore R, Marks A (1989). Refined localisation of the human genome encoding the β subunit of the S100 protein (S100B) and confirmation of a subtle t(9,21) translocation using *in situ* hybridisation. *Cytogen Cell Genet* **50**, 234-235.

Dunn R, Landry C, O'Hanlon D, Dunn J, Allore R, Brown I, Marks A (1987). Reduction in S-100β

subunit mRNA in C6 rat glioma cells following treatment with antimicrotubule drugs. *J Biol Chem* **262**, 3562-3566.

Duro D, Flexor MA, Bernard O, Dagay MF, Berger R, Larsen CJ (1994). Alterations of the putative tumour suppressor gene P16/MTS1 in human haematological malignancies. *CR Acad Sci* **317**, 913-919.

Dynlacht BD, Flores O, Lees JA, Harlow E (1994). Differential regulation of E2F *trans*-activation by cyclin/cdk2 complexes. *Genes Develop* **8**, 1772-1786.

Dyson NP, Howley PM, Munger K, Harlow E (1989). The human papillomavirus-16 E7 oncoprotein is able to bind to the retinoblastoma gene product. *Science* **243**, 934-936.

East JA, Mitchell SD, Hart IR (1992). Transfection of AKR mouse thymoma cells with CD44 variants. *Clin Exp Metastasis* **10** (Suppl. 1), 43.

Easton DF, Bishop DT, Ford D, Crockford GP (1993). Genetic linkage analysis in familial breast and ovarian cancer. Results from 214 families. *Amer J Hum Genet* **52**, 678-701.

Ebert W, Knoch H, Werle B, Trefz G, Muley T, Spiess E (1994). Prognostic value of increased lung tumour tissue cathepsin B. *Anticancer Res* **14**, 895-899.

Ebralidze A, Tulchinsky E, Grigorian M, Afanasyeva A, Senin V, Revazova E, Lukanidin E (1989). Isolation and characterisation of a gene specifically expressed in different metastatic cells and whose deduced gene product has a high degree of homology to Ca^{2+} binding protein family. *Genes Develop* **3**, 1086-1093.

Ebralidze A, Florene, VA, Lukanidin E, Fostad O (1990). The murine *mts1* gene is highly expressed in metastatic but not in non-metastatic human tumour lines. *Clin Exp Metastasis* **8** (Suppl. 1), 35.

Eddington KG, Loughran OP, Berry IJ, Parkinson EK (1995). Cellular immortality: A late event in the progression of human squamous cell carcinoma of the head and neck associated with p53 alteration and a high frequency of allele loss. *Mol Carcinogen* **13**, 254-265.

Edelman GM, Murray BA, Mege RM, Cunningham BA, Gallin WJ (1987). Cellular expression of liver and neural cell adhesion molecules after transfection with their cDNAs results in specific cell-cell binding. *Proc Natl Acad Sci USA* **84**, 8502-8506.

Edvardsen K, Pedersen PH, Bjerkvig R, Hermann GG, Zeuthen J, Laerum OD, Walsh FS, Bock E (1994). Transfection of glioma cells with the neural cell adhesion molecule NCAM. Effect on glioma cell invasion and growth *in vivo*. *Int J Cancer* **58**, 116-122.

Edward M, MacKie RM (1989). Retinoic acid-induced inhibition of lung colonisation and changes in the synthesis of properties of glycosaminoglycans of metasatic B16 melanoma cells. *J Cell Sci* **94**, 537-543.

Edward M, Grant AW, MacKie RM (1992). Human melanoma cell derived factor(s) stimulate fibroblast glycosaminoglycans. *Int J Cancer* **52**, 499-503.

Edwards DR, Murphy G, Reynods JJ, Whitham SE, Docherty AJF, Angel P, Heath JK (1987). Transforming growth factor beta modulates the expression of collagenase and metallo-proteinase inhibitor. *EMBO J* **6**, 1899-1904.

Egan SE, McClarty GA, Jarolin L, Wright JA, Spiro I, Hager G, Greenberg AH (1987). Expression of H-*ras* correlates with metastatic potential: evidence for direct regulation of the metastatic phenotype in 10T1/2 and NIH-3T3 cells. *Mol Cell Biol* **7**, 830-837.

Egan SE, Broere JJ, Jarolin L, Wright JA, Greenberg H (1989). Co-regulation of metastatic and transforming activity of normal and mutant *ras* genes. *Int J Cancer* **43**, 443-449.

Egawa S, Uchida T, Suyama K, Wang CX, Ohori M, Irie S, Iwamura M, Koshiba K (1995). Genomic instability of microsatellite repeats in prostate cancer. Relationship to clinicopathological variables. *Cancer Res* **55**, 2418-2421.

Eisinger F, Stoppalyonnet D, Longy M, Kerangueven F, Noguchi T, Bailly C, Vincent-Salomon A,

Jacquemier J, Birnbaum D, Sobol H (1996). Germline mutation at BRCA1 affects the histoprognostic grade in hereditary breast cancer. *Cancer Res* **56**, 471-474.

El-Azouzi M, Chung RY, Farmer GE, Martuza RL, Black PM, Rouleau GA, Hettlich C, Hedley-White ET, Zervas NT, Panagopoulos K, Nakamura Y, Gusella JF, Seizinger BR (1989). Loss of distinct region on the short arm of chromosome 17 associated with tumorigenesis of human astrocytomas. *Proc Natl Acad Sci USA* **86**, 7186-7190.

El-Deiry WS, Kern SE, Pietenpol JA, Kinzler KW, Vogelstein B (1992). Human genomic DNA sequences define a consensus binding site for p53. *Nature Genet* **1**, 45-49.

El-Deiry WS, Tokino T, Velculescu VE, Levy DB, Parsons R, Trent JM, Lin D, Mercer WE, Kinzler KW, Vogelstein B (1993). WAF1, a potential mediator of p53 tumour suppression. *Cell* **75**, 817-825.

El-Deiry WS, Harper JM, O'Connor PM, Velculescu VE, Canman CE, Jackman J, Pietenpol JA, Burrell M, Hill DE, Wang YS, Wiman KG, Mercer WE, Kastan MB, Kohn KW, Elledge SFJ, Kinzler KW, Vogelstein B (1994). Waf1/cip1 is induced in p53-mediated G1 arrest and apoptosis. *Cancer Res* **54**, 1169-1174.

El-Deiry WS, Tokino T, Waldman T, Oliner JD, Velculescu VE, Burrell M, Hill DE, Healy E, Ress JL, Hamilton SR, Kinzler KW, Vogelstein, B (1995). Topological control of p21 (waf1/cip1) expression in normal and neoplastic tissues. *Cancer Res* **13**, 2910-2919.

Eliyahu D, Michalovitz D, Eliyahaum S, Pinhasi-Kimhi O, Oren M (1989). Wild type p53 can inhibit oncogene-mediated focus formation. *Proc Natl Acad Sci USA* **86**, 8763-8767.

Elledge RM, Clark GM, Fuqua SAW, Yu YY, Allred DC (1994). P53 protein accumulation detected by five different antibodies. Relationship to prognosis and heat shock protein 70 in breast cancer. *Cancer Res* **54**, 3752-3757.

Ellis C, Moran M, McCormick F, Pawson T (1990). Phosphorylation of GAP and GAP associated proteins by transforming and mitogenic kinases. *Nature* **343**, 377-381.

Ellison DW, Gatter KC, Steart PV, Lane DP, Weller RO (1992). Expression of the p53 protein in a spectrum of astrocytic tumours. *J Pathol* **168**, 383-386.

Emonard H, Grimaud JA (1990). Matrix metalloproteinases. A review. *Cell Mol Biol* **36**, 131-153.

Engelkamp E, Schafer BW, Mattei MG, Erne P, Heizmann CW (1993). Six *S100* genes are clustered on human chromosome 1q21: Identification of two genes coding for the two previously unreported calcium-binding proteins S100D and S100E. *Proc Natl Acad Sci USA* **90**, 6547-6551.

Englert C, Hou X, Maheswaran S, Bennett P, Ngwu C, Re GG, Garvin AJ, Rosner MR, Haber DA (1995). Wt1 suppresses synthesis of the epidermal growth factor receptor and induces apoptosis. *EMBO J* **14**, 4662-4675.

Enomoto T, Inoue M, Perantoni AO, Terakawa N, Tanizawa O, Rice JM (1990). K-*ras* activation in neoplasms of the human female reproductive tract. *Cancer Res* **50**, 6139-6145.

Enomoto T, Weghorst CM, Inoue M, Tanizawa O, Rice JM (1991). K-*ras* activation occurs frequently in mucinous adenocarcinomas and rarely in other common epithelial tumours of the ovary. *Am J Path* **139**, 777-785.

Enomoto T, Fujita M, Cheng C, Nakashima R, Ozaki M, Inoue M, Nomura T (1995). Loss of expression and loss of heterozygosity in the DCC gene in neoplasms of the human female reproductive tract. *Br J Cancer* **71**, 462-467.

Escot C, Zhao Y, Puech C, Rochefort H (1996). Cellular localisation by *in situ* hybridization of cathepsin D, stromelysin-3, and urokinase plasminogen activator RNAs in breast cancer. *Breast Cancer Res Treat* **38**, 217-226.

Eshleman JR, Markowitz D (1995). Microsatellite instability in inherited and sporadic neoplasms. *Curr Opin Oncol* **7**, 83-89.

Eshleman JR, Leng EZ, Bowerfind GK, Parsons R, Vogelstein B, Willson JKV, Veigl ML, Sedwick WD, Markowitz SD (1995). Increased mutation rate at the HPRT locus accompanies microsatellite instability in colon cancer. *Oncogene* **10**, 33-57.

Eshleman JR, Markowitz SD, Donover PS, Lang EZ, Lutterbaugh JD, Li GM, Longley M, Modrich P, Veigl ML, Sedwick WD (1996). Diverse hypermutability of multiple expressed sequence motifs present in a cancer with microsatellite instability. *Oncogene* **12**, 1425-1432.

Esteve A, Lehman T, Jiang W, Weinstein IB, Harris CC, Ruol A, Peracchia A, Montesano R, Hollstein M (1993). Correlation of p53 mutations with epidermal growth factor receptor over-expression and absence of *mdm2* amplification in human oesophageal carcinomas. *Mol Carcinogen* **8**, 306-311.

Etzoni A (1994). Adhesion molecules in host defence. *Clin Diagn Lab Immunol* **1**, 1-4.

Eustace W, Johnson B, Jones NA, Rowlands DC, Williams A, Guest SS, Brown G (1995). Down-regulation but not phosphorylation of stathmin is associated with induction of HL-60 cells growth arrest and differentiation by physiological agents. *FEBS Lett* **364**, 309-313.

Evan GI, Wyllie AH, Gilbert CS, Littlewood TD, Land H, Brooks M, Waters CM, Penn LZ, Hancock DC (1992). Induction of apoptosis in fibroblasts by c-myc protein. *Cell* **69**, 119-128.

Ewen ME, Sluss HK, Sherr CJ, Matsushime H, Kato JY, Livingston DM (1993a). Functional interactions of the retinoblastoma protein with mammalian D-type cyclins. *Cell* **73**, 487-497.

Ewen ME, Sluss HK, Whitehouse LL, Livingstone DM (1993b). TGF beta inhibition of cdk4 synthesis is linked to cell cycle arrest. *Cell* **74**, 1009-1020.

Ewing CM, Ru N, Morton RA, Robinson JC, Wheelock MJ, Johnson KR, Barrett JC, Isaacs WB (1995). Chromosome 5 suppresses tumorigenicity of PC prostate cancer cells. Correlation with re-expression of alpha catenin and restoration E-cadherin function. *Cancer Res* **55**, 4813-4817.

Faille A, Decremoux P, Extra JM, Linares G, Espie M, Bourstyn E, Derocquancourt A, Giacchetti S, Marty M, Calvo F (1994). P53 mutations and overexpression in locally advanced breast cancers. *Br J Cancer* **69**, 1145-1150.

Fajac A, Benard J, Lhomme C, Rey A, Duvillard P, Rochard F, Bernaudin JF, Riou G (1995). C-ERBB2 gene amplification and protein expression in ovarian epithelial tumours. Evaluation of their prognostic significance by multivariate analysis. *Int J Cancer* **64**, 146-151.

Fakharzadeh SS, Trusko SP, George DL (1991). Tumorigenic potential associated with enhanced expresssion of a gene that is amplified in a mouse tumour cell line. *EMBO J* **10**, 1565-1569.

Fanti V, Brookes S, Smith S, Casey G, Barnes D, Johnstone G, Peters G, Dickson C (1989). Characterisation of the proto-oncogene *int-2* and its potential for diagnosis of human breast cancer. In: *Cancer Cells*, Vol 2, Greaves M, Furth M (eds). Cold Spring Harbor Laboratory Press, Cold Spring Harbor, NY, pp. 283-287.

Farmer G, Bargonetti J, Zhu H, Friedman P, Prywes R, Prives C (1992). Wild type p53 activates transcription *in vitro*. *Nature* **358**, 83-86.

Farrow SN, White JHM, Martinou I, Raven T, Pun KT, Grinham CJ, Martinou JC, Brown R (1995). Cloning of a *bcl-2* homologue by interaction with adenovirus E1B 19K. *Nature* **374**, 731-733.

Faust JB, Meeker TC (1992). Amplification and expression of *bcl-1* gene in human solid tumour cell lines. *Cancer Res* **52**, 2460-2463.

Fazely F, Ledinko N (1990). Retinoic acid and epidermal growth factor binding in retinoid-mediated invasion suppressed lung carcinoma cells. *Anticancer Res* **10**, 667-670.

Fearon ER, Jones PA (1992). Progressing toward a molecular description of colorectal cancer development. *FASEB J* **6**, 2783-2790.

Fearon ER, Vogelstein B (1990). A genetic model for colorectal tumorigenesis. *Cell* **61**, 759-767.

Fearon ER, Vogelstein B, Feinberg AP (1984). Somatic deletion and duplication of genes on chromosome 11 in Wilms tumours. *Nature* **309**, 176-178.

Fearon ER, Cho KR, Nigro JM, Kern SE, Simons JW, Rupert JM, Hamilton SR, Preisinger AC, Thomas G, Kinzler KW, Vogelstein B (1990). Identification of a chromosome 18q gene that is altered in colorectal cancer. *Science* **247**, 49-56.

Feinstein E, Cimino G, Gale RP, Alimena G, Berthier R, Kishi K, Goldman J, Zaccaria A, Berrebi A, Canaani E (1991). p53 in chronic myelogenous leukaemia in acute phase. *Proc Natl Acad Sci USA* **88**, 6293-6297.

Feng J, Funk WD, Wang SS, Weinrich SL, Avilion AA, Chiu CP, Adams RR, Chang E, Allsopp RC, Yu J, Le S, West MD, Harley DB, Andrews WH, Greider CW, Villeponteau B (1995). The RNA component of human telomerase. *Science* **269**, 1236-1241.

Ferdeghini M, Gaducci A, Prontera C, Annicchiarico C, Gagetti O, Bianchi M, Facchini V, Genazzani AR (1995). Pre-operative serum intercellular adhesion molecule-1 (ICAM) and E-selectin (endothelial cell leukocyte adhesion molecule, ELAM-1) in patients with epithelial ovarian cancer. *Anticancer Res* **15**, 2255-2260.

Ferno M, Baldetorpe B, Borg A, Olsson H, Sigurdsson H, Killander D (1992). Flow cytometric DNA index and S-phase fraction in breast cancer in relation to other prognostic variable and to clinical outcome. *Acta Oncol* **31**, 157-165.

Ferrandina G, Scambia G, Marone M, Panici PB, Giannitelli C, Pernisco S, Coronetta F, Mancuso S (1996). Nm23 in ovarian cancer. *Ann NY Acad Sci* **784**, 509-512.

Ferrando AA, Balbin M, Pendas AM, Vizoso F, Velasco G, Lopezotin C (1996). Mutational analysis of the human cyclin-dependent kinase inhibitor p27 (kip1) in primary breast carcinomas. *Hum Genet* **97**, 91-94.

Ferrara N, Henzel WJ (1989). Pituitary follicular cells secrete a novel heparin-binding growth factor specific for vascular endothelial cells. *Biochem Biophys Res Commun* **161**, 851-858.

Ferrara N, Houck KA, Jakeman LB, Winer J, Leung DW (1991). The vascular endothelial growth factor family of polypeptides. *J Cell Biochem* **47**, 211-218.

Ferrara N, Carver-Moore K, Chen H, Down M, Lu L, O'Shea KS, Powell-Braxton L, Hillan KJ, Moore MW (1996). Heterozygous embryonic lethality induced by targeted inactivation of the VEGF gene. *Nature* **380**, 439-442.

Ferris DK, Harel-Bellan A, Morimoto RI, Welch W, Farrar WL (1988). Mitogen and lymphokine stimulation of heat shock proteins in T lymphocytes. *Proc Natl Acad Sci USA* **85**, 3850-3854.

Fett JW, Strydom DJ, Lobb RR, Alderman EM, Bethune JL, Riordan JF, Vallee BL (1985). Isolation and characterisation of angiogenin, an angiogenic protein from human carcinoma cells. *Biochemistry* **24**, 5480-5486.

Fialkow PJ (1976). Clonal origin of human tumours. *Biochim Biophys Acta* **458**, 283-321.

Fialkow PJ, Martin GM, Klein G, Clifford P, Singh S (1972). Evidence for a clonal origin of head and neck tumours. *Int J Cancer* **9**, 133-142.

Fialkow PJ, Jackson CE, Block MA, Greenawald KA (1977). Multicellular origin of parathyroid adenomas. *N Engl J Med* **297**, 696-698.

Fidler IJ, Ellis LM (1994). The implications of angiogenesis for the biology and therapy of cancer metastasis. *Cell* **79**, 185-188.

Fidler IJ, Gersten DM, Budmen MB (1976). Characterisation in vivo and in vitro of tumour cells selected for resistance to syngeneic lymphocyte-mediated cytotoxicity. *Cancer Res* **36**, 3160-3165.

Field JK, Spandidos DA (1990). The role of *ras* and *myc* oncogenes in human solid tumours and their relevance in diagnosis and prognosis. *Anticancer Res* **10**, 1-22.

Field JK, Spandidos DA, Malliri A, Gosney JR, Yiagnisis M, Stell PM (1991). Elevated p53 expression correlates with a history of heavy smoking in squamous cell carcinoma of the head and neck. *Br J Cancer* **64**, 573-577.

Field JK, Spandidos DA, Stell PM (1992). Overexpression of p53 gene in head and neck cancer, linked with heavy smoking and drinking. *Lancet* **339**, 502-503.

Fink K, Zeuther E (1978). Heat shock proteins in *Tetrahymena*. *Mol Cell Biol* **12**, 103-115.

Finlay CA (1993). The mdm-2 oncogene can overcome wild type p53 suppression of transformed cell growth. *Mol Cell Biol* **13**, 301-306.

Finlay CA, Hinds PW, Tan T, Eliyahu D, Oren M, Levine AJ (1988). Activating mutations for transformation by p53 produce a gene product that forms an hsc70-p53 complex with an altered half-life. *Mol Cell Biol* **8**, 531-539.

Finlay CA, Hinds PW, Levine AJ (1989). The p53 proto-oncogene can act as a suppressor of transformation. *Cell* **57**, 1083-1093.

Finley D, Varshavsky A (1985). The ubiquitin system: functions and mechanisms. *Trends Biochem Sci* **10**, 343-346.

Finley D, Ozkaynak E, Varshavsky A (1987). The yeast polyubiquitin is essential for resistance to high temperatures, starvation, and other stresses. *Cell* **48**, 1035-1046.

Finn GK, Kurz BW, Cheng RZ, Shmookler RRJ (1989). Homologous plasmid recombination is elevated in immortally transformed cells. *Mol Cell Biol* **9**, 4009-4017.

Finnerty H, Kelleher K, Morris GE, Bean K, Mergerb DFM, Kriz R, Morris JC, Soojkdeo H, Turner KJ, Wood CR (1993). Molecular cloning of murine flt and flt4. *Oncogene* **8**, 2293-2298.

Firpo EJ, Koff A, Solomon MJ, Roberts JM (1994). Inactivation of a cdk2 inhibitor during interleukin 2-induced proliferation of human T-lymphocytes. *Mol Cell Biol* **14**, 4889-4901.

Firsching A, Nickel P, Mora P, Allolio B (1995). Anti-proliferative and angiostatic activity of suramin analogues. *Cancer Res* **55**, 4957-4961.

Fishel R, Lescoe MK, Rao MRS, Copeland NG, Genkins NA, Garber J, Kane M, Kolodner R (1993). The human mutator gene homolog MSH2 and its association with hereditary non-polyposis colon cancer. *Cell* **75**, 1027-1038.

Flaman JM, Waridel F, Estreicher A, Vannier A, Limacher JM, Gilbert D, Iggo R, Frebourg T (1996). The human tumour suppressor gene p53 is alternatively spliced in normal cells. *Oncogene* **12**, 813-818.

Florenes VA, Aamdal S, Myklebost O, Maelandsmo GM, Bruland OS, Fodstad O (1992). Levels of nm23 messenger RNA in metastatic malignant melanomas: Inverse correlation to disease progression. *Cancer Res* **52**, 6088-6091.

Florenes VA, Oyjord T, Holm R, Skrede M, Borresen AL, Nesland JM, Fodstad O (1994). Tp53 allele loss, mutations and expression in malignant melanoma. *Br J Cancer* **69**, 253-259.

Folkman J (1972). Anti-angiogenesis: New concept for therapy of solid tumours. *Ann Surg* **175**, 409-416.

Folkman J (1974). Tumour angiogenesis. *Adv Cancer Res* **19**, 331-365.

Folkman J (1975). Tumour angiogenesis. In: *Cancer. A Comprehensive Treatise*, Becker FF (ed.). Plenum Press, New York, pp. 355-365.

Folkman J, Mersler E, Abernathy C, Williams G (1971). Isolation of a tumour factor responsible for angiogenesis. *J Exp Med* **133**, 275-288.

Fong KM, Zimmerman PV, Smith PJ (1994). Correlation of loss of heterozygosity at 11p with tumour progression and survival in non-small cell lung cancer. *Genes Chrom Cancer* **10**, 183-189.

Fong KM, Zimmerman PV, Smith PJ (1995a). Microsatellite instability and other molecular abnormalities in non-small cell lung cancer. *Cancer Res* **55**, 28-30.

Fong KM, Zimmerman PV, Smith PJ (1995b). Tumour progression and loss of heterozygosity at 5q and 18q in non-small cell lung cancer. *Cancer Res* **55**, 220-223.

Fontana X, Ferrari P, Abbes M, Monticelli J, Namer M, Bussiere F (1994). Mdm2 gene amplification in primary breast cancer. *Bull Cancer* **81**, 587-592.

Fontanini G, Bigini D, Vignati S, Basolo F, Mussi A, Lucchi M, Chine S, Angeletti CA, Harris AL, Bevilacqua G (1995). Microvessel count predicts metastatic disease and survival in non-small cell lung cancer. *J Pathol* **177**, 57-63.

Fornace AJ, Nebert DW, Hollander MC, Luethy JD, Papathanasiou M, Fargnoli J, Holbrook NJ (1989). Mammalian genes coordinately regulated by growth arrest signals and DNA damaging agents. *Mol Cell Biol* **9**, 4196-4203.

Forrester K, Almoguera C, Han K, Grizzle WE, Perucho M (1987). Detection of high incidence of K-*ras* oncogenes during colorectal tumorigenesis. *Nature* **327**, 298-303.

Forus A, Florenes VA, Maelandsmo GM, Fodstad O, Myklebost O (1994). The protooncogene CHOP GADD153, involved in growth arrest and DNA damage response, is amplified in a subset of human sarcomas. *Cancer Genet Cytogenet* **78**, 165-171.

Foulds L (1949). Mammary tumours in hybrid mice: Growth and progression of spontaneous tumours. *Br J Cancer* **3**, 345-375.

Foulds L (1969). *Neoplastic Development*, Vol. 1. Academic Press, London.

Foulkes WD, Stamp GWH, Afzal A, Lalani N, McFarlane CP, Trowsdale J, Campbell IG (1995). Mdm2 over-expression is rare in ovarian carcinoma irrespective of p53 mutation status. *Br J Cancer* **72**, 883-888.

Fountain JW, Bale SJ, Housman DE, Dracopoli NC (1990). Genetics of melanoma. *Cancer Surveys* **9**, 645-671.

Fox PL, Sa G, Dobrowolski SF, Stacey DW (1994). The regulation of endothelial cell motility by p21 ras. *Oncogene* **9**, 3519-3526.

Fox SB, Fawcett J, Jackson DG, Collins I, Gatter KC, Harris AL, Gearing A, Simmons DL (1994). Normal human tissues, in addition to some tumours, express multiple different CD44 isoforms. *Cancer Res* **54**, 4539-4546.

Fox SB, Gatter KC, Harris AL, Bicknell R (1995a). Thymidine phosphorylase is angiogenic and promotes tumour growth. *Proc Natl Acad Sci USA* **92**, 998-1002.

Fox SB, Moghaddam A, Westwood M, Turley H, Bicknell R, Gatter KC, Harris AL (1995b). Platelet-derived endothelial cell growth factor thymidine phosphorylase expression in normal tissues. An immunohistochemical study. *J Pathol* **176**, 183-190.

Fox SB, Turner GDH, Gatter KC, Harris AL (1995c). The increased expression of adhesion molecules ICAM-3, E-selectin and P-selectin on breast cancer endothelium. *J Pathol* **177**, 369-376.

Fox SB, Westwood M, Moghaddam A, Comley M, Turley H, Whitehouse RM, Bicknell R, Gatter KC, Harris AL (1996). The angiogenic factor platelet-derived endothelial cell growth factor thymidine phosphorylase is up-regulated in breast cancer epithelium and endothelium. *Br J Cancer* **73**, 275-280.

Francke U, Holmes LB, Atkins L, Riccardi VM (1979). Aniridia-Wilms tumour association: evidence for specific deletion of 11p13. *Cell Genet* **24**, 185-192.

Frank JL, Bur ME, Garb JL, Kay S, Ware JL, Sismanis A, Neifeld JP (1994). p53 tumour suppressor oncogene expression in squamous cell carcinoma of hypopharynx. *Cancer* **73**, 181-186.

Frankel RH, Bayona W, Koslow M, Newcomb EW (1992). p53 mutations in human malignant gliomas. Comparison of loss of heterozygosity with mutation frequency. *Cancer Res* **52**, 1427-1433.

Frater-Schroder M, Risau W, Hallmann R, Gautschi P, Bohlen P (1987). Tumour necrosis factor type α, a potent inhibitor of endothelial cell growth *in vitro* is angiogenic *in vivo*. *Proc Natl Acad Sci USA* **84**, 5277-5281.

Frebourg T, Friend SH (1992). Cancer risks from germline p53 mutations. *J Clin Invest* **90**, 1637-1641.

Fridman R, Fuerst TR, Bird RE, Hoyhtya M, Oelkuct M, Kraus S, Komarek D, Liotta LA, Berman ML, Stetler-Stevenson WG (1992). Domain structure of human 72-kDa gelatinase/type IV collagenase. Characterisation of proteolytic activity and identification of the tissue inhibitor of metalloproteinase-2 (TIMP-2). *J Biol Chem* **267**, 15398-15405.

Friedman LS, Ostermeyer EA, Szabo CI, Dowd P, Lynch ED, Rowell SE, King MC (1994). Confirmation of BRCA1 lay analysis of germline mutations linked to breast and ovarian cancer in 10 families. *Nature Genet* **8**, 399-404.

Friedman LS, Ostermeyer EA, Lynch ED, Welcsh P, Szabo CI, Meza JE, Anderson LA, Dowd P, Lee MK, Rowell SE, Ellison J, Boyd J, King MC (1995). 22 genes from chromosome 17q21. Cloning, sequencing, and characterisation of mutations in breast cancer families and tumours. *Genomics* **25**, 256-263.

Friedman PN, Chen XB, Bargonetti J, Prives C (1993). The p53 protein is an unusually shaped tetramer that binds directly to DNA. *Proc Natl Acad Sci USA* **90**, 3319-3323.

Friedrichs K, Gluba S, Eidtmann H, Jonat W (1993). Overexpression of p53 and prognosis in breast cancer. *Cancer* **72**, 3641-3647.

Friend SH, Bernards R, Rogelj S, Weinberg RA, Rapport JM, Albert DM, Dryja TP (1986). A human DNA segment with properties of the gene that predisposes to retinoblastoma and osteosarcoma. *Nature* **323**, 643-646.

Friend SH, Horowitz JM, Gerber MR, Wang XF, Bogenman E, Li FP, Weinberg RA (1987). Deletions of a DNA sequence in retinoblastoma and mesenchymal tumours: Organisation of the sequence and its encoded protein. *Proc Natl Acad Sci USA* **84**, 9059-9063.

Frisch SM, Ruley HE (1987). Transcription from the stromelysin promoter is induced by interleukin-1 and repressed by dexamethasone. *J Biol Chem* **262**, 16300-16304.

Frixen UH, Behrens J, Sachs M, Eberle G, Voss B, Warda A, Lochner D, Birchmeier W (1991). E-cadherin mediated cell–cell adhesion prevents invasiveness of human carcinoma cells. *J Cell Biol* **113**, 173-185.

Froggatt NJ, Leveson SH, Garner RC (1995). Low frequency and late occurrence of p53 and DCC aberrations in colorectal tumours. *J Cancer Res Clin Oncol* **121**, 7-15.

Frohlich E, Schaumburger-Lever G, Klessen C (1995). Immunocytochemical and immunoelectron microscopic demonstration of cathepsin B in human malignant melanoma. *Br J Dermatol* **132**, 867-875.

Fujita M, Inoue M, Tanizawa O, Iwamoto S, Enomoto T (1992). Alterations of the p53 gene in human primary cervical carcinoma with and without human papilloma virus infection. *Cancer Res* **52**, 5323-5328.

Fujita M, Enomoto T, Yoshino K, Nomura T, Buzard GS, Inoue M, Okudaira Y (1995). Microsatellite instability and alterations in the HMSH2 gene in human ovarian cancer. *Int J Cancer* **64**, 361-366.

Fults D, Trippets RH, Thomas GA, Nakamura Y, White R (1989). Loss of heterozygosity for loci on chromosome 17p in human malignant astrocytoma. *Cancer Res* **49**, 6572-6577.

Fults D, Brockmeyer D, Tullous MW, Pedone CA, Cawthon RM (1992). p53 mutations and loss of heterozygosity on chromosome 17 and 10 during human astrocytoma progression. *Cancer Res* **52**, 674-679.

Fung YT, Murphree AL, T'Ang A, Qian J, Hinrichs SH, Benedict WF (1987). Structural evidence for the authenticity of the human retinoblastoma gene. *Science* **236**, 1657-1661.

Funk WD, Pak DT, Karas RH, Wright WE, Shay JW (1992). A transcriptionally active DNA binding site for human p53 protein complexes. *Mol Cell Biol* **12**, 2866-2871.

Furukawa Y, DeCaprio JA, Belvin M, Griffin JD (1991). Heterogenous expression of the product of the retinoblastoma susceptibility gene in primary human leukaemia cells. *Oncogene* **6**, 1343-1346.

Futreal PA, Liu Q, Shattuck-Eidens CC, Harshman K, Tavtigian S, Bennett LM, Haugen-Strano A, Swensen J, Miki Y, Eddington K, McClure M, Frye C, Weaver-Feldhaus J, Ding W, Gholami Z, Soderkvist P, Terry L, Jhanwar S, Berchuck A, Inglehart JD, Marks J, Ballinger DG, Barrett JC, Skolnick MH, Kamb A, Wiseman R (1994). *BRCA1* mutations in primary breast and ovarian carcinomas. *Science* **266**, 120-122.

Gage JR, Meyers C, Wettstein FO (1990). The E7 protein of the nononcogenic human papilloma virus type 6b (HPV-6b) and of the oncogenic HPV-16 differ in retinoblastoma protein binding and other properties. *J Virol* **64**, 723-730.

Galland F, Karamysheva A, Pebusque MJ, Borg JP, Rottapel R, Dubreuil P, Rosnet O, Birnbaum D (1993). The *flt4* gene encodes a transmembrane tyrosine kinase related to the vascular endothelial growth factor receptor. *Oncogene* **8**, 1233-1240.

Gallo G, Voci A, Schwarze PE, Fugassa E (1987). Effects of triiodothyronine on protein turnover in rat hepatocyte primary culture. *J Endocrinol* **113**, 173-177.

Galtier de Reure F, Capony F, Maudelonde T, Rochefort H (1992). Estradiol stimulates cell growth and secretion of procathepsin D and a 120 kilodalton protein in the human ovarian cancer cell line BG-1. *J Clin Endocrinol Metab* **75**, 1497-1502.

Gamallo C, Palacios J, Suarez A, Pizarro A, Navarro P, Quintanilla M, Cano A (1993). Correlation of E-cadherin expression with differentiation grade and histological type in breast carcinoma. *Amer J Pathol* **142**, 987-993.

Ganesh S, Sier CFM, Griffioen G, Vloedgraven HJM, De Boer A, Welvaart K, van De Velde CJH, van Krieken JHJM, Verheijen JH, Lamers CBHW, Verspaget HW (1994). Prognostic relevance of plasminogen activators and their inhibitors in colorectal cancers. *Cancer Res* **54**, 4065-4071.

Gao C, Wang LC, Voss WC (1988). The role of v-*mos* in transformation, oncogenicity and metastatic potential of mink lung cells. *Oncogene* **3**, 267-273.

Gao X, Chen YQ, Wu N, Grignon DJ, Sakr W, Porter AT, Honn KV (1995a). Somatic mutations of the *waf1/cip1* gene in primary prostate cancer. *Oncogene* **11**, 1395-1398.

Gao X, Zacharek A, Salkowski A, Grignon DJ, Sakr W, Porter AT, Honn KV (1995b). Loss of heterozygosity of the BRCA1 and other loci on chromosome 17q in human prostate cancer. *Cancer Res* **55**, 1002-1005.

Garinchesa P, Sanzmoncasi MP, Campbell IG, Rettig WJ (1994). Non-polarised expression of basal cell adhesion molecule B-CAM in epithelial ovarian cancers. *Int J Oncol* **5**, 1261-1266.

Garver RI, Goldsmith KT, Rodu B, Hu PC, Sorscher EJ, Curiel DT (1994). Strategy for achieving selective killing of carcinomas. *Gene Ther* **1**, 46-50.

Gasparini G, Bevilacqua P, Boracchi P, Maluta S, Pozza F, Barbareschi M, Palma PD, Mezzetti M, Harris AL (1994). Prognostic value of p53 expression in early stage breast carcinoma compared with tumour angiogenesis, epidermal growth factor receptor, c-erbB-2, cathepsin D, DNA ploidy, parameters of cell kinetics and conventional features. *Int J Oncol* **4**, 155-162.

Gasparini G, Bevilacqua P, Bonoldi E, Testolin A, Galassi A, Verderio P, Boracchi P, Gugliemi RB, Pezzella F (1995). Predictive and prognostic markers in a series of patients with head and neck squamous cell invasive carcinoma treated with concurrent chemoradiation therapy. *Clin Cancer Res* **1**, 1375-1383.

Gehlsen KR, Davis GE, Siramarao P (1992). Integrin expression in human melanoma cells with differing invasive and metastatic properties. *Clin Exp Metastasis* **10**, 111-120.

Gessler M, Bruns GAP (1989). A detailed physical map of the WAGR region. *Cytogenet Cell Genet* **51**, 1003-1004.

Gessler M, Thomas GH, Couillin P, Junien C, McGillvray BC, Hayden H, Jaschek G, Bruns GAP (1989a). A deletion map of the WAGR region on human chromosome 11. *Amer J Genet* **44**, 486-495.

Gessler M, Simola KQJ, Bruns GAP (1989b). Cloning of break points of a chromosome in translocation identifies the AN2 locus. *Science* **244**, 1575-1578.

Gessler M, Poustka A, Cavenee W, Neve RL, Orkin SH, Bruns GAP (1990). Homozygous deletion in Wilms tumours of a zinc finger gene identified by chromosome jumping. *Nature* **343**, 774-778.

Gessler M, Konig A, Moore J, Qualman S, Arden K, Cavenee W, Bruns G (1993). Homozygous inactivation of *wt1* in a Wilms tumour associated with the WAGR syndrome. *Genes Chrom Cancer* **7**, 131-136.

Gessler M, Konig A, Arden K, Grundy P, Orkin S, Sallan S, Peters C, Ruyle S, Mandell J, Li F, Cavenee W, Bruns G (1994). Infrequent mutation of the *wt1* gene in 77 Wilms tumours. *Human Mut* **3**, 212-222.

Gherardi E, Stoker M (1990). Hepatocyte and scatter factor. *Nature* **346**, 228.

Gherardi E, Gray J, Stoker M, Perryman M, Furlong R (1989). Purification of scatter factor, a fibroblast-derived basic protein that modulates epithelial interactions and movement. *Proc Natl Acad Sci USA* **86**, 5844-5848.

Ghose T, Lee CLY, Fernandez LA, Lee SHS, Raman R, Colp P (1990). Role of 1q trisomy in tumorigenicity, growth, and metastasis of human leukaemic B cell clones in nude mice. *Cancer Res* **50**, 3737-3742.

Gibbs FEM, Wilkinson MC, Rudland PS, Barraclough R (1994). Interactions *in vitro* of p9Ka, the rat S-100 related metastasis-inducing, calcium-binding protein. *J Biol Chem* **268**, 18992-18999.

Gilhus NE, Jones M, Turley H, Gatter KC, Nagvekar N, Newsom-Davis J, Willcox N (1995). Oncogene proteins and proliferation antigens in thymomas. Increased expression of epidermal growth factor receptor and Ki67 antigen. *J Clin Pathol* **48**, 447-455.

Gilles AM, Presecan E, Vonica A, Lasacu I (1991). Nucleoside diphosphate kinase from human erythrocytes, structural characterisation of the two polypeptide chains responsible for heterogeneity of the hexameric enzyme. *J Biol Chem* **266**, 8784-8789.

Gima T, Kato H, Honda T, Imamura T, Sasazuki T, Wake N (1994). DCC gene alteration in human endometrial carcinoma. *Int J Cancer* **57**, 480-485.

Gimbrone MA, Jr, Gullino PM (1976). Angiogenic capacity of preneoplastic lesions of the murine mammary gland as a marker of neoplastic transformation. *Cancer Res* **36**, 2611-2620.

Gimbrone MA, Jr, Leapman SB, Cotran RS, Folkman J (1972). Tumour dormancy *in vivo* by prevention of neovascularisation. *J Exp Med* **136**, 261-276.

Ginsberg D, Mechta F, Yaniv M, Oren M (1991). Wild type p53 can down-modulate the activity of various promoters. *Proc Natl Acad Sci USA* **88**, 9979-9983.

Girod SC, Cesarz D, Fischer U, Kruaeger GRF (1995). Detection of p53 and mdm2 protein expression in head and neck carcinogenesis. *Anticancer Res* **15**, 1453-1457.

Gladson CL, Cheresh DA (1991). Glioblastoma expression of vitronectin and the $\alpha_v\beta_3$ integrin. Adhesion mechanism for transformed glial cells. *J Clin Invest* **88**, 1924-1932.

Glaser T, Lewis WH, Bruns GAP, Watkins PC, Rogler CE, Shows TB, Powers VE, Willard HF, Goguen JM, Simola KOJ, Housman DE (1986). The β subunit of follicle stimulating hormone is deleted in patients with aniridia and Wilms tumour, allowing a further definition of the WAGR locus. *Nature* **321**, 882-887.

Glaser T, Jones C, Call KM, Lewis WH, Bruns GAP, Junien C, Waziri M, Housman DE (1987). Mapping the WAGR region of chromosome 11p: somatic cell hybrids provide a fine structure map. *Cytogenet Cell Genet* **46**, 620.

Gleeson NC, Gonsalves R, Bonnar J (1993). Plasminogen activator inhibitors in endometrial adenocarcinoma. *Cancer* **72**, 1670-1672.

Glinsky GV, Glinsky VV (1996). Apoptosis and metastasis. A superior resistance of metastatic cancer cells to programmed cell death. *Cancer Lett* **101**, 43-51.

Goldberg AF, Tisschler M, De Martino G, Griffin G (1980). Hormonal regulation of protein degradation and synthesis in skeletal muscle. *Fed Proc* **39**, 31-36.

Goldman CK, Kim J, Wong WL, King V, Brock T, Gillespie GY (1993). Epidermal growth factor stimulates vascular endothelial growth factor production by human malignant glioma cells. A model of glioblastoma multiforme pathophysiology. *Mol Biol Cell* **4**, 121-133.

Gonzalez-Garcia M, Perez-Ballestero R, Ding LY, Duan L, Boise LH, Thompson CB, Nunez G (1994). Bcl-x(L) is the major bcl-x messenger RNA form expressed during murine development and its product localises to mitochondria. *Development* **120**, 3033-3042.

Gonzalez-Garcia M, Garcia I, Ding LY, O'Shea S, Boise LH, Thompson CB, Nunez G (1995). Bcl-x is expressed in embryonic and post-natal neural tissues and functions to prevent neuronal cell death. *Proc Natl Acad Sci USA* **92**, 4304-4308.

Goodrich DW, Lee WH (1990). The molecular genetics of retinoblastoma. *Cancer Surveys* **9**, 529-554.

Gordon P, Brookers S, Smith R, Dickson C (1983). Tumorigenesis by mouse mammary tumour virus: evidence for a common region for provirus integration in mammary tumours. *Cell* **33**, 369-377.

Gorr SU, Shioi J, Cohn DV (1989). Interaction of calcium with procine adrenal chromogranin A (secretory protein I) and chromogranin B (secretogranin I). *Amer J Physiol* **257**, E247-E254.

Gospodarowicz D, Massoglia S, Cheng J, Fujii DK (1986). Effect of fibroblast growth factor and lipoproteins on the proliferation of endothelial cells derived from bovine adrenal cortex, brain cortex, and corpus luteum capillaries. *J Cell Physiol* **127**, 121-136.

Gotley DC, Fawcett J, Walsh MD, Reeder JA, Simmons DL, Antalis TM (1996). Alternatively spliced variants of the cell adhesion molecule CD44 and tumour progression in colorectal cancer. *Br J Cancer* **74**, 342-351.

Goto K, Endo, H, Fijiyoshi T (1988). Cloning of the sequences expressed abundantly in established cell lines: Identification of a cDNA clone highly homologous to S-100, a calcium binding protein. *J Biochem* **103**, 48-53.

Gotsch U, Jager U, Dominis M, Vestweber D (1994). Expression of P-selectin on endothelial cells up-regulated by LPS and TNA-α *in vivo*. *Cell Adhesion Commun* **2**, 7-14.

Goubin F, Ducommun B (1995). Identification of binding domains on the p21 (cip1) cyclin-dependent kinase inhibitor. *Oncogene* **10**, 2281-2287.

Gould VE, Koukoulis GK, Virtanen I (1990). Extracellular matrix proteins and their receptors in the normal hyperplastic and neoplastic breast. *Cell Diff Develop* **32**, 409-416.

Graf J, Iwamoto Y, Sasaki M, Martin GR, Kleinman HK, Robey FA, Yamada Y (1987). Identification of an amino acid sequence in laminin mediating cell attachment, chemotaxis and receptor binding. *Cell* **48**, 989-996.

Graham FL, van der Eb AJ (1973). A new technique for the assay of infectivity of adenovirus 5 DNA. *Virology* **52**, 456-467.

Graninger WB, Seto M, Boutain B, Goldman P, Korsmeyer SJ (1987). Expression of bcl-2 and bcl-2-Ig fusion transcript in normal and neoplastic cells. *J Clin Invest* **80**, 1512-1515.

Grant MFX, Blijham G, Reiner A, Reynder SM, Shutte B, van Asche C, Steger G, Jakesz R (1992). DNA ploidy and other results of DNA flow cytometry as prognostic factors in operable breast cancer: 10-year results of a randomised study. *Eur J Cancer* **28**, 711-716.

Green DR, McGahon A, Martin SJ (1996). Regulation of apoptosis by oncogenes. *J Cell Biochem* **60**, 33-38.

Green MR (1989). When the products of oncogenes and anti-oncogenes meet. *Cell* **56**, 1-3.

Green MR (1991). Biochemical mechanisms of constitutive and regulated pre-mRNA splicing. *Annu Rev Cell Biol* **7**, 559-593.

Greenblatt M, Shubik P (1968). Tumour angiogenesis: Transfilter diffusion studies in the hamster by transparent chamber technique. *J Natl Cancer Inst* **41**, 111-124.

Greider CW, Blackburn EH (1987). The telomere terminal transferase of *Tetrahymena* is a ribonucleoprotein enzyme with two kinds of primer specificity. *Cell* **51** 887-898.

Griffiths TRL, Brotherick I, Bishop RI, White MD, McKenna DM, Horne CHW, Shenton BK, Neal DE, Mellon JK (1996). Cell adhesion molecules in bladder cancer. Soluble serum E-cadherin correlates with predictors of recurrence. *Br J Cancer* **74**, 579-584.

Grigioni WF, Biagini G, D'Errico A, Milani M, Villanacci V, Garbisa S, Mattioli S, Gozzetti G, Mancini AM (1986). Behaviour of basement membrane antigens in gastric and colorectal cancer. Immunohistochemical study. *Acta Path Jpn* **36**, 173-184.

Grigorian MS, Tulchinsky EM, Zain S, Ebralidze AK, Kramerov DA, Kriajevska MV, Georgiev GP, Lukanidin EM (1993). The *mts1* gene and control of tumour metastasis. *Gene* **135**, 229-238.

Grigorian M, Tulchinsky E, Burrone O, Tarabykina S, Georgiev G, Lukanidin E (1994). Modulation of *mts1* expression in mouse and human normal tumour cells. *Electrophoresis* **15**, 463-468.

Grimm T, Johnson JP (1995). Ectopic expression of carcinoembryonic antigen by a melanoma leads to changes in the transcription of two additional cell adhesion molecules. *Cancer Res* **55**, 3254-3257.

Grizzle WE, Myers RB, Arnold MM, Srivastava S (1994). Evaluation of biomarkers in breast and prostate cancer. *J Cell Biochem* **S19**, 259-266.

Groden J, Thliveris A, Samowitz W, Carlson M, Gelbert L, Albertsen H, Joslyn G, Stevens J, Spirio L, Robertson M, Sargeant L, Krapcho K, Wolff E, Burt R, Hughes JP, Warrington J, McPherson J, Wasmuth J, Lepaslier D, Adberrahim H, Cohen D, Leppert M, White R (1991). Identification and characterisation of the familial adenomatous polyposis gene. *Cell* **66**, 589-600.

Groden J, Joslyn G, Samowitz W, Jones D, Bhattacharya N, Spirio L, Thliveris A, Robertson M, Egan S, Meuth M, White R (1995). Response of colon cancer cell lines to the introduction of APC, a colon-specific tumour suppressor gene. *Cancer Res* **55**, 1531-1539.

Grondahl-Hansen J, Christensen IJ, Rosenquist C, Brunner N, Mouridsen HT, Dano K, Blicherttoft M (1993). High levels of urokinase type plasminogen activator and its inhibitor PAI-1 in cytosolic extracts of breast carcinoma are associated with poor prognosis. *Cancer Res* **53**, 2513-2521.

Gross N, Beck D, Beretta C, Jackson D, Perruisseau G (1995). CD44 expression and modulation on human neuroblastoma tumours and cell lines. *Eur J Cancer* **31A**, 471-475.

Gross RH, Sheldon LA, Fletcher CF, Brinckerhoff CE (1984). Isolation of a collagenase cDNA clone and measurement of changing collagenase mRNA levels during induction in rabbit synovial fibroblasts. *Proc Natl Acad Sci USA* **81**, 1981-1985.

Groves RW, Allen MH, Ross EL, Ahsan G, Barker JNWN, MacDonald DfM (1993). Expression of selectin ligands by cutaneous squamous cell carcinoma. *Amer J Pathol* **143**, 1220-1225.

Grubb GR, Yun K, Reeve AE, Eccles MR (1995). Exclusion of the Wilms tumour gene (*wt1*) promoter as a site of frequent mutation in Wilms' tumour. *Oncogene* 10, 1677-1681.

Grumet M, Friedlander DR, Edelman GM (1993). Evidence for the binding of NG-CAM to laminin. *Cell Adhesion Commun* 1, 177-190.

Gu Y, Turck CW, Morgan D (1993). Inhibition of CDK2 activity in vivo by an associated 20K regulatory unit. *Nature* 366, 707-710.

Guan JL, Shalloway D (1992). Regulation of focal adhesion-associated protein tyrosine kinase by both cellular adhesion and oncogenic transformation. *Nature* 358, 690-692.

Guan JL, Trevithick JE, Hynes RO (1991). Fibronectin/integrin interaction induces tyrosine phosphorylation of a 120 kDa protein. *Cell Reg* 2, 951-964.

Gudas JM, Nguyen H, Klein RC, Katayose D, Seth P, Cowan KH (1995a). Differential expression of multiple mdm2 messenger RNAs and proteins in normal and tumorigenic breast epithelial cells. *Clin Cancer Res* 1, 71-80.

Gudas JM, Nguyen H, Li T, Cowan KH (1995b). Hormone dependent regulation of BRCA1 in human breast cancer cells. *Cancer Res* 55, 4561-4565.

Gudas JM, Li T, Nguyen H, Jensen D, Rauscher FJ, Cowan KH (1996). Cell cycle regulation of BRCA1 messenger RNA in human breast epithelial cells. *Cell Growth Differen* 7, 717-723.

Guidal C, Gerard B, Cave H, Elion J, Vilmer E, Grandchamp B (1994). Absence of mutations of the p16/ink4 gene in childhood acute lymphoblastic leukemia even when blasts display loss of heterozygosity. *Blood* 84 (suppl. 1), 1175.

Guidi AJ, Abujawdeh G, Tognazzi K, Dvorak HF, Browth LF (1996). Expression of vascular permeability factor (vascular endothelial growth factor) and its receptors in endometrial carcinoma. *Cancer* 78, 454-460.

Guillouf C, Grana X, Selvakumaran M, Deluca A, Giordano A, Hoffman B, Liebermann DA (1995). Dissection of the genetic programs of p53-mediated G1 growth arrest and apoptosis. Blocking p53-induced apoptosis unmasks G1 arrest. *Blood* 85, 2691-2698.

Gulbis B, Galand P (1993). Immunodetection of the p21-*ras* products in human normal and preneoplastic tissues and solid tumours. *Human Pathol* 24, 1271-1285.

Gum R, Wang SW, Ernst LY, Yu DH, Hung MC, Juarez J, Boyd D (1995). Up-regulation of urokinase type plasminogen activator expression by the HER2/*neu* proto-oncogene. *Anticancer Res* 15, 1167-1172.

Gunthert U, Hofmann M, Rudy W, Reber W, Zoller M, Haussmann I, Matzku S, Wenzel A, Ponta H, Herrlich P (1991). A new variant of glycoprotein CD44 confers metastatic potential to rat carcinoma cells. *Cell* 65, 13-24.

Guo YJ, Liu GL, Wang XN, Jin D, Wu MC, MA J, Sy MS (1994). Potential use of soluble CD44 in serum as indicator of tumour burden and metastasis in patients with gastric or colon cancer. *Cancer Res* 54, 422-426.

Gupta RS (1990). Microtubules, mitochondria and molecular chaperones: a new hypothesis for *in vivo* assembly of microtubules. *Biochem Cell Biol* 68, 1352-1363.

Guttinger M, Sutti F, Barnier C, Mackay C, Berti E (1995). Expression of CD44 standard and variant forms in skin tumours. Loss of CD44 correlates with aggressive potential. *Eur J Dermatol* 5, 398-406.

Haas-Kogan DA, Kogan SC, Levi D, Dazin P, Tang A, Fung YKT, Israel MA (1995). Inhibition of apoptosis by the retinoblastoma gene product. *EMBO J* 14, 461-472.

Habuchi T, Kinoshita H, Yamada H, Kakehi Y, Ogawa O, Wu WJ, Takahashi R, Sugiyama T, Yoshida O (1994). Oncogene amplification in urothelial cancers with p53 gene mutation or *mdm2* amplification. *J Natl Cancer Inst* 86, 1331-1335.

Hachiya T, Nakano H, Wake N, Sueishi R (1995). *In vitro* invasiveness of human breast cancer cells through plasminogen activator activity independently regulated by hormones and transforming growth factor β-1. *Cancer J* **8**, 13-20.

Hackett RW, Lis JT (1983). Localisation of the hsp83 transcript within the 3292 nucleotide sequence from the 63B heat shock locus of *Drosophila melanogaster. Nucl Acids Res* **11**, 7011-7030.

Hagiwara M, Ochiai M, Owada K, Tanaka T, Hidak H (1988). Modulation of tyrosine phosphorylation of p36 and other substrates by the S-100 protein. *J Biol Chem* **263**, 6438-6441.

Hague A, Moorghen M, Hicks D, Chapman N, Paraskeva C (1994). Bcl-2 expression in human colorectal adenomas and carcinomas. *Oncogene* **9**, 3367-3370.

Hahn SA, Seymour AB, Hoque ATMS, Schutte M, da Costa LT, Redston MS, Caldas C, Weinstein CL, Fischer A, Yeo CJ, Hruban RH, Kern SE (1995). Allelotype of pancreatic adenocarcinoma using xenograft enrichment. *Cancer Res* **55**, 4670-4675.

Hahn SA, Schutte M, Hoque ATMS, Moskaluk CA, da Costa LT, Rozenblum E, Weinstein CL, Fischer A, Yeo CJ, Hruban RH, Kern SE (1996a). *DPC4*, a candidate tumour suppressor gene at human chromosome 18q21.1. *Science* **271**, 350-353.

Hahn SA, Hoque ATMS, Moskaluk CA, da Costa LT, Schutte M, Rozenblum E, Seymour AB, Weinstein CL, Yeo CJ, Hruban RH, Kern SE (1996b). Homozygous deletion map at 18q21.1. in pancreatic cancer. *Cancer Res* **56**, 490-494.

Hahnel AC, Gifford DJ, Heikkila JJ, Schultz GA (1986). Expression of the major heat shock protein (HSP70) family during early mouse embryo development. *Teratogen Carcinogen Mutagen* **6**, 493-510.

Hahnel R, Harvey J, Robbins P, Sterrett G (1993). Cathepsin D in human breast cancer. Correlation with vascular invasion and other clinical and histopathological characteristics. *Anticancer Res* **13**, 2131-2135.

Hailat N, Keim DR, Melhem RF, Zhu X, Eckerskorn C, Brodeur GM, Reynolds CP, Seeger RC, Lottspeich F, Strahler JR, Hanash SM (1991). High levels of p19/nm23 protein in neuroblastoma are associated with advanced stage disease and with N-*myc* gene amplification. *J Clin Invest* **88**, 341-345.

Haimoto H, Hosada S, Kato K (1987). Differential distribution of immunoreactive S100α and S100β proteins in normal nonnervous human tissues. *Lab Invest* **57**, 489-498.

Hainaut P, Milner J (1992). Interaction of heat shock protein 70 with p53 translated *in vitro*: evidence for interaction with dimeric p53 and for a role in the regulation of p53 conformation. *EMBO J* **11**, 3513-3520.

Haines DS, Landers JE, Engle LJ, George DL (1994). Physical and functional interaction between wild type p53 and mdm2 proteins. *Mol Cell Biol* **14**, 1171-1178.

Hainsworth PJ, Henderson MA, Stillwell RG, Bennett RC (1991). Comparison of EGFr, c-*erbB-2* product and *ras* p21 immunohistochemistry as prognostic markers in primary breast cancer. *Eur J Surg Oncol* **17**, 9-15.

Hakamori S, Anderson M (1994). Novel endothelial cell activation factor(s) released from activated platelets which induce E-selectin expression and tumour cell adhesion to endothelial cells. A preliminary note. *Biochem Biophys Res Commun* **203**, 1605-1613.

Hakem R, Delapompa JL, Sirard C, Mo R, Woo M, Hakem A (1996). The tumour suppressor gene BRCA1 is required for embryonic cellular proliferation in the mouse. *Cell* **85**, 1009-1023.

Hakim JP, Levine AJ (1994). Absence of p53 point mutations in parathyroid adenoma and carcinoma. *J Clin Endocrinol Metab* **78**, 103-106.

Halazonetis TD, Kandil AN (1993). Conformational shifts propagate from the oligomerisation domain of p53 to its tetrameric DNA binding domain and restore DNA binding to select p53 mutants. *EMBO J* **12**, 5057-5064.

Halazonetis TD, Davis LJ, Kandil AN (1993). Wild type p53 adopts a 'mutant'-like conformation when bound to DNA. *EMBO J* **12**, 1021-1028.

Haldane JS, Hird V, Hughes CM, Gullick WJ (1990). c-*erbB-2* oncogene expression in ovarian cancer. *J Pathol* **162**, 231-237.

Halevy O, Novitch BG, Spicer DB, Skapek SX, Rhee J, Hannon GJ, Beach D, Lassar AB (1995). Correlation of terminal cell cycle arrest of skeletal muscle with induction of p21 by MyoD. *Science* **267**, 1018-1021.

Hall M, Bates S, Peters G (1995). Evidence for different modes of action of cyclin dependent kinase inhibitors p15 and p16 bind to kinases and p21 and p27 bind to cyclins. *Oncogene* **11**, 1581-1588.

Hamada K, Alemany R, Zhang WW, Hittelman WN, Lotan R, Roth JA, Mitchell MF (1996). Adenovirus-mediated transfer of a wild type p53 gene and induction of apoptosis in cervical cancer. *Cancer Res* **56**, 3047-3054.

Hamelin R, Laurent-Puig P, Olschwang S, Jego N, Asselain B, Remvikos Y, Girodet J, Salmon R, Thomas G (1994a). Association of p53 mutations with short survival in colorectal cancer. *Gastroenterol* **106**, 42-48.

Hamelin R, Zucman J, Melot T, Delattre O, Thomas G (1994b). p53 mutations in human tumours with chimeric EWS/FLI-1 genes. *Int J Cancer* **57**, 336-340.

Hamilton TB, Barilla KC, Romaniuk PJ (1995). High affinity binding sites for the Wilms tumour suppressor protein wt1. *Nucl Acids Res* **23**, 277-284.

Hampl M, Hampl J, Frank S, Hahn M, Nagel M, Ockert D, Schackert G, Saeger HD, Schackert HK (1996). Loss of heterozygosity (LOH) in breast cancer susceptibility genes (BRCA1, BRCA2, AT, p53) in breast carcinomas and their metastases. *Langenbecks Arch Chir* **S1**, 201-204.

Han HJ, Yanagisawa A, Kato Y, Park JG, Nakamura Y (1993). Genetic instability in pancreatic cancer and poorly differentiated type of gastric cancer. *Cancer Res* **53**, 5087-5089.

Handa K, White T, Ito K, Fang H, Wang SS, Hakamori SI (1995). P-selectin dependent adhesion of human cancer cells. Requirement for co-expression of a PSGL-1-like core protein and the glycosylation process for a sialosyl-Le(x) or sialosyl-Le(a). *Int J Oncol* **6**, 773-781.

Hannon GJ, Beach D (1994). P15 (ink4B) is a potential effector of TGF beta-induced cell cycle arrest. *Nature* **371**, 257-261.

Harada M, Dosaka-Akita H, Miyamoto H, Kuzumaki N, Kawakami Y (1992). Prognostic significance of the expression of *ras* oncogene product in non-small cell lung cancer. *Cancer* **69**, 72-77.

Harada S, Nagy JA, Sullivan KA, Thomas KA, Endo N, Rodan GA, Rodan SB (1994). Induction of vascular endothelial growth factor expression by prostaglandin E(2) and E(1) in osteoblasts. *J Clin Invest* **93**, 2490-2496.

Harbour JW, Lai SH, Whang-Peng J, Gazdar AF, Minna JD, Kaye FJ (1988). Abnormalities in structure and expression of the human retinoblastoma gene in SCLC. *Science* **241**, 353-357.

Harley CB, Futcher AB, Greider CW (1990). Telomeres shortened during ageing of human fibroblasts. *Nature* **345**, 458-460.

Harlow E, Willamson NM, Ralston R, Halfman DM, Adams TE (1985). Molecular cloning and *in vitro* expression of a cDNA clone for human cellular tumour antigen p53. *Mol Cell Biol* **5**, 1601-1610.

Harn HJ, Ho LI, Chang JY, Wu CW, Jiang SFY, Lee HS, Lee WH (1995). Differential expression of the human metastasis adhesion molecule CD44v in normal and carcinomatous mucosa of Chinese subjects. *Cancer* **75**, 1065-1071.

Harn HJ, Ho LI, Liu CA, Liu GC, Lin FG, Lin JJ, Lee WH (1996). Down-regulation of *bcl-2* by p53 in nasopharyngeal carcinoma and lack of detection of its specific t(14;18) chromosomal translocation in fixed tissues. *Histopathology* **28**, 317-323.

Harper JW, Adami GR, Wei N, Keyomarsi K, Elledge SJ (1993). The p21 CDK-interacting protein CIP1 is a potent inhibitor of G1 cyclin-dependent kinases. *Cell* **75**, 805-816.

Harper JW, Elledge SJ, Keyomarsi K, Dynlacht B, Tsai LH, Zhang PM, Dobrowolski S, Bai C, Connell-Crowley L, Swindell E, Fox MP, Wei N (1995). Inhibition of cyclin dependent kinases by p21. *Mol Biol Cell* **6**, 387-400.

Harris AL, Nicholson S (1988). Epidermal growth factor receptors in human breast cancer. In: *Breast Cancer: Cellular and Molecular Biology*, Lipmann ME, Dickson RB (eds). Kluwer Academic Publishers, Boston, pp. 93-118.

Harris AL, Zhang HT, Moghaddam A, Fox S, Scott P, Pattison A, Gatter K, Stratford I, Bicknell R (1996). Breast cancer angiogenesis. New approaches to therapy via antiangiogenesis, hypoxic activated drugs and vascular targeting. *Breast Cancer Res Treat* **38**, 97-108.

Harris H, Miller OJ, Klein G, Worst P, Tachebana T (1969). Suppression of malignancy by cell fusion. *Nature* **223**, 363-368.

Harris JF, Chambers AF, Hill RP, Ling V (1982). Metastatic variants are generated spontaneously at a high rate in mouse KHT tumour. *Proc Natl Acad Sci USA* **79**, 5547-5551.

Hartman LC, Podratz KC, Keeney GL, Kamel NA, Edmonson JH, Grill JP, Su JQ, Katzman JA, Roche PC (1994). Prognostic significance of p53 immunostaining in epithelial ovarian cancer. *J Clin Oncol* **12**, 64-69.

Hastie ND, Dempster M, Dunlop MG, Thompson AM, Green DK, Allshire RG (1990). Telomere reduction in human colorectal carcinoma and with ageing. *Nature* **346**, 866-868.

Haupt Y, Barak Y, Oren M (1996). Cell type specific inhibition of p53-mediated apoptosis by mdm2. *EMBO J* **15**, 1596-1606.

Hauser S, Weich HA (1993). A heparin-binding form of placental growth factor (PLGF-2) is expressed in human umbilical vein endothelial cells and in placenta. *Growth Factors* **9**, 259-268.

Haut M, Steeg, PS, Willson JKV, Markowitz SD (1991). Induction of nm23 expression in human colonic neoplasms and equal expression in colon tumours of a high and low metastatic potential. *J Natl Cancer Inst* **83**, 712-716.

Haverstick DM, Engelhard VH, Gray LS (1991). Three intracellular signals for cytotoxic T lymphocyte mediated killing. Independent roles for protein kinase C, Ca^{2+} influx and Ca^{2+} release from internal stores. *J Immunol* **146**, 3303-3313.

Hayashi N, Ito I, Yanagisawa A, Kato Y, Nakamori S, Imaoka S, Watanabe H, Ogawa M, Nakamura Y (1995). Genetic diagnosis of lymph node metastasis in colorectal cancer. *Lancet* **345**, 1257-1259.

Hayashi N, Sugimoto Y, Tsuchiya E, Ogawa M, Nakamura Y (1994). Somatic mutations of the MTS (multiple tumour suppressor)-1 CDK4I (cyclin-dependent kinase-4 inhibitor) gene in human primary non-small cell lung carcinomas. *Biochem Biophys Res Commun* **202**, 1426-1430.

Haynes BF, Telen MJ, Hale LP, Dennings SM (1989). CD44 - A molecule involved in leukocyte adherence and T-cell activation. *Immunol Today* **10**, 423-428.

He CY, Merrick BA, Patterson RM, Selkirk JK (1995). Altered protein synthesis in p53 null and hemizygotic transgenic mouse embryonic fibroblasts. *Appl Theor Electrophoresis* **5**, 15-24.

Healy KC (1995). Telomere dynamics and telomerase activation in tumour progression. Prospects for prognosis and therapy. *Oncol Res* **7**, 121-130.

Hearing VJ, Law LW, Corti A, Appella E, Blasi F (1988). Modulation of metastatic potential by cell surface urokinase of murine melanoma cells. *Cancer Res* **48**, 1270-1278.

Hebert J, Cayuela JM, Berkeley J, Sigaux F (1994). Candidate tumour suppressor genes MTS1 (P16/INK4A) and MTS2 (P15/INK4B) display frequent homozygous deletions in primary cells from T cell but not from B cell lineage. *Blood* **84**, 4038-4044.

Hedley D, Rugg CA, Gelber RD (1987). Association of DNA index and S-phase fraction with prognosis of node-positive early breast cancer. *Cancer Res* **47**, 4729-4735.

Hedrick JP, Hartl FU (1993). Molecular chaperone functions of heat shock proteins. *Annu Rev Biochem* **62**, 349-384.

Heermeier K, Benedict M, Li ML, Furth P, Nunez G, Henning-Hausen L (1996). Bar and bcl-x(S) are induced at the onset of apoptosis in involuting mammary epithelial cells. *Mech Develop* **56**, 197-207.

Heider KH, Hoffman M, Hors E, van den Berg F, Ponta H, Herrlich P, Pals ST (1993). A human homologue of rat metastasis associated variant of CD44 is expressed in colorectal carcinomas and adenomatous polyps. *J Cell Biol* **120**, 227-233.

Heidtmann HH, Salge U, Havemann K, Kirschke H, Wiederanders B (1993). Secretion of a latent, acid activatable cathepsin L precursor by human non-small cell lung cancer cell lines. *Oncol Res* **5**, 441-451.

Heikkila JJ, Darasch SP, Mosser DD, Bols NC (1987). Heat and sodium arsenite act synergistically on the induction of heat shock gene expression in *Xenopus laevis* A6 cells. *Biochem Cell Biol* **65**, 310-316.

Heim S, Mitelman F (1987). *Cancer Cytogenetics*. Alan R Liss, New York.

Heinen CD, Richardson D, White R, Groden J (1995). Microsatellite instability in colorectal adenocarcinoma cell lines that have full-length adenomatous polyposis coli protein. *Cancer Res* **55**, 4797-4799.

Helin K, Lees JA, Vidal M, Dyson N, Harlow E, Fattaey A (1992). A cDNA encoding a pRb-binding protein with properties of the transcription factor E2F. *Cell* **70**, 337-350.

Helin K, Wu CL, Fattaey AR, Lees JA, Dynlacht BD, Ngwu C, Harlow E (1993). Heterodimerisation of the transcription factors E2F-1 and DP-1 leads to cooperative *trans*-activation. *Genes Devel* **7**, 1850-1861.

Hemler ME, Crouse C, Sonnenberg A (1989). Association of the VLA α_6 subunit with a novel protein. *J Biol Chem* **264**, 6529-6535.

Hemmings HC, Greengard P, Tung HYL, Cohen P (1984). DARPP-32 a dopamine regulated neuronal phosphoprotein, is a potent inhibitor of protein phosphatase 1. *Nature* **310**, 503-505

Hendrick L, Cho KR, Fearon ER, Wu TC, Kinzler KW, Vogelstein B (1994). The DCC gene product in cellular differentiation and colorectal tumorigenesis. *Genes Devel* **8**, 1174-1183.

Hengartner M, Horvitz HR (1994). *C. elegans* cell survival gene ced-9 encodes a functional homologue of the mammalian proto-oncogene bcl-2. *Cell* **76**, 665-676.

Hengartner M, Ellis RE, Hortitz HR (1992). *Caenorhabditis elegans* gene ced-9 protects cells from programmed cell death. *Nature* **356**, 494-499.

Hennessy C, Henry JA, May FEB, Westley BR, Angus B, Lennard TWJ (1991). Expression of the antimetastatic gene *nm23* in human breast cancer: an association with good prognosis. *J Natl Cancer Inst* **83**, 281-285.

Hennig G, Behrens J, Truss M, Frisch S, Reichmann E, Birchmeier W (1995). Progression of carcinoma cells is associated with alterations in chromatin structure and factor binding at the E-cadherin promoter *in vivo*. *Oncogene* **11**, 476-484.

Henry I, Grandjouan S, Couillin P, Barichard F, Huerre-Jeanpierre C, Glaser T, Phillips T, Lenoir

G, Chaussain JL, Junien C (1989). Tumour specific loss of 11p15.5 allele in del11p13 Wilms tumour and in familial adrenocortical carcinoma. *Proc Natl Acad Sci USA* **86**, 3247-3251.

Hensel CH, Hsieh CL, Gazdar AF, Johnson BE, Sakaguchi AY, Naylor SL, Lee WH, Lee EYHP (1990). Altered structure and expression of the human retinoblastoma susceptibility gene in small cell lung cancer. *Cancer Res* **50**, 3067-3072.

Henzen-Logmans SC, Fieret EJH, Berns EMJJ, Van der burg MEL, Klijn JGM, Foekens JA (1994). Ki-67 staining in benign, borderline, malignant primary and metastatic ovarian tumours. Correlation with steroid receptor status, epidermal growth factor receptor and cathepsin D. *Int J Cancer* **57**, 468-472.

Herron GS, Banda MJ, Clark EJ, Gavrilovic J, Werb Z (1986a). Secretion of metalloproteinases by stimulated capillary endothelial cells. 2. Expression of collagenase and stromelysin activities is regulated by endogenous inhibitors. *J Biol Chem* **261**, 2814-2818.

Herron GS, Werb Z, Dwyer K, Banda MJ (1986b). Secretion of metalloproteinases by stimulated capillary endothelial cells. 1. Production of procollagenase and prostromelysin exceeds expression of proteolytic activity. *J Biol Chem* **261**, 2810-2813.

Hertig CM, Eppenberger-Eberhardt M, Koch S, Eppenberger HM (1996). *N*-cadherin in adult rat cardiomyocytes in culture. 1. Functional role of *N*-cadherin and impairment of cell-cell contact by a truncated *N*-cadherin mutant. *J Cell Sci* **109**, 1-10.

Hewitt RE, Leach IH, Powe DG, Clark IM, Cawston TE, Turner DR (1991). Distribution of collagenase and tissue inhibitor of metalloproteinases (TIMP) in colorectal tumours. *Int J Cancer* **49**, 666-672.

Hewitt SM, Hamada S, McDonnell TJ, Rauscher FJ, Saunders GF (1995). Regulation of proto-oncogenes *bcl-2* and c-*myc* by the Wilms tumour suppressor gene. *Cancer Res* **55**, 5386-5389.

Hidaka H, Mizutani A (1993). Function and structure of two family of Ca^{2+}-receptive protein, annexin and EF-hand protein calcyclin and its target protein CAP-50. *Biomed Res* **14**, 53-55.

Hiebert SW, Chellappan SP, Horowitz JM, Nevins JR (1992). The interaction of Rb with E2F coincides with an inhibition of the transcriptional activity of E2F. *Genes Develop* **6**, 177-185.

Higashio K, Shima N, Goto M, Itagaki Y, Nagao M, Yasuda H, Morinaga T (1990). Identity of a tumour cytotoxic factor from human fibroblasts and hepatocyte growth factor. *Biochem Biophys Res Commun* **170**, 397-404.

Higashiyama M, Doi O, Yokouchi H, Kodama K, Nakamori S, Tateishi R, Kimura N (1992). Immunohistochemical analysis of *nm23* gene product/NDP kinase expression in pulmonary adenocarcinoma: lack of prognostic value. *Br J Cancer* **66**, 533-536.

Higuchi M, Ohnishi T, Arita N, Hiraga S, Hayakawa T (1993). Expression of tenascin in human gliomas. Its relation to histological malignancy, tumour dedifferentiation and angiogenesis. *Acta Neuropathol* **85**, 481-487.

Hijmans EM, Voorhoeve PM, Beijersbergen RL, Van'T Veer LJ, Bernards R (1995). E2F-5, a new E2F family member that interacts with p130 *in vivo*. *Mol Cell Biol* **15**, 3082-3089.

Hildenbrand R, Dilger I, Horlin A, Stutte HJ (1995a). Urokinase and macrophages in tumour angiogenesis. *Br J Cancer* **72**, 818-823.

Hildenbrand R, Dilger I, Horlin A, Stutte JH (1995b). Urokinase plasminogen activator induces angiogenesis and tumour vessel invasion in breast cancer. *Pathol Res Pract* **191**, 403-409.

Hinck L, Nelson WJ, Papkoff J (1994). Wnt-1 modulates cell-cell adhesion in mammalian cells by stabilising beta catenin binding to the cell adhesion protein cadherin. *J Cell Biol* **124**, 729-741.

Hinds PW, Mittnacht S, Dulic V, Arnold A, Reed SI, Weinberg RA (1992). Regulation of retinoblastoma protein functions by ectopic expression of human cyclins. *Cell* **70**, 993-1006.

Hirano S, Kimoto N, Shimoyama V, Hirohashi S, Takeichi M (1992). Identification of a neural α-catenin as a key regulator of cadherin function and multicellular organisation. *Cell* **70**, 293-301.

Hiscox S, Jiang WG (1996). Regulation of expression of the hepatocyte growth factor scatter factor receptor, c-met, by cytokines. *Oncol Rep* **3**, 553-557.

Hiyama E, Yokoyama T, Tatsumoto N, Hiyama K, Imamura Y, Murakami Y, Kodama T, Piatyszek MA, Shay JW, Matsuura Y (1995a). Telomerase activity in gastric cancer. *Cancer Res* **55**, 3248-3262.

Hiyama E, Hiyama K, Yokoyama T, Matsuura Y, Piatyszek MA, Shay JW (1995b). Correlating telomerase activity levels with human neuroblastoma outcomes. *Nature Med* **1**, 249-255.

Hiyama E, Gollahon L, Kataoka T, Kuroi K, Yokoyama T, Gazdar AF, Hiyama K, Piatyszek MA, Shay JW (1996). Telomerase activity in human breast cancer. *J Natl Cancer Inst* **88**, 116-122.

Hiyama K, Ishioka S, Shirotani Y, Inai K, Hiyama E, Murakami I, Isobe T, Inamizu T, Yamakido M (1995a). Alterations in telomeric repeat length in lung cancer are associated with loss of heterozygosity in p53 and rb. *Oncogene* **10**, 937-944.

Hiyama K, Hiyama E, Ishioka S, Yamakido M, Inai K, Gazdar AF, Piatyszek MA, Shay JW (1995b). Telomerase activity in small cell and non-small cell lung cancers. *J Natl Cancer Inst* **87**, 895-902.

Hockenbery DM, Nunez G, Milliman C, Schreiber RD, Korsmeyer SJ (1990). Bcl-2 is an inner mitochondrial membrane protein that blocks programmed cell death. *Nature* **348**, 334-336.

Hockenbery DM, Zutter M, Hickey W, Nahm M, Korsmeyer SJ (1991). Bcl-2 protein is topographically restricted in tissues characterised by apoptotic cell death. *Proc Natl Acad Sci USA* **88**, 6961-6965.

Hockenbery DM, Oltvai ZN, Yin XM, Lilliman CL, Korsmeyer SJ (1993). Bcl-2 functions in an antioxidant pathway to prevent apoptosis. *Cell* **75**, 241-251.

Hoffman R, Paper DH, Donaldson J, Vogl H (1996). Inhibition of angiogenesis and murine tumour growth by laminarin sulphate. *Br J Cancer* **73**, 1183-1186.

Hoffmann M, Rudy W, Zoller H, Tolg C, Ponta H, Herrlich P, Gunthert U (1991). CD44 splice variants confer metastatic behaviour in rats: Homologous sequences are expressed in human tumour cell lines. *Cancer Res* **51**, 5292-5297.

Hoffmann M, Rudy W, Gunthert U, Zimmer SG, Zawadzki V, Zoller M, Lichtner RB, Herrlich P, Ponta H (1993). A link between *ras* and metastatic behaviour of tumour cells. *ras* induces CD44 promoter activity and leads to a low-level expression of metastasis-specific variants of CA44 in CREF cells. *Cancer Res* **53**, 1516-1521.

Hogg N, Bates PA, Harvey J (1991). Structure and function of intercellular adhesion molecule-1. *Chem Immunol* **50**, 98-115.

Hollas W, Blasi F, Boyd D (1991). Role of the urokinase receptor in facilitating extracellular matrix invasion by cultured colon cancer. *Cancer Res* **51**, 3690-3695.

Hollstein M, Sidransky D, Vogelstein B, Harris CC (1991). p53 mutations in human cancers. *Science* **253**, 49-53.

Hollyday M, McMahon JA, McMahon AP (1995). Wnt expression patterns in chick embryo nervous system. *Mech Develop* **52**, 9-25.

Holme TC, Kellie S, Wyke JA, Crawford N (1986). Effect of transformation of Rous sarcoma virus on the character and distribution of actin in rat fibroblasts. *Br J Cancer* **53**, 465-476.

Holmgren L, O'Reilly MS, Folkman J (1995). Dormancy of micrometastases. Balanced proliferation and apoptosis in the presence of angiogenesis suppression. *Nature Med* **1**, 149-153.

Holt JT, Thompson ME, Szabo C, Robinson-Benion C, Arteaga CL, King MC, Jensen RA (1996). Growth retardation and tumour inhibition by *BRCA1*. *Nature Genet* **12**, 298-302.

Hong RL, Pu YS, Chu JS, Lee WJ, Chen YC, Wu CW (1995). Correlation of expression of CD44 isoforms and E-cadherin with differentiation in human urothelial cell lines and transitional cell carcinoma. *Cancer Lett* **89**, 81-87.

Honore B, Rasmussen HH, Celis A, Leffers H, Madsen P, Celis JE (1994). The molecular chaperones HSP28, GRP78, endoplasmin and calnexin exhibit strikingly different levels in quiescent keratinocytes as compared to their proliferating normal and transformed counterparts - cDNA cloning and expression of calnexin. *Electrophoresis* **15**, 482-490.

Horak E, Smith K, Bromley L, LeJeune S, Greenall M, Lane D, Harris AL (1991). Mutant p53, EGF receptor and c-*erb*B2 expression in human breast cancer. *Br J Cancer* **6**, 2277-2284.

Horak E, Leek R, Klenk N, LeJeune S, Smith K, Stuart N, Greenall M, Stepniewsak K, Harris AL (1992). Angiogenesis, assessed by platelet/endothelial cell adhesion molecule antibodies as indicator of node metastases and survival in breast cancer. *Lancet* **340**, 1120-1124.

Hori A, Sasada R, Matsutani E, Waito K, Sakura Y, Fujita T, Kozai Y (1991). Suppression of solid tumour growth by immunoneutralising monoclonal antibody against human basic fibroblast growth factor. *Cancer Res* **51**, 6180-6184.

Horii A, Nakatsuru S, Ichii S, Nagase H, Nakamura Y (1993). Multiple forms of the APC gene transcripts and their tissue specific expression. *Human Mol Genet* **2**, 283-287.

Horowitz JM, Park SH, Bogenmann E, Cheng JC, Yandell DW, Kaye FJ, Minna JD, Dryja TP, Weinberg RA (1990). Frequent inactivation of the retinoblastoma anti-oncogene is restricted to a subset of human tumour cells. *Proc Natl Acad Sci USA* **87**, 2775-2779.

Hosking L, Trowsdale J, Nicolai H, Solomon E, Foulkes W, Stamp G, Signer E, Jeffreys A (1995). A somatic BRCA1 mutation in an ovarian tumour. *Nature Genet* **9**, 343-344.

Houck KA, Ferrara N, Winer J, Cachianes G, Li B, Leung DW (1991). The vascular endothelial growth factor family. Identification of a 4th molecular species and characterisation of alternative splicing of RNA. *Mol Endocrinol* **5**, 1806-1814.

Houck KA, Leung DW, Rowland AM, Winer J, Ferrara N (1992). Dual regulation of vascular endothelial growth factor bioavailability by genetic and proteolytic mechanisms. *J Biol Chem* **267**, 26031-26037.

Hoyhtya M, Hujanen E, Turpeenniemi-Hujanen T, Thorgeirsson U, Liotta LA, Tryggvason K (1990). Modulation of type-IV collagenase activity and invasive behaviour of metastatic human melanoma (A2058) cells *in vitro* by monoclonal antibodies to type-IV collagenase. *Int J Cancer* **46**, 282-286.

Hsieh LL, Huang YC (1995). Loss of heterozygosity of APC/MCC gene in differentiated and undifferentiated gastric carcinomas in Taiwan. *Cancer Lett* **96**, 169-174.

Hsu DW, Efird JT, Hedley-White ET (1995). Prognostic role of urokinase type plasminogen activator in human gliomas. *Amer J Pathol* **147**, 114-123.

Hsu SH, Luk GD, Krush AJ, Hamilton SR, Hoover HH, Jr (1983). Multiclonal origin of polyps in Gardner syndrome. *Science* **221**, 951-953.

Hu L, Aizawa S, Tokuhisa T (1995). P53 controls proliferation of early B-lineage cells by a p21 (waf1/cip1)-independent pathway. *Biochem Biophys Res Commun* **206**, 948-954.

Huang FL, Glinsmann WH (1976). Separation and characterisation of two phosphorylase inhibitors from rabbit skeletal muscle. *Eur J Biochem* **70**, 419-426.

Huang HJS, Yee JK, Shew JY, Chen PL, Bookstein R, Friedmann T, Lee EYHP, Lee WE (1988). Suppression of the neoplastic phenotype by replacement of the RB gene in human cancer cells. *Science* **242**, 1563-1566.

Huang J, Lufa M, Gutman N, Xie S, Bar-Eli M (1996). Molecular mechanism of melanoma metastasis. *Proc 9th Int Conf Soc Diff*, Pisa, Italy, p. 79.

Huang THM, Yeh PLH, Martin MB, Straub RE, Gilliam TC, Caldwell CW, Skibba JL (1995).

Genetic alterations of microsatellites on chromosome 18 in human breast carcinoma. *Diag Mol Pathol* **4**, 66-72.

Huang YQ, Li YY, Moscatelli D, Basilico C, Nicolaides A, Zhang WG, Poiesz B, Friedman-Kien AE (1993). Expression of *int-2* oncogene in Kaposi's sarcoma lesion. *J Clin Invest* **91**, 1191-1197.

Hubbard MJ, Cohen P (1989). Regulation of protein phosphatase I_G from rabbit skeletal muscle. *Eur J Biochem* **186**, 701-709.

Huet S, Groux H, Caillou B, Valentin H, Prieur AM, Bernard A (1989). CD44 contributes to T cell activation. *J Immunol* **143**, 798-801.

Huguet EL, McMahon JA, McMahon AP, Bicknell R, Harris AL (1994). Differential expression of human wnt gene-2, gene-3, gene-4 and gene-7b in human breast cell lines and normal disease states of human breast tissue. *Cancer Res* **54**, 2615-2621.

Huibregtse JM, Scheffner M, Howley PM (1993). Cloning and expression of the cDNA for E6-AP, a protein that mediates the interaction of the human papilloma virus E6 oncoprotein with p53. *Mol Cell Biol* **13**, 775-784.

Hulsken J, Birchmeier W, Behrens J (1994). E-cadherin and APC compete for the interaction with beta catenin and the cytoskeleton. *J Cell Biol* **6**, 2061-2069.

Hume CR, Dodd J (1993). Cwnt-8c – A novel wnt gene with a potential role in primitive streak formation and hindbrain organisation. *Development* **119**, 1147-1160.

Humphrey PA, Zhu XP, Zarnegar R, Swanson PE, Ratliff TL, Vollmer RT, Day ML (1995). Hepatocyte growth factor and its receptor (c-met) in prostatic carcinoma. *Amer J Pathol* **147**, 386-396.

Hung MC, Schechter AL, Chevray PYM, Stern DF, Weinberg RA (1986). Molecular cloning of the neu gene. Absence of gross structural alterations in oncogenic alleles. *Proc Natl Acad Sci USA* **83**, 261-264.

Hunt C, Morimoto RI (1985). Conserved features of eukaryotic hsp70 genes revealed by comparison with nucleotide sequence of human hsp70. *Proc Natl Acad Sci USA* **82**, 6455-6459.

Hunter T (1993). Braking the cycle. *Cell* **75**, 839-841.

Hupp TR, Meek DW, Midgley CA, Lane DP (1992). Regulation of the specific DNA binding function of p53. *Cell* **71**, 875-886.

Huttner WB, Gerdes HH, Rosa P (1991). The granin (chromogranin/secretogranin) family. *Trends Biochem Sci* **16**, 27-30.

Hynes NE, Stern DF (1994). The biology of *erbB2/neu/HER-2* and its role in cancer. *Biochim Biophys Acta* **1198**, 165-184.

Ichikawa A, Hotta T, Takagi N, Tsushita T, Kinoshita T, Nagai H, Murakami Y, Hayashi K, Saito H (1992). Mutations of p53 gene and their relation to disease progression in B-cell lymphoma. *Blood* **79**, 2701-2707.

Ichikawa T, Ichikawa Y, Dong J, Hawkins AL, Griffin CA, Isaacs WB, Oshimura M, Barrett JC, Issacs JT (1992). Localisation of metastasis suppressor gene(s) for prostatic cancer to the short arm of human chromosome 11. *Cancer Res* **52**, 3486-3490.

Ichikawa W (1994). Positive relationship between expression of CD44 and hepatic metastases in colorectal cancer. *Pathobiology* **62**, 172-179.

Igawa M, Rukstalis DB, Tanabe T, Chodak GW (1994). High levels of nm23 expression are related to cell proliferation in human prostate cancer. *Cancer Res* **54**, 1313-1318.

Iino H, Fukayama M, Maeda Y, Koike M, Mori T, Takahashi T, Kikuchiyanoshita R, Miyaki M, Mizuno S, Watanabe S (1994). Molecular genetics for clinical management of colorectal carcinoma. *Cancer* **73**, 1324-1331.

Ikeda E, Achen MG, Brier G, Risau W (1995). Hypoxia-induced transcriptional activation and increased messenger RNA stability of vascular endothelial growth factor in C6 glioma cells. *J Biol Chem* **270**, 19761-19766.

Imai Y, Leung CKH, Frieson HG, Shiu RPC (1982). Epidermal growth factor receptor and effect of epidermal growth factor on growth of human breast cancer cells in long term tissue culture. *Cancer Res* **42**, 4394-4398.

Imamura T, Arima T, Kato H, Miamoto S, Sasazuki T, Wake N (1992). Chromosomal deletions and K-*ras* gene mutations in human endometrial carcinomas. *Int J Cancer* **51**, 47-52.

Ingolia TD, Slater MR, Craig EA (1982). *Saccharomyces cerevisiae* contains a complex multigene family related to the major heat shock inducible gene of *Drosophila*. *Mol Cell Biol* **2**, 1388-1398.

Inoue A, Torigoe T, Sogahata K, Kamiguchi K, Takahashi S, Sawada Y, Saijo M, Taya Y, Ishii S, Sato N, Kikuchi K (1995). 70-kDa heat shock cognate protein interacts directly with the *N*-terminal region of the retinoblastoma gene product pRB. Identification of a novel region of pRB-mediating protein interaction. *J Biol Chem* **270**, 22571-22576.

Inoue K, Furihata M, Ohtsuki Y, Fujita Y (1993). Distribution of S-100 protein-positive dendritic cells and expression of HLA-DR antigen in transitional cell carcinoma of the urinary bladder in relation to tumour progression and prognosis. *Virchows Arch A* **422**, 351-355.

Inoue T, Ishida T, Sugio K, Sugimachi K (1994). Cathepsin B expression and laminin degradation as factors influencing prognosis of surgically treated patients with lung adenocarcinoma. *Cancer Res* **54**, 6133-6136.

Ionov Y, Peinado MA, Malkhosyan S, Shibata D, Perucho M (1993). Ubiquitous somatic mutations in simple repeated sequences reveal a new mechanism for colonic carcinogenesis. *Nature* **363**, 558-561.

Ishikawa J, Xu JH, Hu SX, Yandell DW, Maeda S, Kamidono S, Benedict WF, Takahashi R (1991). Inactivation of the retinoblastoma gene in human bladder and renal cell carcinoma. *Cancer Res* **51**, 5736-5743.

Ishimaru G, Adachi J, Shiseki M, Yamaguchi N, Muto T, Yokota J (1995). Microsatellite instability in primary and metastatic colorectal cancers. *Int J Cancer* **64**, 153-157.

Isobe T, Okuyama T (1978). The amino acid sequence of S100 protein (PAP-1-b protein) and its relation to the calcium binding proteins. *Eur J Biochem* **89**, 379-388.

Isobe T, Okuyama T (1981). The aminoacid sequence of the α subunit of bovine brain S100a protein. *Eur J Biochem* **116**, 79-86.

Itoh, N, Yokota S, Takagishi U, Hatta A, Okamoto H (1987). Thiol proteinase inhibitor in the ascitic fluid of sarcoma 180. *Cancer Res* **47**, 5560-5565.

Iuzzolino P, Ghimenton C, Nocolato A, Giorgiutti F, Fina P, Doglioni C, Barbareschi M (1994). p53 protein in low grade astrocytomas: a study with long term follow-up. *Br J Cancer* **69**, 586-591.

Iwai K, Ishikura H, Kaji M, Sugiura H, Ishizu A, Takahashi C, Kato H, Tanabe T, Yoshiki T (1993). Importance of E-selectin (ELAM-1) and sialyl Lewis (a) in the adhesion of pancreatic carcinoma cells to activated endothelium. *Int J Cancer* **54**, 972-977.

Iwamoto Y, Robey FA, Graf J, Sasaki M, Kleinman HK, Yamada Y, Martin GR (1987). TIGSR, a synthetic laminin pentapeptide inhibits experimental metastasis formation. *Science* **238**, 1132-1134.

Iwamoto Y, Graf J, Sasaki M, Kleinman HK, Martin GR, Robey FA, Yamada Y (1988). A synthetic peptide from the B1 chain of laminin is chemotactic for B16 F10 melanoma cells. *J Cell Physiol* **134**, 287-291.

Iwamoto Y, Nomizu M, Yamada Y, Ito Y, Tanaka K, Sugioka Y (1996). Inhibition of angiogenesis, tumour growth and experimental metastasis of human fibrosarcoma cells HT1080 by a multimeric form of the laminin sequence Tyr-Ile-Gly-Ser-Arg (YIGSR). *Br J Cancer* **73**, 589-595.

Iwaya K, Tsuda H, Fujita S, Suzuki M, Hirohashi S (1995). Natural state of mutant p53 protein and heat shock protein 70 in breast cancer. *Lab Invest* **72**, 707-714.

Izumi Y, Taniuchi Y, Tsuji T, Smith CW, Nakamori S, Fidler IJ, Irimura T (1995). Characterisation of human colon carcinoma variant cells selected for sialyl Le(x) carbohydrate antigen. Liver colonisation and adhesion to vascular endothelial cells. *Exp Cell Res* **216**, 215-221.

Jaakkola S, Salmikangas P, Nylund S, Partanen J, Armstrong E, Pyrhonen S, Lehtovirta P, Nevanlinna H (1993). Amplification of FGFR4 gene in human breast and gynecological cancers. *Int J Cancer* **54**, 378-382.

Jackson DG, Schenker T, Waibel R, Bell JI, Stahel RA (1994). Expression of alternatively spliced forms of the CD44 extracellular matrix receptor on human lung carcinomas. *Int J Cancer* **S8**, 110-115.

Jackson-Grusby L, Swiergiel J, Linzer DIH (1988). A growth related mRNA in cultured mouse cells encodes a placental calcium binding protein. *Nucl Acids Res* **15**, 6677-6690.

Jacobs IJ, Kohler MF, Wiseman RW, Marks JR, Whitaker R, Kerns BAJ, Humphrey P, Berchuk A, Ponder BAJ, Bast RC, Jr (1992). Clonal origin of epithelial ovarian cancer: Analysis by loss of heterozygosity, p53 mutation and X-chromosome inactivation. *J Natl Cancer Inst* **84**, 1793-1798.

Jacobson MD, Raff MC (1995). Programmed cell death and bcl-2 protection in very low oxygen. *Nature* **374**, 814-816.

Jacobson MD, Burne JF, King MP, Miyashita T, Reed JC, Raff MC (1993). Bcl-2 blocks apoptosis in cells lacking mitochondrial DNA. *Nature* **361**, 365-369.

Jacobson MD, Burne JF, Raff MC (1994). Programmed cell death and bcl-2 protection in the absence of a nucleus. *EMBO J* **13**, 1899-1910.

Jacques G, Auerbach B, Pritsch M, Wolf M, Madry N, Havemann K (1993). Evaluation of serum neural cell adhesion molecule as a new tumour marker in small cell lung cancer. *Cancer* **72**, 418-425.

Jakobovits A, Shackleford G, Varmus H, Martin G (1986). Two proto-oncogenes implicated in mammary carcinogenesis, int-1 and int-2, are independently regulated during mouse development. *Proc Natl Acad Sci USA* **83**, 7806-7810.

Jamal HH, Cano-Gauci DF, Buick RN, Filmus J (1994). Activated *ras* and *src* genes induce CD44 overexpression in rat epithelial cells. *Oncogene* **9**, 417-423.

James CD, Carlbom E, Nordenskjold M, Collins VP, Cavenee WK (1989). Mitotic recombination of chromosome 17 in astrocytes. *Proc Natl Acad Sci USA* **89**, 2858-2862.

Janicke F, Schmitt M, Pache L, Ulm K, Harbeck N, Hofler H, Graeff H (1993). Urokinase (uPA) and its inhibitor PAI-1 are strong and independent prognostic factors in node negative breast cancer. *Breast Cancer Res Treat* **24**, 195-208.

Janis RA, Silver PJ, Triggle DJ (1987). Drug action and cellular calcium regulation. *Adv Drug Res* **16**, 309-591.

Jares P, Fernandez PL, Campo E, Nadal A, Bosch F, Aiza G, Nayach I, Traserra J, Cardesa A (1994). PRAD-1 cyclin D1 gene amplification correlates with messenger RNA overexpression and tumour progression in human laryngeal carcinomas. *Cancer Res* **54**, 4813-4817.

Jaros E, Perry RH, Adam L, Kelly PJ, Crawford PJ, Kalbag RM, Mendelow AD, Sengupta RP, Pearson ADJ (1992). Prognostic implications of p53 protein, epidermal growth factor receptor and ki-67 labelling in brain tumours. *Br J Cancer* **66**, 373-385.

Jarosz DE, Hamer PJ, Tenney DY, Zabrecky JR (1995). Elevated levels of pro-cathepsin D in the plasma of breast cancer patients. *Int J Oncol* **6**, 859-865.

Jeanpierre C, Antignac C, Beroud C, Lavedan C, Henry I, Saunders G, Williams B, Glaser T, Junien C (1990). Constitutional and somatic deletions of two different regions of maternal chromosome 11 in Wilms tumour. *Genomics* **7**, 434-438.

Jenkins JR, Rudge K, Chumakov P, Currie GA (1985). The cellular oncogene p53 can be activated by mutagenesis. *Nature* **317**, 816-818.

Jensen RA, Thompson ME, Jetton TL, Szabo CI, van der Meer R, Helou B, Tronick SR, Page DL, King MC, Holt JT (1996). BRCA1 is secreted and exhibits properties of a granin. *Nature Genet* **12**, 303-308.

Jetten AM (1985). Retinoids and their modulation of cell growth. In: *Growth and Maturation Factors*, Guroff G (ed.), **3**, 221-293.

Jhanwar SC, Gerdes H, Chen Q, Winawer SJ (eds) (1992). *Hereditary Colon Cancer*. Elsevier, North Holland, Amsterdam.

Jiang HP, Lin J, Su ZZ, Collart FR, Huberman E, Fisher PB (1994). Induction of differentiation in human promyelocytic HL-60 leukaemic cells activates p21, WAF1/CIP1, expression in the absence of p53. *Oncogene* **9**, 3397-3406.

Jimenez M, Kameyama K, Maloy WL, Tomita Y, Hearing VJ (1988). Mammalian tyrosinase: Biosynthesis, processing and modulation by melanocyte stimulating hormone. *Proc Natl Acad Sci USA* **85**, 3830-3834.

Johnson DG, Schwarz JK, Cress WD, Nevins JR (1993). Expression of transcription factor E2F1 induces quiescent cells to enter S phase. *Nature* **365**, 349-352.

Johnson MD, Torri JA, Lippman ME, Dickson RB (1993). The role of cathepsin D in the invasiveness of human breast cancer cells. *Cancer Res* **53**, 873-877.

Johnson MD, Kim HRC, Chesler L, Tsaowu G, Bouck N, Polverini PJ (1994). Inhibition of angiogenesis by tissue inhibitor of metalloproteinase. *J Cell Physiol* **160**, 194-202.

Jones CE, Davis MB, Darlin JL, Geddes JF, Thomas DGT, Harding AE (1995). Loss of heterozygosity for DNA polymorphism mapping to chromosome 10 and chromosome 17 and prognosis in patients with gliomas. *J Neurol Neurosurg Psych* **58**, 218-221.

Jonsson M, Johannsson O, Borg A (1995). Infrequent occurrence of microsatellite instability in sporadic and familial breast cancer. *Eur J Cancer* **31A**, 2330-2334.

Jonveaux P, Fenaux P, Quiquandon I, Pignon JM, Lai JL, Loucheux-Lefebre MH, Goosens M, Bauters F, Berger R (1991). Mutations in the p53 gene in myelodysplastic syndromes. *Oncogene* **6**, 2243-2247.

Joslyn G, Carlson M, Thliveris A, Albertsen H, Gelbert L, Samowitz W, Groden J, Stevens J, Spirio L, Robertson M, Sargeant L, Krapcho K, Wolff E, Burt R, Hughes JP, Warrington J, McPherson J, Wasmuth J, Lepaslier D, Abderrahim H, Cohen D, Leppert M, White R (1991). Identification of deletion mutations and 3 new genes at the familial polyposis locus. *Cell* **66**, 601-613.

Jue SF, Bradley RS, Rudnicki JA, Varmus HE, Brown AMC (1992). The mouse wnt-1 gene can act via paracrine mechanism in transformation of mammary epithelial cells. *Mol Cell Biol* **12**, 321-328.

Juliano RL, Haskill S (1993). Signal transduction from the extracellular matrix. *J Cell Biol* **120**, 577-585.

Jung JM, Li H, Kobayashi T, Kyritsis AP, Langford LA, Bruner JM, Levin VA, Zhang W (1995a). Inhibition of human glioblastoma cell growth by waf1/cip1 can be attenuated by mutant p53. *Cell Growth Differen* **6**, 909-913.

Jung JM, Bruner JM, Ruan SB, Langford LA, Kyritsis AP, Kobayashi T, Levin VA, Zhang W

(1995b). Increased levels of p21 (waf1/cip1) in human brain tumours. *Oncogene* **11**, 2021-2028.

Kaddurah-Daouk R, Greene JM, Baldwin AS, Jr, Kinsgston RE (1987). Activation and repression of mammalian gene expression by the c-myc protein. *Genes Develop* **1**, 347-357.

Kaden D, Gadi IK, Bardwell L, Gelman R, Sager R (1989). Spontaneous mutation rates of tumorigenic and non-tumorigenic CHEF cell lines. *Cancer Res* **49**, 3374-3379.

Kaelin WGJ, Krek W, Sellers WR, DeCaprio JA, Ajchenbaum F, Fuchs CS, Chittenden T, Li Y, Farnham PJ, Blanar MA, Livingston DM, Fleminton EK (1992). Expression cloning of a cDNA encoding a retinoblastoma-binding protein with E2F-like properties. *Cell* **70**, 351-364.

Kahn H, Marks A, Thorn RT, Baumal R (1983). Role of antibody to S100 protein in diagnostic pathology. *Amer J Clin Pathol* **79**, 341-347.

Kahn P, Graf T (1986). *Oncogenes and Growth Control*. Springer Verlag, Berlin, New York.

Kainz C, Kohlberger P, Sliutz G, Tempfer C, Heinzl H, Reinthaller A, Breitenecker G, Koelbl H (1995). Splice variants of CD44 in human cervical cancer stage IB to IIB. *Gynaecol Oncol* **57**, 383-387.

Kajiji S, Tamura RN, Quaranta V (1989). A novel integrin ($\alpha_E\beta_4$) from human epithelial cells suggests a fourth family of integrin adhesion receptors. *EMBO J* **8**, 673-680.

Kamata T, Wright R, Takada Y (1995). Critical threonine and aspartic acid residues within the I-domains of beta-2 integrins for interactions with intercellular adhesion molecule-1 (ICAM-1) and C3Bi. *J Biol Chem* **270**, 12531-12535.

Kamb A, Gruis NA, Weaver-Feldhaus J, Liu Q, Harshman E, Tavtigian SV, Stockert EL, Day III RS, Johnson BE, Skolnick MH (1994). A cell cycle regulator potentially involved in genesis of many tumour types. *Science* **264**, 436-440.

Kameyama K, Vieira WD, Tsukamoto K, Law LW, Hearing VJ (1990). Differentiation and the tumorigenic and metastatic phenotype of murine melanoma cells. *Int J Cancer* **45**, 1151-1158.

Kantor JD, McCormick B, Steeg PS, Zetter BR (1993). Inhibition of cell motility after nm23 transfection of human and murine tumour cells. *Cancer Res* **53**, 1971-1973.

Kao CC, Yew PR, Berk AJ (1990). Domain required for *in vitro* association between the cellular p53 and the adenovirus 2 E1B 55K proteins. *Virology* **179**, 806-814.

Kapitanovic S, Spaventi R, Vujsic S, Petrovic Z, Kurjak A, Pavelic ZP, Gluckman JL, Stambrook PJ, Pavelic K (1995). Nm23-H1 gene expression in ovarian tumours. A potential tumour marker. *Anticancer Res* **15**, 587-590.

Kaplan DR, Morrison DK, Wong G, McCormick F, Williams LT (1990). PDGFβ receptor stimulates tyrosine phosphorylation of GAP and association of GAP with a signalling complex. *Cell* **61**, 125-133.

Karlseder J, Zeillinger R, Schneeberger C, Czerwenka K, Speiser P, Kubista E, Birnbaum D, Gaudray P, Theillet C (1994). Patterns of DNA amplification at band q13 of chromosome 11 in human breast cancer. *Genes Chrom Cancer* **9**, 42-48.

Karlsson M, Boeryd B, Carstensen J, Kagedal B, Bratel AT, Wingren S (1993). DNA ploidy and S-phase in primary malignant melanoma as prognostic factors for stage III disease. *Br J Cancer* **67**, 134-138.

Kashiwaba M, Tamura G, Ishida M (1994). Aberrations of the APC gene in primary breast carcinoma. *J Cancer Res Clin Oncol* **120**, 727-731.

Kashiwaba M, Tamura G, Ishida M (1995). Frequent loss of heterozygosity at the deleted-in-colorectal carcinoma locus and its association with histologic phenotypes in breast cancer. *Virchows Arch Pathol* **426**, 441-446.

Kastan MB, Onyekwere O, Sidransky D, Vogelstein B, Craig RW (1991). Participation of p53 protein in the cellular response to DNA damage. *Cancer Res* **51**, 6304-6311.

Kastan MB, Zhan QM, El-Deiry WS, Carrier F, Jacks T, Walsh WV, Punkett BS, Vogelstein B, Fornace AJ (1992). A mammalian cell cycle checkpoint pathway utilizing p53 and GADD45 is defective in ataxia telangiectasia. *Cell* **71**, 587-597.

Kastrinakis WV, Ramchurren N, Rieger KM, Hess DT, Loda M, Steele G, Summerhayes IC (1995). Increased incidence of p53 mutations is associated with hepatic metastasis in colorectal neoplastic progression. *Oncogene* **11**, 647-652.

Katayama M, Hirai S, Kamihagi K, Nakagawa K, Yasumoto M, Kato I (1994). Soluble E-cadherin fragments increased in circulation of cancer patients. *Br J Cancer* **69**, 580-585.

Katayose D, Wersto R, Cowan KH, Seth P (1995). Effects of a recombinant adenovirus expressing waf1/cip1 on cell growth, cell cycle, and apoptosis. *Cell Growth Differen* **6**, 1207-1212.

Kato H (1977). Spontaneous and induced sister chromatid exchanges. *Int Rev Cytol* **49**, 55-97.

Kato I, Tominaga N (1979). Trypsin-subtilisin inhibitor from Red Sea turtle egg white consists of two tandem domains, one Kunitz and one a new family. *Fed Proc* **38**, 832.

Kato JY, Matsuoka M, Polyak, K, Massague J, Sherr CJ (1994). Cyclic-AMP induced G1 phase arrest mediated by an inhibitor (p27/kip1) of cyclin dependent kinase-4 activation. *Cell* **79**, 487-496.

Kato K, Kimura S (1985). S100a$_0$ (α,α) protein is mainly located in the heart and striated muscles. *Biochem Biophys Acta* **842**, 146-150.

Katunuma N, Kominami E (1985). Molecular basis of intracellular regulation of thiol proteinase inhibitors. *Curr Top Cell Reg* **27**, 345-360.

Kaufmann M, Heider KH, Sinn HP, Vonminckwitz G, Ponta H, Herrlich P (1995). CD44 variant exon epitopes in primary breast cancer and length of survival. *Lancet* **345**, 615-619.

Kawamata N, Morosetti R, Miller CW, Park D, Spirin KS, Nakamaki T, Takeuchi S, Hatta Y, Simpson J, Wilczynski S, Lee YY, Bartram CR, Koeffler HP (1995). Molecular analysis of the cyclin-dependent kinase inhibitor gene p27/kip1 in human malignancies. *Cancer Res* **55**, 2266-2269.

Kawami H, Yoshida K, Ohsaki A, Kuroi K, Nishiyama M, Toge T (1993). Stromelysin-3 mRNA expression and malignancy: Comparison with clinicopathological features and type IV collagenase mRNA expression in breast tumours. *Anticancer Res* **13**, 2130-2324.

Kawamoto H, Uozumi T, Kawamoto K, Arita K, Yano T and Hirohata T (1995). Analysis of the growth rate and cavernous sinus invasion of pituitary adenomas. *Acta Neurochir* **136**, 37-43.

Kazu I, Bicknell R, Harris AL, Jones M, Gatter KC, Mason DY (1992). Heterogeneity of vascular endothelial cells with relevance to diagnosis of vascular tumours. *J Clin Pathol* **45**, 143-148.

Kearsey JM, Coates PJ, Prescott AR, Warbrick E, Hall PA (1995). GADD45 is a nuclear cell cycle-regulated protein which interacts with p21 (cip1). *Oncogene* **11**, 1675-1683.

Keim D, Hailat N, Melhem R, Zhu XX, Lascu I, Veron M, Strahler J (1992). Proliferation related expression of p19/nm23 nucleoside diphosphate kinase. *J Clin Invest* **89**, 919-924.

Kelly P, Schlesinger MJ (1978). The effect of amino acid analogues and heat shock on gene expression in chicken embryo fibroblasts. *Cell* **15**, 1277-1286.

Kent J, Coriat AM, Sharpe PT, Hastie ND, van Heyningen V (1995). The evolution of *wt1* sequence and expression pattern in the vertebrates. *Oncogene* **11**, 1781-1792.

Keppler D, Waridel P, Abrahamson M, Bachmann D, Berdoz J, Sordat B (1994). Latency of cathepsin B secreted by human colon carcinoma cells is not linked to secretion of cystatin C and is relieved by neutrophil elastase. *Biochem Biophys Acta* **1226**, 117-125.

Kerbel RS, Waghorne C, Man MS, Elliott B, Breitman ML (1987). Alteration of the tumorigenic and metastatic properties of neoplastic cells is associated with the process of calcium phosphate-mediated DNA transfection. *Proc Natl Acad Sci* **84**, 1263-1267.

Keren Z, LeGrue SJ (1988). Identification of cell surface cathepsin B-like activity on murine melanomas and fibrosarcomas. Modulation by butanol extraction. *Cancer Res* **48**, 1416-1421.

Kern SE, Pietenpol JA, Thiagalingam S, Seymour A, Kinzler KW, Vogelstein B (1992). Oncogenic forms of p53 inhibit p53 regulated gene expression. *Science* **256**, 827-830.

Kerr LD, Holt JT, Matrisian LM (1988). Growth factors regulate transin gene expression by c-fos-dependent and c-fos-independent pathways. *Science* **242**, 1424-1427.

Kerr LD, Miller DB, Matrisian LM (1990). TGF-β1 inhibition of transin/stromelysin gene expression is mediated through a fos binding sequence. *Cell* **61**, 267-278.

Keyt BA, Berleau LT, Nguyen HV, Chen H, Heinsohn H, Vandlen R, Ferrara N (1996). The carboxyl terminal domain (111-165) of vascular endothelial growth factor is critical for its mitogenic potency. *J Biol Chem* **271**, 7788-7795.

Khalifa MA, Abdoh AA, Mannel RS, Haraway ST, Walker JL, Min KW (1994). Prognostic utility of epidermal growth factor receptor over-expression in endometrial adenocarcinoma. *Cancer* **73**, 370-376.

Khan P, Graf T (1986). *Oncogenes and Growth Control*. Springer, Berlin and New York.

Khokha R, Waterhouse P, Yagel S, Lala PK, Overall CM, Norton G, Denhardt DT (1989). Antisense RNA-induced reduction in murine TIMP levels confers oncogenicity on Swiss 3T3 cells. *Science* **243**, 947-950.

Kiaris H, Spandidos DA, Jones AS, Field JK (1994). Loss of heterozygosity and microsatellite instability of the H-*ras* gene in cancer of the head and neck. *Int J Oncol* **5**, 579-582.

Kihlman BA, Andersson HC (1985). Synergistic enhancement of the frequency of chromatid aberrations in cultured human lymphocytes by combinations of inhibitors of DNA repair. *Mutation Res* **150**, 313-325.

Kim KJ, Li B, Winer J, Aramanini M, Gillet N, Phillips HS, Ferrara N (1993). Inhibition of vascular endothelial growth factor-induced angiogenesis suppresses tumour growth *in vivo*. *Nature* **362**, 841-844.

Kim SJ, Wagner S, Liu F, O'Reilly MA, Robbins PD, Green MR (1992). Retinoblastoma gene product activates expression of the human TGF beta-2 gene through transcription factor ATF-2. *Nature* **358**, 331-334.

Kim TM, Benedict WF, Xu HJ, Hu SX, Gosewehr J, Veliceson M, Yin E, Zheng J, D'Ablaing G, Dubeau L (1994). Loss of heterozygosity on chromosome 13 is common only in the biologically more aggressive subtypes of ovarian epithelial tumours and is associated with normal retinoblastoma gene expression. *Cancer Res* **54**, 605-609.

Kim WH, Schnaper HW, Nomizu M, Yamada Y, Kleinman HK (1994). Apoptosis in human fibrosarcoma cells is induced by a multimeric synthetic Tyr-Ile-Gly-Ser-Arg (YIGSR)-containing polypeptide from laminin. *Cancer Res* **54**, 5005-5010.

Kimata M, Honma Y, Okayama M, Oguri K, Hozumi M, Suzuki S (1983). Increased synthesis of hyaluronic acid by mouse mammary carcinoma cell variants with high metastatic potential. *Cancer Res* **43**, 1347-1354.

King RC, Swain SM, Porter L, Steinberg SM, Lippman ME, Gelman EP (1989). Heterogeneous expression of erb B2 messenger in human breast cancer. *Cancer Res* **49**, 4185-4191.

King TV, Vallee BL (1991). Neovascularisation of the meniscus with angiogenin: An experimental study in rabbits. *J Bone Joint Surg Br* **73**, 587-590.

Kintner CR, Melton DA (1987). Expression of *Xenopus* NCAM RNA is an early response of ectoderm to induction. *Development* **99**, 311-325.

Kinzler KW, Nilbert MC, Vogelstein B, Bryan TM, Levy DB, Smith KJ, Preisinger AC, Hamilton SR, Hedge P, Markham A, Carlson M, Joslyn G, Groden J, White R, Miki Y, Miyoshi Y, Nishisho I, Nakamura Y (1991a). Identification of a gene located at chromosome 5q21 that is mutated in colorectal cancer. *Science* **251**, 1366-1370.

Kinzler KW, Nilbert MC, Su LK, Vogelstein B, Bryan TM, Levy DB, Smith KJ, Preisinger AC, Hedge P, McKechnie D, Finniear R, Markham A, Groffen J, Boguski MS, Altschul SF, Horii A, Ando H, Miyoshi Y, Miki Y, Nishisho I, Nakamura Y (1991b). Identification of FAP locus genes from chromosome 5q21. *Science* **253**, 661-665.

Kitagawa Y, Ueda M, Anado N, Shiozawa Y, Shimizu N, Abe O (1991). Significance of *int-2/hst-1* coamplification as a prognostic factor in patients with oesophageal squamous carcinoma. *Cancer Res* **51**, 1504-1508.

Klee C, Cohen P (1988). *Aspects of Cellular Regulation.* Elsevier Biomedical Press, Amsterdam, pp. 225-248.

Klee CB (1991). Concerted regulation of protein phosphorylation and dephosphorylation by calmodulin. *Neurochem Res* **16**, 1059-1065.

Klein CL, Kohler H, Bittinger F, Wagner M, Hermanns I, Grant K, Lewis JC, Kirkpatrick CJ (1994). Comparative studies on vascular endothelium *in vitro*. I: Cytokine effects on the expression of adhesion molecules by human umbilical vein, saphenous vein, and femoral artery endothelial cells. *Pathobiology* **62**, 199-208.

Klein CL, Bittinger F, Kohler H, Wagner M, Otto M, Hermanns I, Kirkpatrick CJ (1995). Comparative studies on vascular endothelium *in vitro*. III: Effects of cytokines on the expression of E-selectin, ICAM-1 and VCAM-1 by cultured human endothelial cells obtained from different passages. *Pathobiology* **63**, 83-92.

Kligman D, Hilt CC (1988). The S-100 protein family. *TIBS* **13**, 437-443.

Kligman D, Marshak DR (1985). Purification and characterisation of a neurite extension factor from bovine brain. *Proc Natl Acad Sci USA* **82**, 7136-7139.

Klingelhutz AJ, Hendrick L, Cho KR, McDougall JR (1995). The DCC gene suppresses the malignant phenotype of transformed human epithelial cells. *Oncogene* **10**, 1581-1586.

Kluck RM, McDougall CA, Harmon BV, Halliday JW (1994). Calcium chelators induce apoptosis. Evidence that raised intracellular calcium is not essential for apoptosis. *Biochim Biophys Acta* **1223**, 247-254.

Knudsen KA, Wheelock MJ (1992). Plakoglobin or an 83-kDa homologue distinct from β-catenin, interacts with E-cadherin and N-cadherin. *J Cell Biol* **118**, 671-679.

Knudson AG, Jr (1971). Mutation and cancer: statistical study of retinoblastoma. *Proc Natl Acad Sci USA* **68**, 820-823.

Knudson AG, Jr (1973). Mutation and human cancer. *Adv Cancer Res* **17**, 317-348..

Knudson AG, Jr (1985). Hereditary cancer, oncogenes, and antioncogenes. *Cancer Res* **45**, 1437-1443.

Kobayashi H, Moniwa N, Sugimura M, Shinohara H, Ohi H, Terao T (1993). Effects of membrane associated cathepsin B on the activation of receptor bound pro-urokinase and subsequent invasion of reconstituted basement membranes. *Biochim Biophys Acta* **1178**, 55-62.

Kobayashi H, Gotoh J, Fujie M, Shinohara H, Moniwa N, Terao T (1994). Inhibition of metastasis of Lewis lung carcinoma by a synthetic peptide within growth factor-like domain of urokinase in the experimental and spontaneous metastasis model. *Int J Cancer* **57**, 727-733.

Kobayashi K, Sagae S, Kudo R, Saito H, Koi S, Nakamura Y (1995). Microsatellite instability in endometrial carcinomas. Frequent replication errors in tumours of early onset and/or of poorly differentiated type. *Genes Chrom Cancer* **14**, 128-132.

Kobayashi K, Matsushima M, Koi S, Saito H, Sagae S, Kudo R, Nakamura Y (1996). Mutational analysis of mismatch repair genes, HMLH1 and HMSH2, in sporadic endometrial carcinomas with microsatellite instability. *Jap J Cancer Res* **87**, 141-145.

Kobayashi S, Iwase H, Itoh Y, Fukuoka H, Yamahita H, Kuzushima T, Iwata H, Masaoka A, Kimura N (1992). Estrogen receptor, c-erbB2 and nm23/NDP kinase expression in the intraductal and invasive components of human breast cancers. *Jpn J Cancer Res* **83**, 859-865.

Koch AE, Polverini PJ, Kunkel SL, Harlow LA, DiPietro LA, Elner VM, Elner SG, Strieter RM (1992). Interleukin-8 as a macrophage-derived mediator of angiogenesis. *Science* **258**, 1798-1801.

Koch AE, Harlow LA, Haines GK, Amento EP, Unemori EN, Wong WL, Pope RM, Ferrara N (1994). Vascular endothelial growth factor. A cytokine modulating endothelial function in rheumatoid arthritis. *J Immuno* **152**, 149-152.

Koch AE, Halloran MM, Haskell CJ, Shah MR, Polverini PJ (1995). Angiogenesis mediated by soluble forms of E-selectin and vascular cell adhesion molecule. *Nature* **376**, 517-519.

Koff A, Ohtsuki M, Polyak K, Roberts JM, Massague J (1993). Negative regulation of G1 in mammalian cells. Inhibition of cyclin E-dependent kinase by TGF beta. *Science* **260**, 536-539.

Koga H, Zhang SJ, Kumanishi T, Washiyama K, Ichikawa T, Tanaka R, Mukawa J (1994). Analysis of p53 gene mutations in low grade and high grade astrocytomas by polymerase chain reaction assisted single strand conformation polymorphism and immunohistochemistry. *Acta Neuropath* **87**, 225-232.

Kohler M, Janz I, Wintzer HO, Wagner E, Banknecht T (1989). The expression of EGF receptors, EGF-like factors and c-myc in ovarian and cervical carcinomas and their clinical significance. *Anticancer Res* **9**, 1537-1547.

Kohler MF, Berchuck A, Davidoff AM, Humphrey PA, Dodge RK, Iglehart JD, Soper JT, Clarke-Pearson DL, Bast RC, Jr, Marks JR (1992). Overexpression and mutation of *p53* in endometrial carcinoma. *Cancer Res* **52**, 1622-1627.

Kohn PH (1983). Sister chromatid exchange in cancer. *Ann Clin Lab Sci* **13**, 267-274.

Kolkenbrock H, Orgel D, Hecker-Kia A, Noack W, Ulbrich N (1991). The complex between a tissue inhibitor of metalloproteinases (TIMP-2) and 72-kDa progelatinase is a metalloproteinase inhibitor. *Eur J Biochem* **198**, 775-781.

Kondo E, Nakamura S, Onoue H, Matsuo Y, Yoshino T, Aoki H, Hayashi K, Takahashi K, Minowada J, Nomura S, Akagi T (1992). Detection of bcl-2 protein and bcl-2 messenger RNA in normal and neoplastic lymphoid tissues by immunohistochemistry and *in situ* hybridisation. *Blood* **80** 2044-2051.

Koochekpour S, Pilkington GJ (1996). Vascular and perivascular GD3 expression in human glioma. *Cancer Lett* **104**, 97-102.

Koochekpour S, Merzak A, Pilkington GJ (1995). Vascular endothelial growth factor production is stimulated in response to growth factors in human glioma cells. *Oncol Rep* **2**, 1059-1061.

Koopmann J, Maintz D, Schild S, Schramm J, Louis DN, Wiestler OD, von Deimling A (1995). Multiple polymorphisms, but no mutations, in the *waf1/cip1* gene in human brain tumours. *Br J Cancer* **72**, 1230-1233.

Kornberg LJ, Earp HS, Turner CS, Prockop C, Juliano RL (1991). Signal transduction by integrins: Increased protein tyrosine kinase phosphorylation caused by clustering of β integrins. *Proc Natl Acad Sci USA* **88**, 8392-8396.

Kos J, Smid A, Krasovec M, Svetic B, Lenarcic B, Vrhovec I, Skrk J, Turk V (1995). Lysosomal proteinases cathepsin D, cathepsin B, cathepsin H, cathepsin L and their inhibitors stefin A and stefin B in head and neck cancer. *Biol Chem Hoppe-Seyler* **376**, 401-405.

Kothary R, Perry MD, Moran LA, Rossant J (1987). Cell lineage-specific expression of the mouse HSP68 gene during embryogenesis. *Develop Biol* **121**, 342-348.

Kotovuori P, Tontti E, Pigott R, Shepherd M, Kiso M, Hasegawa A, Renkonen R, Nortamo P, Altieri DC, Gahmberg CG (1993). The vascular E-selectin binds to the leukocyte integrins CD11/CD18. *Glycobiology* **3**, 131-136.

Koufos A, Hansen MF, Lampkin BC, Workman ML, Copeland NG, Jenkins NA, Cavanee WK (1984). Loss of alleles on human chromosome 11 during genesis of Wilms tumour. *Nature* **309**, 170-172.

Kovesdi I, Reichel R, Nevins, JR (1986). Identification of a cellular transcription factor involved in E1A *trans*-activation. *Cell* **45**, 219-228.

Kowalik TF, De Gregori J, Schwarz JK, Nevins JR (1995). E2F1 over-expression in quiescent fibroblasts leads to induction of cellular DNA synthesis and apoptosis. *J Virol* **69**, 2491-2500.

Kraus JA, Bolln C, Wolf HK, Neumann J, Kindermann D, Fimmers R, Forster F, Baumann A, Schlegel U (1994). Tp53 alterations and clinical outcome in low grade astrocytomas. *Genes Chrom Cancer* **10**, 143-149.

Krek W, Livingston DM, Shirodkar S (1993). Binding to DNA and the retinoblastoma gene product by complex formation of different E2F family members. *Science* **262**, 1557-1560.

Krek W, Ewen ME, Shirodkar S, Arany Z, Kaelin, Jr, WG, Livingston DM (1994). Negative regulation of the growth promoting transcription factor E2F-1 by a stably bound cyclin A-dependent protein kinase. *Cell* **78**, 161-172.

Krone PH, Heikkila JJ (1988). Analysis of hsp30, hsp70 and ubiquitin gene expression in *Xenopus laevis* tadpoles. *Develop Biol* **103**, 59-67.

Kros JM, Godschalk JJCJ, Krishnadath KK, van Eden CG (1993). Expresssion of p53 in oligodendrogliomas. *J Pathol* **171**, 285-290.

Kruithof EKO, Tran-Thang C, Gudinchet A, Hauert J, Nocoloso G, Genton C, Welti H, Bachmann F (1987). Fibrinolysis in pregnancy. A study of plasminogen activator inhibitors. *Blood* **69**, 460-466.

Kuczyk MA, Serth J, Bokemeyer C, Hofner K, Allhoff EP, Jonas U (1994). Immunohistochemical detection of cathepsin D expression in prostate cancer. *Oncology Rep* **1**, 1247-1251.

Kudoh T, Ishidate T, Moriyama M, Toyoshima K, Akiyama T (1995). G(1) phase arrest induced by Wilms tumour protein wt1 is abrogated by cyclin/CDK complexes. *Proc Natl Acad Sci USA* **92**, 4517-4521.

Kulesz-Martin MF, Lisafeld B, Huang H, Kisiel ND, Lee L (1994). Endogenous p53 protein generated from wild-type alternatively spliced p53 RNA in mouse epidermal cells. *Mol Cell Biol* **14**, 1698-1708.

Kumar S, Harrison CJ, Heighway J, Marsden HB, West DC, Jones PM (1987). A cell line from Wilms' tumour with deletion in short arm of chromosome 11. *Int J Cancer* **40**, 499-504.

Kuppner MC, van Meir E, Gauthier TH, Hamou MF, De Tribolet N (1992). Differential expression of the CD44 molecule in human brain tumours. *Int J Cancer* **50**, 572-577.

Kupryjanczyk J, Thor AD, Beauchamp R, Merrit V, Edgerton SM, Bell DA, Yandell DW (1993). p53 gene mutations and protein accumulation in human ovarian cancer. *Proc Natl Acad Sci USA* **90**, 4961-4965.

Kupryjanczyk J, Bell DA, Dimeo D, Beauchamp R, Thor AD, Yandell DW (1995). P53 gene analysis of ovarian borderline tumours and stage I carcinomas. *Human Pathol* **26**, 387-392.

Kurtz S, Lindquist S (1984). Changing patterns of gene expression during sporulation in yeast. *Proc Natl Acad Sci USA* **81**, 7323-7327.

Kurtz S, Rossi J, Petko L, Lindquist S (1986). An ancient developmental induction: heat shock proteins induced in sporulation and oogenesis. *Science* **231**, 1154-1157.

Kury F, Sliutz G, Schemper M, Reiner G, Reiner A, Jakesz R, Wrba F, Zeillinger R, Knogler W,

Huber J, Holzner H, Spona J (1990). HER-2 oncogene amplification and overall survival of breast carcinoma patients. *Eur J Cancer* 26, 946-949.

Kushima R, Moritani S, Hattori T (1994). Over-expression of p53 protein in gastric carcinomas. Relationship with development, progression and mucin histochemical differentiation. *Cancer J* 7, 192-197.

Kvanta A (1995). Expression and regulation of vascular endothelial growth factor in choroidal fibroblasts. *Curr Eye Res* 14, 1015-1020.

Kwan H, Pecenka V, Tsukamoto A, Parslow TG, Guzman R, Lin TP, Muller WJ, Lee FS, Leder P, Varmus HE (1992). Transgenes expressing the wnt-1 and int-2 protooncogenes cooperate during mammary carcinogenesis in doubly transgenic mice. *Mol Cell Biol* 12, 147-154.

Kyritsis AP, Bondy MAL, Xiao M, Berman EL, Cunningham JE, Lee PS, Levin VA, Saya H (1994). Germline p53 mutations in subsets of glioma patients. *J Natl Cancer Inst* 86, 344-349.

Lacombe M, Sastre-Garau X, Lascu I, Vonica A, Wallet V, Thiery JP, Veron M (1991). Over-expression of nucleoside diphosphate kinase (nm23) in solid tumours. *Eur J Cancer* 27, 1302-1307.

Lacombe ML, Wallet V, Troll H, Veron M (1990). Functional cloning of nucleoside diphosphate kinase from *Dictyostelium discoideum*. *J Biol Chem* 265, 10112-10118.

Ladanyi M, Lewis R, Jhanwar SC, Gerald W, Huvos AG, Healey JH (1995). Mdm2 and CDK4 gene amplification in Ewings sarcoma. *J Pathol* 175, 211-217.

Ladoux A, Frelin C (1993). Hypoxia is a strong inducer of vascular endothelial growth factor messenger RNA expression in the heart. *Biochem Biophys Res Commun* 195, 1005-1010.

Lah TT, Buck MR, Honn KV, Crissman JD, Rao NC, Liotta LA, Sloane BF (1989). Degradation of laminin by human tumour cathepsin B. *Clin Exp Metastasis* 7, 461-468.

Lah TT, Calaf G, Kalman E, Shinde BG, Russo J, Jarosz D, Zabrecky J, Somers R, Daskal I (1995). Cathepsin D, cathepsin B and cathepsin L in breast carcinoma and in transformed human breast epithelial cells (HBEC). *Biol Chem Hoppe-Seyler* 376, 357-363.

Lah TT, Kokalj-Kunovar M, Turk V (1990). Cysteine proteinase inhibitors in human cancerous tissues and fluids. *Biol Chem Hoppe-Seyler* 371, 199-203.

Lakshmi MS, Sherbet GV (1989). Gene amplification correlates with sister chromatid exchange in B16 murine and human melanoma and human astrocytoma cell lines. *Anticancer Res* 9, 113-114.

Lakshmi MS, Sherbet GV (1990). Genetic recombination in human melanomas and astrocytoma cell lines involves oncogenes and growth factor genes. *Clin Exp Metastasis* 8, 75-87.

Lakshmi MS, Hunt G, Sherbet GV (1988). Spontaneous sister chromatid exchange in metastatic variants of the murine B16 melanoma and human astrocytomas in culture. *Invasion Metastasis* 8, 205-216.

Lakshmi MS, Parker C, Sherbet GV (1991). Chromosomal mapping of the *mts1* gene by *in situ* hybridisation. *Eur J Cancer* 27 (Suppl. 3), 34.

Lakshmi MS, Parker C, Sherbet GV (1993). Metastasis associated *mts1* and *nm23* genes affect tubulin polymerisation in B16 melanomas: A possible mechanism of their regulation of metastatic behaviour. *Anticancer Res* 13, 299-304.

Lala PK, Graham CH (1990). Mechanisms of trophoblast invasiveness and their control: the role of proteases and protease inhibitors. *Cancer Metastasis Rev* 9, 369-379.

Lam EWF, La Thangue NB (1994). DP and E2F proteins: coordinating transcription with cell cycle progression. *Curr Opin Cell Biol* 6, 859-866.

Lam EWF, Watson RJ (1993). An E2F binding site mediates cell cycle regulated repression of mouse B-myb transcription. *EMBO J* 12, 2705-2713.

Lam KT, Calderwood SK (1992). HSP70 binds specifically to a peptide derived from the highly conserved domain I region of p53. *Biochem Biophys Res Commun* **184**, 167-174.

Lamb P, Crawford LV (1986). Characterisation of the human p53 gene. *Mol Cell Biol* **6**, 1379-1385.

Lammie GA, Fantl V, Smith R, Schuuring E, Brookes S, Michalides R, Dickson C, Arnold A, Peters G (1991). D11S287, a putative oncogene on chromosome 11q13, is amplified in squamous cell and mammary carcinomas and linked to BCL-1. *Oncogene* **6**, 439-444.

Lamph WW, Wamsley P, Sassone-Corse P, Verma I (1988). Induction of proto-oncogene *Jun*/AP1 by serum and TPA. *Nature* **334**, 629-631.

Lane DP, Benchimol S (1990). p53: Oncogene or anti-oncogene? *Genes Develop* **4**, 1-8.

Lane DP, Crawford LV (1979). T-antigen is bound to a host protein in SV40 transformed cells. *Nature* **278**, 261-263.

Lane DP (1992). p53, guardian of the genome. *Nature* **358**, 15-16.

Lane TF, Deng CX, Elson A, Lyu MS, Kozak CA, Leder P (1995). Expression of BRCA1 is associated with terminal differentiation of ectodermally and mesodermally derived tissues in mice. *Genes Develop* **21**, 2712-2722.

Lang FF, Miller DC, Pihsarody S, Koslow M, Newcomb EW (1994). High frequency of p53 protein accumulation without p53 gene mutation in human juvenile pilocytic, low grade and anaplastic astrocytomas. *Oncogene* **9**, 949-954.

Langerak AW, Willimson KA, Miyagawa K, Hagemeijer A, Versnel MA, Hastie ND (1995). Expression of the Wilms tumour gene wt1 in human malignant mesothelioma cell lines and relationship to platelet-derived growth factor A and insulin-like growth factor-2 expression. *Genes Chrom Cancer* **12**, 87-96.

Lanigan, DJ, McLean PA, Murphy DM, Donovan MG, Leader M (1992). Image analysis in the determination of ploidy and prognosis in renal cell carcinoma. *Eur J Urology* **22**, 228-234.

Largey JS, Meltzer SJ, Sauk JJ, Hebert CA, Archibald DW (1994). Loss of heterozygosity involving the APC gene in oral squamous cell carcinoma. *Oral Surg Oral Med Oral Pathol* **77**, 260-263.

Larson AA, Kern S, Sommers RL, Yokota J, Cavenee WK, Hampton GM (1996). Analysis of replication error (RER+) phenotypes in cervical carcinoma. *Cancer Res* **56**, 1426-1431.

Larsson N, Melander H, Marklund U, Osterman O, Gullberg M (1995). G2/M transition requires multisite phosphorylation of oncoprotein-18 by 2 distinct protein kinase systems. *J Biol Chem* **270**, 14175-14183.

Larsson SH, Charlieu JP, Miyagawa K, Engelkamp D, Rassoulzadegan M, Ross A, Cuzin F, van Heyningen V, Hastie ND (1995). Subnuclear localisation of wt1 in splicing or transcription factor domains is regulated by alternative splicing. *Cell* **81**, 1-20.

Latham C, Maner S, Blegen H, Eriksson E, Zickert P, Auer G, Zetterberg A (1996). Relationship between oncogene amplification, aneuploidy and altered expression of p53 in breast cancer. *Int J Oncol* **8**, 359-365.

Latil A, Baron JC, Cussenot O, Fournier G, Boccongibod L, Leduc A, Lidereau R (1994). Oncogene amplification in early stage human prostate carcinomas. *Int J Cancer* **59**, 637-638.

Lauri D, Needham L, Martin-Padura I, Gejana E (1991). Tumour cell adhesion to endothelial cells: Endothelial leukocyte adhesion molecule-1 as an inducible adhesive receptor for colon carcinoma cells. *J Natl Cancer Inst* **83**, 1321-1324.

Leach FS, Nicolaides NC, Papadopoulos N, Liu B, Jen J, Parsons R, Peltomaki P, Sistonen P, Aaltonen LA, Nystrom-Lahti M, Guan XY, Zhang J, Meltzer PS, Yu JW, Kao FT, Chen DJ, Cerosaletti KM, Fournier REK, Todd S, Lewis T, Leach RJ, Naylor SL, Green J, Jass J, Watson P,

Lynch HT, Trent JM, De la Chapelle A, Kinzler KW, Vogelstein B (1993). Mutations of a *mut*S homologue in hereditary non-polyposis colorectal cancer. *Cell* **75**, 1215-1225.

Leake R, Carr L, Rinaldi F (1991). Autocrine and paracrine effects in the endometrium. *Ann NY Acad Sci* **622**, 145-148.

Ledermann JA, Pasini F, Olabiran Y, Pelosi G (1994). Detection of the neural cell adhesion molecule (NCAM) in serum of patients with small cell lung cancer (SCLC) with limited or extensive disease, and bone marrow infiltration. *Int J Cancer* **S8**, 49-52.

Lee EYHP, To H, Shew JY, Bookstein R, Scully P, Lee WH (1988). Inactivation of the retinoblastoma susceptibility gene in human breast cancers. *Science* **241**, 218-221.

Lee MH, Reynisdottir I, Massague J (1995). Cloning of p57 (kip2), a cyclin dependent kinase inhibitor with unique domain structure and tissue distribution. *Genes Develop* **9**, 639-649.

Lee WH, Bookstein R, Hong F, Young LJ, Shew JY, Lee EYHP (1987a). Human retinoblastoma susceptibility gene: cloning, identification and sequence. *Science* **235**, 1394-1399.

Lee WH, Shew JY, Hong FD, Sery TW, Donoso LA, Young LJ, Bookstein R, Lee EYHP (1987b). The retinoblastoma susceptibility gene encodes a nuclear phosphoprotein associated with DNA binding activity. *Nature* **329**, 642-645.

Lee WH, Bookstein RE, Lee EYHP (1990). Molecular biology of the human retinoblastoma gene. In: *Tumour Suppressor Genes*, Klein G (ed.). Marcel Dekker, New York, pp. 169-199.

Lee YI, Kim SJ (1996). Transcriptional repression of human insulin-like growth factor II P4 promoter by Wilms tumour suppressor wt1. *DNA Cell Biol* **15**, 99-104.

Lee YY, Wilczynski SP, Cumakov A, Chih D, Koeffler HP (1994). Carcinoma of the vulva: HPV and p53 mutations. *Oncogene* **9**, 1655-1659.

Leek RD, Kaklamanis L, Pezzella F, Gatter KC, Harris AL (1994). *Bcl-2* in normal human breast and carcinoma, association with oestrogen receptor-positive, epidermal growth factor receptor-negative tumours and *in situ* cancer. *Br J Cancer* **69**, 135-139.

Le Febvere V, Peeters-Joris C, Vaes G (1991). Production of gelatin degrading matrix metalloproteinases (type IV collagenases) and inhibitors by articular chondrocytes during their dedifferentiation and serial subcultures and under stimulation by interleukin-1 and tumour necrosis factor-α. *Biochem Biophys Acta* **1094**, 8-18.

Lehmann AR, Norris PG (1989). DNA repair and cancer: Speculations based on studies with xeroderma pigmentosum, Cockayne's syndrome and trocho-thiodystrophy. *Carcinogenesis* **10**, 1353-1356.

Lehrman MA, Goldstein JL, Russel DW, Brown MS (1987). Duplication of seven exons in LDL receptor gene caused by *alu-alu* recombination in a subject with familial hypercholesterolemia. *Cell* **48**, 827-835.

Lehto VP, Wasenius VM, Salven P, Saraste M (1988). Transforming and membrane proteins. *Nature* **334**, 388.

Leibovich SJ, Polverini PJ, Shepard HM, Wiseman DM, Shively V, Nuseir N (1987). Macrophage-induced angiogenesis is mediated by tumour necrosis factor α. *Nature* **329**, 630-632.

Leighton LA, Curmi P, Campbell DG, Cohen P, Sobel A (1993). The phosphorylation of stathmin by MAP kinase. *Mol Cell Biochem* **128**, 151-156.

LeJeune S, Huguet EL, Hamby A, Poulsom R, Harris AL (1995). Wnt-5 alpha cloning, expression and up-regulation in human primary breast cancers. *Clin Cancer Res* **1**, 215-222.

Lemaux PG, Herendeen SL, Bloch PL, Neidhardt FC (1978). Transient rates of synthesis of individual polypeptides in *E. coli* following temperature shifts. *Cell* **13**, 427-434.

Lemoine NR (1994). Molecular biology of breast cancer. *Ann Oncol* **5** (Suppl. S4), 31-37.

Leng P, Brown DR, Deb S, Deb SP (1995). Human oncoprotein mdm2 interacts with the TATA binding protein *in vitro* and *in vivo*. *Int J Oncol* **6**, 251-259.

Leone A, McBride WO, Wang M, Weston A, Anglard P, Lineham MW, Harris CC, Liotta LA, Steeg PA (1990). Allelic loss of nm23 gene in lung and renal carcinomas. *Clin Exp Metastasis* **8** (Suppl. 1), 21-22.

Leone A, McBride OW, Weston A, Wang MG, Anglard P, Cropps CS, Goepel JR, Lindereau R, Callahan R, Lineham WM, Rees RC, Harris CC, Liotta LA, Steeg PS (1991a). Somatic allelic deletion of nm23 in human cancer. *Cancer Res* **51**, 2490-2493.

Leone A, Flatow, U, King CR, Sandeen MA, Margulies IMK, Liotta LA, and Steeg PS (1991b). Reduced tumour incidence, metastatic potential and cytokine responsiveness in nm23-transfected melanoma cells. *Cell* **65**, 25-36

Leone A, Seeger RC, Hong CM, Hu YY, Arboleda J, Brodeur M, Stram D, Slamon DJ, Steeg PS (1993). Evidence for nm23 RNA overexpression, DNA amplification and mutation in aggressive childhood neuroblastomas. *Oncogene* **8**, 855-865.

Lerner AB, McGuire JS (1961). Effect of alpha and beta melanocyte stimulating hormone on the skin colour of man. *Nature* **189**, 176-179.

Lese CM, Rossie KM, Appel BN, Reddy JK, Johnson JT, Myers EN, Gollin SM (1995). Visualisation of int2 and hst1 amplification in oral squamous cell carcinomas. *Genes Chrom Cancer* **12**, 288-295.

Lester DR, Cauchi MN (1990). Point mutations at codon 12 of c-K-*ras* in human endometrial carcinomas. *Cancer Lett* **51**, 7-10.

Leung MF, Sokoloski JA, Sartorelli AC (1992). Changes in microtubules, microtubulc associated proteins, and intermediatc filaments during the differentiation of HL60 leukaemia cells. *Cancer Res* **52**, 949-954.

Levine AJ, Momand J, Finlay CA (1991). The p53 tumour suppressor genc. *Nature* **351**, 453-456.

Levine AJ, Chang A, Dittmer D, Notterman DA, Silver A, Thorn K, Welsh D (1993). The p53 tumour suppressor gene. *J Lab Clin Med* **123**, 817-823.

Levine AJ, Perry ME, Chang A, Silver A, Dittmer D, Wu M, Welsh D (1994). The role of the p53 tumour suppressor gene in tumorigenesis. *Br J Cancer* **69**, 409-416.

Li CY, Suardet L, Little JB (1995). Potential role of waf1/cip1/p21 as a mediator of TGF-beta cytoinhibitory effect. *J Biol Chem* **270**, 4971-4974.

Li H, Hamou MF, Detribolet N, Jaufeerally R, Hofmann M (1993). Variant CD44 adhesion molecules are expressed in human brain metastases but not in glioblastomas. *Cancer Res* **53**, 5345-5349.

Li R, Nortamo P, Kantor C, Kovanen P, Timonen T, Gahmberg CG (1993). A leukocyte integrin binding peptide from intercellular adhesion molecule-2 stimulates T-cell adhesion and natural killer cell activity. *J Biol Chem* **268**, 21474-21477.

Li R, Xie JL, Kantor C, Koistinen V, Altieri DC, Nortamo P, Gahmberg CG (1995). A peptide derived from the intercellular adhesion molecule-2 regulates the avidity of the leukocyte integrins CD11b/CD18 and CD11c/CD18. *J Cell Biol* **129**, 1143-1153.

Li SB, Schwartz PE, Lee W, Yang-Feng TL (1991). Allele loss at the retinoblastoma locus in human ovarian cancer. *J Natl Cancer Inst* **83**, 637-640.

Li XW, Tsuji TS, Wen SM, Sobhan F, Wang ZY, Shinozaki F (1995). Cytoplasmic expression of p53 protein and its morphological features in salivary gland lesions. *J Oral Path Med* **24**, 201-205.

Li YJ, Laurentpuig P, Salmon RJ, Thomas G, Hamelin R (1995). Polymorphisms and probable lack of mutation in the *waf1/cip1* gene in colorectal cancer. *Oncogene* **10**, 599-601.

Lianes P, Orlow I, Zhang ZF, Oliva MR, Sarkis AS, Reuter VE, Cordon-Cardo C (1994). Altered patterns of mdm2 and tp53 expression in human bladder cancer. *J Natl Cancer Inst* **86**, 1325-1330.

Liang XH, Volkman M, Klein R, Herman B, Lockett SJ (1993). Co-localisation of the tumour suppressor protein p53 and human papillomavirus E6 protein in human cervical carcinoma cell lines. *Oncogene* **8**, 2645-2652.

Liberek K, Georgopoulos C, Zylicz M (1988). The role of *E. coli* DnaK and DnaJ heat shock proteins in the initiation of bacteriophase lambda DNA replication. *Proc Natl Acad Sci USA* **85**, 6632-6636.

Lin BTY, Gruenwald S, Moria A, Lee WH, Wang JYJ (1991). Retinoblastoma cancer suppressor gene product is a substrate of the cell cycle regulator cdc2 kinase. *EMBO J* **10**, 857-864.

Lin D, Shields MT, Ullrich SJ, Appella E, Mercer WE (1992). Growth arrest induced by wild type p53 protein blocks cells prior to or near the restriction point in late G1 phase. *Proc Natl Acad Sci USA* **89**, 9210-9214.

Lin D, Fiscella M, O'Connor PM, Jackman J, Chen M, Luo LL, Sala A, Travali S, Appella E, Mercer WE (1994). Constitutive expression of B-myb can bypass p53-induced WAF1/CIP1 mediated G_1 arrest. *Proc Natl Acad Sci USA* **91**, 10079-10083.

Lin E, Orlofsky A, Berger M, Prystowsky M (1993). Characterisation of A1, a novel hemopoietic-specific early response gene with sequence similarity to *bcl-2*. *J Immunol* **151**, 1979-1988.

Lin JT, Wu MS, Shun CT, Lee WJ, Sheu JC, Wang TH (1995). Occurrence of microsatellite instability in gastric carcinoma is associated with enhanced expression of erbB-2 onco-protein. *Cancer Res* **55**, 1428-1430.

Lin JY, Simmons DTJ (1991). The ability of large T antigen to complex with p53 is necessary for the increased life span and partial transformation of human cells by simian virus 40. *J Virol* **65**, 6447-6453.

Lin RS, Turi A, Kwock L, Lu RC (1982). Hyperthermic effect on microtubule organisation. *Natl Cancer Inst Monogr* **61**, 57-61.

Lin Y, Chan SH (1995). Cloning and characterisation of two processed p53 pseudogenes from the rat genome. *Gene* **156**, 183-189.

Lin Y, Miyamoto H, Fujinami K, Uemura H, Hosaka M, Iwasaki Y, Kubota Y (1996). Telomerase activity in human bladder cancer. *Clin Cancer Res* **2**, 929-932.

Lindblom A, Tannergard P, Werelius B, Nordenskjold M (1993). Genetic mapping of a second locus predisposing to hereditary non-polyposis colon cancer. *Nature Genet* **5**, 279-282.

Linzer DIH, Malzman W, Levine AJ (1979). Characterisation of a 54k dalton cellular SV40 tumour antigen present in SV40 transformed cells and uninfected embryonal carcinoma cells. *Cell* **17**, 43-52.

Liotta LA, Tryggvason K, Garbisa S, Hart I, Foltz CM, Shafie S (1980). Metastatic potential correlates with enzymatic degradation of basement membrane collagen. *Nature* **284**, 67-68.

Liotta LA, Goldfarb R. Brundage R, Siegel G, Terranova V, Garbisa S (1981). Effect of plasminogen activator (urokinase), plasmin, and thrombin on glycoprotein and collagenous components of basement membrane. *Cancer Res* **41**, 4629-4636.

Lipponen P, Papinaho S, Eskelinen M, Klemi PJ, Aaltomaa S, Kosma VM, Marin S, Syrjanen K (1992). DNA ploidy, S-phase fraction and mitotic indices as prognostic predictors of female breast cancer. *Anticancer Res* **12**, 1533-1538.

Lipponen P, Saarelainen E, Ji H, Aaltomaa S, Syrjanen K (1994). Expression of E-cadherin (E-cd) as related to other prognostic factors and survival in breast cancer. *J Pathol* **174**, 101-109.

Lipponen P, Piettilainen T, Kosma VM, Aaltomaa S, Eskelinen M, Syrjanen K (1995a). Apoptosis suppressing protein bcl-2 is expressed in well differentiated breast carcinomas with favourable prognosis. *J Pathol* **177**, 49-55.

Lipponen P, Eskelinen M, Syrjanen K (1995b). Expression of tumour suppressor gene RB, apoptosis suppressing protein bcl-2 and c-myc have no independent prognostic value in renal adenocarcinoma. *Br J Cancer* **71**, 863-867.

Lipponen PK (1996). Expression of cathepsin D in transitional cell bladder tumours. *J Pathol* **178**, 59-64.

Lipponen PK, Eskelinen MJ (1995). Reduced expression of E-cadherin is related to invasive disease and frequent recurrence in bladder cancer. *J Cancer Res Clin Oncol* **121**, 303-308.

Lipponen PK, Eskelinen MJ, Kiviranta J, Nordling S (1991). Classic prognostic factors, flow cytometric data, nuclear morphometric variables and mitotic indexes as predictors in transitional cell bladder cancer. *Anticancer Res* **11**, 911-916.

Lithgow T, van Driel R, Bertram JF, Strasser A (1994). The protein product of the oncogene bcl-2 is a component of the nuclear envelope and endoplasmic reticulum and the outer mitochondrial membrane. *Cell Growth Diff* **5**, 411-417.

Little M, Holmes G, Bickmore W, van Heyningen V, Hastie N, Wainwright B (1995). DNA binding capacity of the wt1 protein is abolished by Denys–Drash syndrome wt1 point mutations. *Human Mol Genet* **4**, 351-358.

Liu FS, Kohler MF, Marks JR, Bast RC, Boyd J, Berchuck A (1994). Mutation and overexpression of the p53 tumour suppressor gene frequently occurs in uterine and ovarian sarcomas. *Obs Gynecol* **83**, 118-124

Liu Y, Martindale JL, Gorospe M, Holbrook NH (1996). Regulation of p21 waf/cip1 expression through mitogen activated protein kinase signalling pathway. *Cancer Res* **56**, 31-35.

Liu YJ, Mason DY, Johnson GD, Abbot S, Gregory CD, Hardie DL, Gordon J, MacLennan ICM (1991). Germinal centre cells express bcl-2 protein after activation by signals which prevent their entry into apoptosis. *Eur J Immunol* **21**, 1905-1910.

Llewellyn-Jones CG, Lomas DA, Stockley RA (1994). Potential role of recombinant secretory leukoprotease inhibitor in the prevention of neutrophil-mediated matrix degradation. *Thorax* **49**, 567-572.

Loeb LA (1991). Mutator phenotye may be required for multistage carcinogenesis. *Cancer Res* **51**, 3075-3079.

Loeb LA (1994). Microsatellite instability: Marker of a mutator phenotype in cancer. *Cancer Res* **54**, 5059-5063.

Lohrer HD, Tangen U, Anderson RF, Arrand JE (1994). Characterisation of a hybrid hamster-human cell line complemented for the ataxia telangiectasia DNA repair defects. *Pathobiology* **62**, 140-148.

Lokeshwar VB, Bourguignon LYW (1992). The lymphoma transmembrane glycoprotein GP85 (CD44) is a novel guanine nucleotide binding protein which regulates GP85 (CD44) ankyrin interaction. *J Biol Chem* **267**, 22073-22078.

Lombardi D, Sacchi A, D'Agostino G, Tibursi G (1995). The association of the nm23-Mi protein and β-tubulin correlates with cell differentiation. *Exp Cell Res* **217**, 267-271.

Loskutoff DJ, Ny T, Sawdey M, Lawrence D (1986). Fibrinolytic system of cultured endothelial cells: Regulation by plasminogen activator inhibitor. *J Cell Biochem* **32**, 273-280.

Lotem J, Sachs L (1993). Regulation by bcl-2, c-myc and p53 of susceptibility to induction of apoptosis by heat shock and cancer chemotherapy compounds in differentiation-competent and differentiation-defective myeloid leukaemia cells. *Cell Growth Diff* **4**, 41-47.

Lotem J, Sachs L (1995). Regulation of bcl-2, bcl-x(L) and bax in the control of apoptosis by haematopoietic cytokines and dexamethasone. *Cell Growth Diff* **6**, 647-653.

Lothe RA, Peltomaki P, Tommerup N, Fossa SD, Stenwig AE, Borresen AL, Nesland JM (1995). Molecular genetic changes in human male germ cell tumours. *Lab Invest* **73**, 606-614.

Louis DN, von Deimling A, Chung RY, Rubio M, Whaley JM, Eibl RH, Ohgaki H, Wiestler OD, Thor AD, Seizinger BR (1993). Comparative study of p53 gene and protein alterations in human astrocytic tumours. *J Neuropath Exp Neurol* **52**, 31-38.

Lovec H, Grzeschiczek A, Kowalski MB, Moroy T (1994a). Cyclin D1 Bcl-1 cooperates with myc genes in the generation of B-cell lymphoma in transgenic mice. *EMBO J* **13**, 3487-3495.

Lovec H, Sewing A, Lucibello FC, Muller R, Moroy T (1994b). Oncogenic activity of cyclin D1 revealed through co-operation with Ha-ras: link between cell cycle control and malignant transformation. *Oncogene* **9**, 323-326.

Lowe JB, Stoolman LM, Nair RP, Larsen RD, Berhend TL, Marks RM (1990). ELAM-1-dependent cell adhesion to vascular endothelium determined by a transfected human fucosyltransferase cDNA. *Cell* **63**, 475-484.

Lowe SW, Ruley HE (1993). Stabilization of the p53 tumour suppressor is induced by adenovirus 5 E1A and accompanies apoptosis. *Genes Develop* **7**, 535-545.

Lowe SW, Schmitt EM, Smith SW, Osborne BA, Jacks T (1993). P53 is required for radiation-induced apoptosis in mouse thymocytes. *Nature* **362**, 847-849.

Lowry WS, Atkinson RJ (1993). Tumour suppressor genes and risk of metastasis in ovarian cancer. *Br Med J* **307**, 542.

Lotz M, Guerne PA (1991). Interleukin-6 induces the synthesis of tissue inhibitor of metallo-proteinase-1/erythroid potentiating activity (TIMP-1/EPA). *J Biol Chem* **266**, 2017-2020.

Lu QL, Elia G, Lucas S, Thomas JA (1993). Bcl-2 proto-oncogene expression in Epstein–Barr virus associated nasopharyngeal carcinoma. *Int J Cancer* **53**, 29-35.

Lucas JM, Mountain RE, Gramza AW, Schullelr DE, Wilkie NM, Lang JC (1994). Expression of cyclin D1 in squamous cell carcinomas of the head and neck. *Int J Oncol* **5**, 469-472.

Ludlow JW, De Capria JA, Huang CM, Lee WH, Paucha E, Livingston DM (1989). SV 40 large T antigen binds preferentially to an underphosphorylated member of the retinoblastoma susceptibility gene product family. *Cell* **56**, 57-65.

Ludlow JW, Shon J, Pipas JM, Livingston DM, De Caprio JA (1990). The retinoblastoma susceptibility gene product undergoes cell cycle dependent phosphorylation and binding to and release from SV40 large T. *Cell* **60**, 387-396.

Lunec J, Pieron C, Sherbet GV, Thody AJ (1990). Alpha melanocyte stimulating hormone immunoreactivity in melanoma cells. *Pathobiology* **58**, 193-197.

Luo Y, Hurwitz J, Massague J (1995). Cell cycle inhibition by independent cdk and PCNA binding domains in p21 (cip1). *Nature* **375**, 159-161.

Luthgens K, Ebert W, Trefz G, Barijelcic D, Turk V, Lah T (1993). Cathepsin B and cysteine proteinase inhibitors in bronchoalveolar lavage fluid of lung cancer patients. *Cancer Detection Prevention* **17**, 387-397.

McCann AH, Dervan PA, O'Regan M, Codd MB, Gullick WJ, Tobin BMJ, Carney DN (1991). Prognostic significance of c-erbB2 and oestrogen receptor status in human breast cancer. *Cancer Res* **51**, 3296-3303.

McCann AH, Kirley A, Carney DN, Corbally N, Magee HM, Keating G, Dervan PA (1995). Amplification of the mdm2 gene in human breast cancer and its association with mdm2 and p53 protein status. *Br J Cancer* **71**, 981-985.

McCann S, Sullivan J, Guerra J, Arcinas M, Boxer LM (1995). Repression of the c-myb gene by wt1 protein in T-cell and B-cell lines. *J Biol Chem* **270**, 23785-23789.

McCarty LP, Karr SM, Harris BZ, Michelson SG, Leith JT (1995). Comparison of basic fibroblast growth factor levels in clone A human colon cancer cells *in vitro* with levels in xenografted tumours. *Br J Cancer* **72**, 10-16.

McConkey DJ, Hartzell P, Nicotera P, Orrenius S (1989). Calcium-activated DNA fragmentation kills immature thymocytes. *FASEB J* **3**, 1843-1849.

McCormick D (1993). Secretion of cathepsin D by human gliomas *in vitro*. *Neuropath Appl Neurobiol* **19**, 146-151.

McCrea PD, Gumbiner BM (1991). Purification of a 92 kDa cytoplasmic protein tightly associated with the cell-cell adhesion molecule E-cadherin (uvomorulin). *J Biol Chem* **266**, 4514-4520.

Macdonald NJ, Delarosa A, Benedict MA, Freije JMP, Krutsch H. and Steeg PS (1993). A serine phosphorylation of nm23, and not its nucleoside diphosphate kinase activity, correlates with suppression of tumour metastatic potential. *J Biol Chem* **268**, 25780-25789.

McDonnell SE, Kerr LD, Matrisian LM (1990). Epidermal growth factor stimulation of mRNA in rat fibroblasts requires induction of proto-oncogene c-fos and c-jun and activation of protein kinase C. *Mol Cell Biol* **10**, 4284-4293.

McDonnell SE, Navre M, Coffey RJ, Matrisian LM (1991). Expression and localisation of the matrix metalloproteinase pump-1 (MMP-7) in human gastric and colon carcinomas. *Molec Carcinogen* **4**, 527-533.

McDonnell TJ, Troncoso P, Brisbay S, Logothetis C, Leland WK, Hsieh JC, Tu S, Campbell M (1992). Expression of the proto-oncogene *bcl-2* in the prostate and its association with the emergence of androgen independent prostate cancer. *Cancer Res* **52**, 6940-6944.

McGregor JM, Yu CCW, Dublin EA, Barnes DM, Levison DA, Macdonald DM (1993). p53 immunoreactivity in human malignant melanoma and dysplastic naevi. *Br J Dermatol* **128**, 606-611.

Machida CM, Rodland KD, Matrisian L, Magun BE, Ciment G (1989). NGF induction of the gene encoding the protease transin accompanies neuronal differentiation in PC12 cells. *Neuron* **2**, 1587-1596.

Machida CM, Scott JD, Ciment G (1991). NGF-induction of the metalloproteinase transin-Stromelysin in PC12 cells: Involvement of multiple protein kinases. *J Cell Biol* **114**, 1037-1048.

Macias A, Azavedo E, Hagerstrom T, Klintenberg C, Perez R, Skoog L (1991). Prognostic significance of the receptor for epidermal growth factor in human mammary carcinomas. *Anticancer Res* **3**, 217-222.

Mackay AR, Corbitt RH, Hartzier JL, Thorgeirsson U (1990). Basement membrane type IV collagen degradation: evidence for the involvement of a proteolytic cascade independent of metalloproteinases. *Cancer Res* **50**, 5997-6001.

Madden SL, Cook DM, Morris JF, Gashler A, Sukhatme VP, Rauscher FJ, III (1991). Transcriptional repression mediated by the wt1 Wilms tumour gene product. *Science* **253**, 1550-1553.

Maeda K, Chung YS, Takatsuka S, Ogawa Y, Onoda N, Sawada T, Kato Y, Nitta A, Arimoto Y, Kondo Y, Sowa M (1995). Tumour angiogenesis and tumour cell proliferation as prognostic indicators in gastric carcinoma. *Br J Cancer* **72**, 319-323.

Maehle L, Metcalf RA, Ryberg D, Bennett WP, Harris CC, Haugen A (1992). Altered p53 gene structure and expression in human epithelial cells after exposure to nickel. *Cancer Res* **52**, 218-221.

Maestro R, Gloghini A, Doglioni C, Gasparotto D (1995). Mdm2 over-expression does not account for stabilization of wild type p53 protein in non-Hodgkin's lymphoma. *Blood* **85**, 3239-3246.

Magee AI, Buxton RS (1991). Transmembrane molecular assemblies regulated by the greater cadherin family. *Curr Opin Cell Biol* **3**, 854-861.

Maglione D, Guerriero V, Viglietto G, Ferraro MG, Aprelikova O, Alitalo K, Delvecchio S, Lei KJ,

Chou JY, Persico MG (1993). Two alternative messenger RNAs coding for the angiogenic factor, placental growth factor (PIGF), are transcribed from a single gene of chromosome 14. *Oncogene* **8**, 925-931.

Maguchi S, Taniguchi N, Makita A (1988). Elevated activity and increased mannose-6-phosphate in the carbohydrate moiety of cathepsin D from human hepatoma. *Cancer Res* **48**, 362-367.

Maheswaran S, Park S, Bernard A, Morris JF, Rauscher FJ, Hill DE, Haber DA (1993). Physical and functional interaction between wt1 and p53 proteins. *Proc Natl Acad Sci USA* **90**, 5100-5104.

Maheswaran S, Englert C, Bennett P, Heinrich G, Haber DA (1995). The *wt1* gene product stabilises and inhibits p53-mediated apoptosis. *Genes Develop* **9**, 2143-2156.

Maier R, Ganu V, Lotz M (1993). Interleukin-11, an inducible cytokine in human articular chondrocytes and synoviocytes, stimulates the production of the tissue inhibitor of metalloproteinases. *J Biol Chem* **268**, 21527-21532.

Maiorana A, Gullino PM (1978). Acquisition of angiogenic capacity and neoplastic transformation in the rat mammary gland. *Cancer Res* **38**, 4409-4414.

Majuri ML, Niemela R, Tiisala S, Renkonen O, Renkonen R (1995). Expression and induction of alpha-2, 3-sialyl transferases and alpha-1,3/1,4-fucosyl transferases in colon adenocarcinoma. *Int J Cancer* **63**, 551-559.

Makar R, Mason A, Kittelson JM, Bowden GT, Cress AE, Nagle RB (1994). Immunohistochemical analysis of cathepsin D in prostate carcinoma. *Modern Pathol* **7**, 747-751.

Malkin D, Sexsmith E, Yeger H, Williams BRG, Coppes MJ (1994). Mutations of the p53 tumour suppressor gene occur infrequently in Wilms tumour. *Cancer Res* **54**, 2077-2079.

Mandai M, Konishi I, Koshiyama M, Mori T, Arao S, Tashiro H, Okamura H, Nomura H, Hiai H, Fukumoto M (1994). Expression of metastasis-related nm23-H1 and nm23-H2 genes in ovarian carcinomas. Correlation with clinicopathology, EGFR, c-erbB2, and c-erbB3 genes, and sex steroid receptor expression. *Cancer Res* **54**, 1825-1830.

Mandriota SJ, Menoud PA, Pepper MS (1996). Transforming growth factor β-1 down-regulates vascular endothelial growth factor receptor 2/flk-1 expression in vascular endothelial cells. *J Biol Chem* **271**, 11500-11505.

Maniatis T (1991). Mechanisms of alternative pre-mRNA splicing. *Science* **251**, 33-34.

Mann JS, Kindy MS, Edwards DR, Curry TE, Jr (1991). Hormonal regulation of matrix metalloproteinase inhibitors in rat granulosa cells and ovaries. *Endocrinol* **128**, 1825-1832.

Mannens M, Slater RM, Heytig C, Bliek J, De Kraker J, Coad N, de Pagter-Holthuizen P, Pearson PL (1988). Molecular nature of genetic changes resulting in loss of heterozygosity of chromosome 11 in Wilms tumours. *Human Genet* **81**, 41-48.

Mannens M, Devilee P, Bliek J, Mandjes I, De Kraker J, Heytig C, Slater RM, Westerveld A (1990). Loss of heterozygosity in Wilms tumours studied for six putative tumour suppressor regions is limited to chromosome 11. *Cancer Res* **50**, 3279-3283.

Mansour EG, Ravdin PM, Dressler L (1994). Prognostic factors in early breast carcinoma. *Cancer* **74**, 381-400.

Mantell LL, Greider CW (1994). Telomerase activity in germline and embryonic cells of *Xenopus. EMBO J* **13**, 3211-3217.

Mantenhorst E, Danen EHJ, Smith L, Snoek M, Lepoole IC, Vanmuijen GNP, Pals ST, Ruiter DJ (1995). Expression of CD44 splice variants in human cutaneous melanoma and melanoma cell lines is related to tumour progression and metastatic potential. *Int J Cancer* **64**, 182-188.

Marchetti A, Buttitta F, Pellegrini S, Merlo G, Chella A, Angeletti CA, Bevilacqua G (1995a). Mdm2 gene amplification and over-expression in non-small cell lung carcinomas with accumulation of the p53 protein in the absence of p53 mutation. *Diag Mol Pathol* **4**, 93-97.

Marchetti A, Buttitta F, Girlando S, Dallapalma P, Pellegrini S, Fina P, Doglioni C, Bevilacqua G, Barbareshi M (1995b). Mdm2 gene alteration and mdm2 protein expression in breast carcinomas. *J Pathol* **175**, 31-38.

Marchetti A, Buttitta F, Pellegrini S, Bertacca G, Lori A, Bevilacqua G (1995c). Absence of somatic mutations in the coding region of the *waf1/cip1* gene in human breast, lung and ovarian carcinomas. A polymorphism at codon-31. *Int J Oncol* **6**, 187-189.

Marchisio PC, Cirillo D, Teti A, Zambonin-Zallone A, Tarone A (1987). Rous sarcoma virus transformed fibroblasts and cell of monocytic origin display a peculiar dot-like organisation of cytoskeletal proteins involved in microfilament membrane interaction. *Exp Cell Res* **169**, 202-214.

Marcus JN, Watson P, Page DL, Narod SA, Lenoir GM, Tonin P, Linder-Stephenson L, Salerno G, Conway TA, Lynch HT (1996). Hereditary breast cancer. Pathobiology, prognosis, and BRCA1 and BRCA2 gene linkage. *Cancer* **77**, 697-709.

Mareel MM, Behrens J, Birchmeier W, De Bruyne GK, Vleminckx K, Hoogewijs A, Fiers WC, van Roy FM (1991). Down regulation of E-cadherin expression in Madin Darby canine kidney (MDCK) cell tumours of nude mice. *Int J Cancer* **47**, 922-928.

Margolis B, Silvennoinen O, Comoglio F, Roonprapunt C, Skolnik E, Ullrich A, Schlessinger J (1992). Higher efficiency expression/cloning of epidermal growth factor receptor binding proteins with src homology 2 domains. *Proc Natl Acad Sci USA* **89**, 8894-8898.

Marin MC, Hsu B, Stephens LC, Brisbay S, McDonnell TJ (1995). The functional basis of c-*myc* and *bcl-2* complementation during multistep lymphomagenesis *in vivo*. *Expt Cell Res* **217**, 240-247.

Markert CL (1968). Neoplasia: a disease of cell differentiation. *Cancer Res* **28**, 1908-1914.

Markowitz S, Wang J, Mycroff L, Parsons R, Sun L, Lutterbaugh J, Fan RS, Zborowska E, Kinzler KW, Vogelstein B, Brattain M, Willson JKV (1995). Inactivation of the type II TGF-β receptor in colon cancer with microsatellite instability. *Science* **268**, 1336-1338.

Marks A, Petsche D, O'Hanlon D, Kwong PC, Sted R, Dunn R, Baumal R, Liao SK (1990). S-100 protein expression in human melanoma cells: Comparison of levels of expression among different cell lines and individual cells in different phases of the cell cycle. *Exp Cell Res* **187**, 59-64.

Marques AL, Franco ELF, Torloni H, Brentani MM, Da Silva-Neto JB, Brentani RR (1990). Independent prognostic value of laminin receptor expression in breast cancer survival. *Cancer Res* **50**, 1479-1483.

Marquis ST, Rajan JV, Wynshaw-Boris A, Xu TJ, Yin GY, Abel KJ, Weber BL, Chodosh LA (1995). The developmental pattern of BRCA1 expression implied a role in differentiation of the breast and other tissues. *Nature Genet* **11**, 17-26.

Mars WM, Zarnegar R, Michalopoulos GK (1993). Activation of hepatocyte growth factor by the plasminogen activators uPA and tPA. *Amer J Pathol* **143**, 949-958.

Marston NJ, Crook T, Vousden KH (1994). Interaction of p53 with mdm2 is independent of E6 and does not mediate wild type transformation suppressor function. *Oncogene* **9**, 2707-2716.

Martin A, Hung MC (1994). The retinoblastoma gene product, Rb, represses *neu* expression through two regions within the *neu* regulatory sequence. *Oncogene* **9**, 1333-1339.

Martin DW, Munoz RM, Subler MA, Deb S (1993). P53 binding to the TATA binding protein-TATA complex. *J Biol Chem* **268**, 13062-13067.

Martin E, Cacheux V, Cave H, Lapierre JM, Lepaslier D, Grandchamp B (1995). Localisation of the CDKN4/p27 (kip1) gene to human chromosome 12p12.3. *Human Genet* **96**, 668-670.

Martin K, Akinwunmi J, Rooprai HK, Kennedy AJ, Linke A, Ognjenovic N, Pilkington GJ (1995).

Non-expression of CD15 by neoplastic glia. A barrier to metastasis. *Anticancer Res* **15**, 1159-1165.

Martin-Padura I, Mortarini R, Lauri D, Beanasconi S, Sanchez-Madrid F, Parmiani G, Mantovani A, Anichini A, Dejana E (1991). Heterogeneity in human melanoma cell adhesion to cytokine activated endothelial cells correlate with VLA-4 expression. *Cancer Res* **51**, 2239-2241.

Marx J (1994a). New tumour suppressor may rival p53. *Science* **264**, 344-345.

Marx J (1994b). A challenge to p16 gene as a major tumour suppressor. *Science* **264**, 1846.

Mashal R, Shtalrid M, Talpaz M, Kantarjian H, Smith L, Beran M, Cork A, Trujillo J, Gutterman J, Deisseroth A (1990). Rearrangement and expression of p53 in the chronic phase and blast crisis of chronic myelogenous leukaemia. *Blood* **75**, 180-189.

Mashiyama S, Murakami Y, Yoshimoto T, Sekiya T, Hayashi K (1991). Detection of p53 mutations in human brain tumours by single strand conformation polymorphism analysis of polymerase chain reaction products. *Oncogene* **6**, 1313-1318.

Masiakowski P, Shooter EM (1988). Nerve growth factor induces genes for two proteins related to a family of calcium-binding proteins in PC12 cells. *Proc Natl Acad Sci USA* **85**, 1277-1281.

Mason PJ, Hall LMC, Gausz CH (1984). The expression of heat shock genes during normal development in *Drosophila melanogaster. Mol Cell Genet* **194**, 73-78.

Massague J (1987). The TGF beta family of growth and differentiation factors. *Cell* **49**, 437-438.

Massague J (1990). The transforming growth factor beta family. *Annu Rev Cell Biol* **6**, 597-641.

Matlashweski G, Lamb P, Pim D, Peacock J, Crawford L, Benchimole S (1984). Isolation and characterisation of a human p53 cDNA clone: Expression of the human p53 gene. *EMBO J* **3**, 3257-3262.

Matrisian LM, Bowden GT (1990). Stromelysin/transin and tumour progression. *Sem Cancer Biol* **1**, 107-115.

Matrisian LM, Glaichenhaus N, Gesnel MC, Breathnach R (1985). Epidermal growth factor and oncogenes induce transcription of the same cellular mRNA in rat fibroblasts. *EMBO J* **4**, 1435-1440.

Matrisian LM, Bowden GT, Krieg P, Furstenberger G, Briand JP, Leroy P, Breathnach R (1986a). The mRNA coding for the secreted protein transin is expressed more abundantly in malignant than in benign tumours. *Proc Natl Acad Sci USA* **83**, 9413-9417.

Matrisian LM, Leroy P, Ruhlmann C, Gesnel MC, Breathnach R (1986b). Isolation of the oncogene and epidermal growth factor-induced transin gene: complex control in rat fibroblasts. *Mol Cell Biol* **6**, 1679-1686.

Matsuda H, Strebel FR, Kaneko T, Stephens LC, Danhauser LL, Jenkins GN, Toyota N, Bull JMC (1996). Apoptosis and necrosis occurring during different stages of primary and metastatic tumour growth of a rat mammary adenocarcinoma. *Anticancer Res* **16**, 1117-1122.

Matsumoto H, Shimura M, Omatsu T, Okaichi K, Majima H, Ohnishi T (1994). P53 proteins accumulated by heat stress associate with heat shock proteins HSP72/HSC73 in human glioblastoma cell lines. *Cancer Lett* **87**, 39-46.

Matsuo K, Kobayashi I, Tsukuba T, Kiyoshima T, Ishibashi Y, Miyoshi A, Yamamoto K, Sakai H (1996). Immunohistochemical localisation of cathepsin D and cathepsin E in human gastric cancer. A possible correlation with local invasive and metastatic activities of carcinoma cells. *Human Pathol* **27**, 184-190.

Matsuoka S, Edwards MC, Bai C, Parker S, Zhang PM, Baldini A, Harper JW, Elledge SJ (1995). P57 (kip2), a structurally distinct member of the p21 (cip1) cdk inhibitor family, is a candidate tumour-suppressor gene. *Genes Develop* **9**, 650-662.

Mattern J, Koomagi R, Volm M (1996). Association of vascular endothelial growth factor expression with intratumoral microvessel density and tumour cell proliferation in human epidermoid lung carcinoma. *Br J Cancer* **73**, 931-934.

Matthews JB, Scully C, Jovanovic A, van der Waal, I, Yeudall WA, Prime SS (1993). Relationship of tobacco/alcohol use to p53 expression in patients with lingual squamous cell carcinoma. *Oral Oncol Eur J Cancer* **29B**, 285-289.

Matthews W, Jordan CT, Gavin M, Jenkins NA, Copeland NG, Lemischka IR (1991). A receptor tyrosine kinase cDNA isolated from a population of enriched primitive hematopoietic cells and exhibiting close genetic linkage to c-kit. *Proc Natl Acad Sci USA* **88**, 9026-9030.

Mattsbybaltzer I, Jakobsson A, Sorbo J, Norrby K (1994). Endotoxin is angiogenic. *Int J Expt Pathol* **75**, 191-196.

Maw MA, Grundy PE, Millow LJ, Eccles MR, Dunn RS, Smith PJ, Feinberg AP, Law DJ, Paterson MC, Telzerow PE, Callen DF, Thompson AD, Richards RI, Reeve AE (1992). A third Wilms tumour locus on chromosome 16q. *Cancer Res* **52**, 3094-3098.

Maxwell SA (1994). Selective compartmentalization of different mdm2 proteins within the nucleus. *Anticancer Res* **14**, 2541-2547.

Maxwell SA, Ames SK, Sawai ET, Decker GL, Cook RG, Butel JS (1991). Simian virus 40 large T antigen and p53 are microtubule-associated proteins in transformed cells. *Cell Growth Diff* **2**, 115-127.

Mayer B, Lorenz C, Babic R, Jauch KW, Schildberg FW, Funke I, Johnson JP (1995). Expression of leukocyte cell adhesion molecule on gastric carcinomas. Possible involvement of LFA-3 expression in the development of distant metastases. *Int J Cancer* **64**, 415-423.

Mayerhofer A, Lahr G, Frohlich U, Zienecker R, Sterzik K, Gratzl M (1994). Expression and alternative splicing of the neural cell adhesion molecule NCAM in human granulosa cells during luteinisation. *FEBS Lett* **346**, 207-212.

Mazars P, Barboule N, Baldin V, Vidal S, Ducommun B, Valette A (1995). Effects of TGF beta 1 (transforming growth factor beta 1) on the cell cycle regulation of human breast adenocarcinoma (MCF-7) cells. *FEBS Lett* **362**, 295-300.

Mazars R, Pujol P, Maudelonde T, Jeanteur P, Theillet C (1991). *p53* mutations in ovarian cancer: a late event? *Oncogene* **6**, 1685-1690.

Means AL, Slansky JE, McMahon SL, Knuth MW, Farnham PJ (1992). The HIP1 binding site is required for growth regulation of the dihydrofolate reductase gene promoter. *Mol Cell Biol* **12**, 1054-1063.

Medeiros AC, Nagai MA, Neto MM, Brentani RR (1994). Loss of heterozygosity affecting the APC and MCC genetic loci in patients with primary breast cancer. *Cancer Epidemiol Biomarkers Prevention* **3**, 331-333.

Meijerink JPP, Smetsers TFCM, Sloetjes AW, Linders EHP (1995). Bax mutations in cell lines derived from haematological malignancies. *Leukaemia* **9**, 1828-1832.

Meijers MHM, Aisa CM, Billingham MEJ, Russell RGG, Bunning RAD (1994). The effect of interleukin-1-beta and transforming growth factor beta on cathepsin B activity in human articular chondrocytes. *Agents Actions* **41**, C198-C200.

Meltzer SJ, Yin J, Manin B, Rhyu MG, Cottrell J, Hudson E, Redd JL, Krasna MJ, Abraham JM, Reid BJ (1994). Microsatellite instability occurs frequently and in both diploid and aneuploid populations of Barrett's-associated oesophageal adenocarcinomas. *Cancer Res* **54**, 3379-3382.

Menssen HD, Renkl HJ, Rodeck U, Maurer J, Notter M, Schwartz S, Reinhardt R, Thiel E (1995). Presence of Wilms tumour gene (*wt*1) transcripts and the wt1 nuclear protein in the majority of human acute leukaemias. *Leukaemia* **9**, 1060-1067.

Merajver SD, Pham TM, Carduff RF, Chen M, Poy EL, Cooney KA, Weber BL, Collins FS, Johnston

C, Frank TS (1995). Somatic mutations in the BRCA1 gene in sporadic ovarian tumours. *Nature Genet* **9**, 439-443.

Merlo A, Mabry M, Gabrielson E, Vollmer R, Baylin SB, Sidransky D (1994). Frequent microsatellite instability in primary small cell lung cancer. *Cancer Res* **54**, 2098-2101.

Merzak A, Raynal S, Rogers JP, Lawrence D, Pilkington GJ (1994a). Human wild type p53 inhibits cell proliferation and elicits dramatic morphological changes in human glioma cell lines *in vitro. J Neurol Sci* **127**, 125-133.

Merzak A, Parker C, Koocheckpour S, Sherbet GV, Pilkington GJ (1994b). Overexpression of *18A2/mts1* gene and down-regulation of TIMP2 gene in invasive glioma cells *in vitro. Neuropath App Neurobiol* **6**, 614-619.

Merzak A, Koocheckpour S, Pilkington GJ (1994c). CD44 mediates human glioma cell adhesion and invasion *in vitro. Cancer Res* **54**, 3988-3992.

Metaye T, Millet C, Kraimps JL, Aubouin B, Barbier J, Begon F (1993). Estrogen receptors and cathepsin D in human thyroid tissue. *Cancer* **72**, 1991-1996.

Meyer MB, Bastholm L, Nielsen MH, Elling F, Rygaard J, Chen WC, Obrink B, Bock E, Edvardsen K (1995). Localisation of NCAM on NCAM-B expressing cells with inhibited migration on collagen. *APMIS* **103**, 197-208.

Meyne J, Ratliff RL, Moyzis RK (1989). Conservation of the human telomere sequence (TTA GGA)n among vertebrates. *Proc Natl Acad Sci USA* **86**, 7049-7053.

Michalides R, Volberg T, Geiger B (1994). Augmentation of adherence junction formation in mesenchymal cells by co-expression of NCAM or short term stimulation of tyrosine phosphorylation. *Cell Adh Commun* **2**, 481-490.

Michalowitz D, Halevy O, Oren M (1990). Conditional inhibition of transformation and cell proliferation by a temperature sensitive mutant of p53. *Cell* **62**, 671-680.

Michieli P, Chedid M, Lin D, Pierce JH, Mercer WE, Givol D (1994). Induction of *waf1/cip1* by a p53-independent pathway. *Cancer Res* **54**, 3391-3395.

Mietz JA, Unger T, Huibregtse JM, Howley PM (1992). The transcriptional transactivation function of wild type p53 is inhibited by SV40 large T-antigen and by HPV-16 E6 oncoprotein. *EMBO J* **11**, 5013-5020.

Miki Y, Swensen J, Shaatuck-Eidens D, Futreal PA, Harshman K, Tavtigian S, Liu QY, Cochran C, Bennett LM, Ding W, Bell R, Rosenthal J, Hussey C, Tran T, McClure M, Frye C, Hattier T, Phelps R, Haugenstrano A, Katcher H, Yakumo K, Gholami Z, Shaffer D, Stone S, Bayer S, Wray C, Bogden R, Dayananth P, Ward J, Tonin P, Narod S, Bristow PK, Norris FH, Helvering L, Morrison P, Rosteck P, Lai M, Barrett JC, Lewis C, Neuhausen S, Cannon-Abright L, Goldgar D, Wiseman R, Kamb A, Skolnick MH (1994). A strong candidate for the breast and ovarian cancer susceptibility gene BRCA1. *Science* **266**, 66-71.

Mikkelsen T, Yan PS, Ho KL, Sameni M, Sloane BF, Rosenblum ML (1995). Immunolocalisation of cathepsin B in human glioma. *J Neurosurg* **83**, 285-290.

Mikulski SM (1994). Pathogenesis of cancer in view of mutually opposing apoptotic and anti-apoptotic growth signals. *Int J Oncol* **4**, 1257-1263.

Milarski K, Morimoto RI (1986). Expression of human HSP70 during the synthetic phase of the cell cycle. *Proc Natl Acad Sci USA* **83**, 9517-9521.

Milbrandt J (1987). A nerve growth factor-induced gene encodes a possible transcriptional regulatory factor. *Science* **238**, 797-799.

Mileo AM, Fanuele M, Battaglia F, Scambia G, Benedetti-Panici C, Mattei E, Mancuso S, Delphino A (1992). Preliminary evaluation of HER-2/neu oncogene and epidermal growth factor receptor expression in normal and neoplastic human ovaries. *Int J Biol Markers* **7**, 47-51.

Miliaras D, Kamas A, Kalekou H (1995). Angiogenesis in invasive breast carcinoma. Is it associated with parameters of prognostic significance? *Histopathol* **26**, 165-169.

Millauer B, Longhi MP, Plate KH, Shawver LK, Risau W, Ullrich A, Strawn LM (1996). Dominant negative inhibition of Flk-1 suppresses the growth of many tumour types *in vivo*. *Cancer Res* **56**, 1615-1620.

Miller CW, Aslo A, Campbell M, Koeffler HP (1994). Alterations of p16 common in sarcoma cell lines but rare in tumours. *Blood* **84** (Suppl. 1), 298a.

Miller FR (1983). Tumour subpopulation interactions in metastasis. *Invasion Metastasis* **3**, 234-242.

Miller RW, Fraumeni JF, Jr, Manning MD (1964). Association of Wilms tumour with aniridia hemihypertrophy, and other congenital malformations. *New Eng J Med* **270**, 922-927.

Milner J, Medcalf EA (1991). Co-translation of activated mutant p53 with wild type drives the wild type p53 protein into the mutant conformation. *Cell* **65**, 765-774.

Milner J, Medcalf EA, Cook A (1991). Tumour suppressor p53: analysis of wild type and mutant p53 complexes. *Mol Cell Biol* **11**, 12-19.

Minami H, Tokumitsu H, Mizutani A, Watanabe Y, Watanabe M, Hidaka H (1992). Specific binding of CAP-50 to calcyclin. *FEBS Lett* **305**, 217-219.

Minn AJ, Rudin CM, Boise LH, Thompson CB (1995). Expression of bcl-x(L) can confer multidrug resistance phenotype. *Blood* **86**, 1903-1910.

Minn AJ, Boise LH, Thompson CB (1996). Bcl-x(S) antagonises the protective effects of bcl-x(L). *J Biol Chem* **271**, 6306-6312.

Minna JD, Carney DN, Alvarez R, Bunn PAJ, Cuttita F, Ihde DC, Matthews MJ, Oie H, Rosen S, Whang-Peng J, Gazdar AF (1982). Heterogeneity and homogeneity of human small cell lung cancer. In: *Tumour Cell Heterogeneity, Origins, Implications*, Owens AH, Jr, Coffey DS, Baylin SB (eds). Academic Press, New York, London, pp. 29-52.

Mitra AB, Murty VVVS, Pratap M, Phelps WC, Harlow E, Howley PM (1994). *ERBB2 (HER2/neu)* oncogene is frequently amplified in squamous cell carcinoma of the uterine cervix. *Cancer Res* **54**, 637-639.

Mitsudomi T, Oyama T, Kusano T, Osaki T, Nakanishi R, Shirakusa T (1993). Mutations of the p53 gene as a predictor of poor prognosis in patients with non-small cell lung cancer. *J Natl Cancer Inst* **85**, 2018-2023.

Mittnacht S, Lees JA, Desai D, Harlow E, Morgan DO, Weinberg RA (1994). Distinct sub-populations of the retinoblastoma protein show a distinct pattern of phosphorylation. *EMBO J* **13**, 118-127.

Miwa K, Miyamoto S, Kato H, Imamura T, Nishida M, Yoshikawa Y, Nagata Y, Wake N (1995). The role of p53 inactivation in human cervical cell carcinoma development. *Br J Cancer* **71**, 219-226.

Miyagawa K, Kent J, Schedl A, Van Heyningen V, Hastie ND (1994). Wilms tumour. A case of disrupted development. *J Cell Sci* **S18**, 1-5.

Miyajima Y, Ota S, Yasukawa H, Zenmyou M, Morimatsu M, Kashiwagi S, Hirano M (1996). Neural cell adhesion molecule expression in thyroid cancer. A clinico-pathological study. *Oncol Rep* **3**, 63-67.

Miyake K, Underhill CB, Lesley J, Kincade PW (1990). Hyaluronate can function as a cell adhesion molecule and CD44 participates in hyaluronate recognition. *J Exp Med* **172**, 69-75.

Miyake S, Nagai K, Yoshino K, Oto M, Endo M, Yuasa Y (1994). Point mutations and allelic deletion of tumor suppressor gene DCC in human oesophageal squamous cell carcinomas and their relation to metastasis. *Cancer Res* **54**, 3007-3010.

Miyaki M, Tanaka K, Kikuchiyanoshita R, Muraoka M, Konishi M (1995). Familial polyposis. Recent advances. *Crit Rev Oncol Haematol* **19**, 1-31.

Miyashiro I, Senda T, Matsumine A, Baeg GH, Kuroda T, Shimano T, Miura S, Noda T, Kobayashi S, Monden M, Toyoshima K, Akiyama, T (1995). Subcellular localisation of the APC protein. Immunoelectron microscopic study of the association of the APC protein with catenin. *Oncogene* **11**, 89-96.

Miyashita T, Krajewski S, Krajewska M, Wang HG, Lin HK, Liebermann DA, Hoffman B, Reed JC (1994). Tumour suppressor p53 is a regulator of *bcl-2* and *bax* gene expression *in vitro* and *in vivo*. *Oncogene* **9**, 1799-1805.

Moberg KH, Tyndall WA, Hall DJ (1992). Wild type murine p53 represses transcription from the murine c-*myc* promoter in a human glial cell line. *J Cell Biochem* **49**, 208-215.

Moch H, Torhorst J, Durmuller U, Feichter GE, Sauter G, Gudat F (1993). Comparative analysis of the expression of tenascin and established prognostic factors in human breast cancer. *Pathol Res Pract* **189**, 510-514.

Moe RE, Moe KS, Porter P, Gown AM, Ellis G, Tapper D (1991). Expression of Her-2/neu oncogene protein product and epidermal growth factor receptors in surgical specimens of human breast cancers. *Amer J Surg* **161**, 580-583.

Moghaddam A, Zhang HT, Fan TPD, Hu DE, Lees VC, Turley H, Fox SB, Gatter KC, Harris AL, Bicknell R (1995). Thymidine phosphorylase is angiogenic and promotes tumour growth. *Proc Natl Acad Sci USA* **92**, 998-1002.

Mohanam S, Sawaya RE, Yamamoto M, Bruner JM, Nicolson GL, Rao JS (1994). Proteolysis and invasiveness of brain tumour. Role of urokinase type plasminogen activator receptor. *J Neuro-oncol* **22**, 153-160.

Moll UM, Riou G, Levine AJ (1992). Two distinct mechanisms alter p53 in breast cancer. Mutation and nuclear exclusion. *Proc Natl Acad Sci USA* **89**, 7262-7266.

Moller LB (1993). Structure and function of the urokinase receptor. *Blood Coag Fibrinolysis* **4**, 293-303.

Molloy CJ, Bottaro DP, Fleming TP, Marshall MS, Gibbs JB, Aaronson SA (1989). PDGF induction of tyrosine phosphorylation of GTPase activating protein. *Nature* **342**, 711-714.

Momand J, Zambetti GP, Olson DC, George D, Levine AJ (1992). The mdm2 oncogene product forms a complex with the p53 protein and inhibits p53-mediated transactivation. *Cell* **69**, 1237-1245.

Momosaki S, Yano H, Ogasawara S, Higaki K, Hisaka T, Kojiro M (1995). Expression of intercellular adhesion molecule-1 in human hepatocellular carcinoma. *Hepatology* **22**, 1708-1713.

Monaghan P, Robertson D, Amos TAS, Dyer MJS, Mason DY, Greaves MF (1992). Ultrastructural localisation of bcl-2 protein. *J Histochem Cytochem* **40**, 1819-1825.

Montazeri A, Kanitakis J, Zambruno G, Bourchany D, Schmitt D, Claudy A (1995). Expression of ICAM-3/CD50 in normal and diseased skin. *Br J Dermatol* **133**, 377-384.

Montcourrier P, Valembois C, Rochefort H (1993). Large acidic vesicles are correlated in *in vitro* invasive potential of breast cancer cells. *CR Acad Sci* **316**, 421-424.

Montcourrier P, Mangeat PH, Valenbois C, Salazar G, Sahuquet A, Duperray C, Rochefort H (1994). Characterisation of very acidic phagosomes in breast cancer cells and their association with invasion. *J Cell Sci* **107**, 2381-2391.

Montpetit M, Lawless KR, Tenniswood M (1986). Androgen-repressed messages in the rat ventral prostate. *Prostate* **8**, 25-36.

Moore BW (1965). A soluble protein characteristic of the nervous system. *Biochem Biophys Res Commun* **19**, 739-744.

Mooy CM, Luyten GPM, DeJong PTVM, Jensen OA, Luider TM, Vanderham F, Bosman FT (1995). Neural cell adhesion molecule distribution in primary and metastatic uveal melanoma. *Human Pathol* **26**, 1185-1190.

Moran M, Koch CA, Anderson D, Ellis C, England L, Martin GS, Pawson T (1990). Src homology region 2 domains direct protein–protein interactions in signal transduction. *Proc Natl Acad Sci USA* **87**, 8622-8626.

Morgenbesser SD, Williams BO, Jacks T, DePinho RA (1994). *p53*-dependent apoptosis produced by *rb*-deficiency in the developing mouse lens. *Nature* **371**, 72-74.

Mori N, Yokota J, Akiyama T, Sameshima Y, Okamoto A, Mizoguchi H, Toyoshima K, Sugimura T, Terada M (1990). Variable mutation of the *RB* gene in small cell lung carcinoma. *Oncogene* **5**, 1713-1717.

Mori T, Miura K, Aoki T, Nishihira T, Mori S, Nakamura Y (1994). Frequent somatic mutations of the MTS1/CDK4I (multiple tumour suppressor cyclin-dependent kinase-4 inhibitor) gene in oesophageal squamous cell carcinoma. *Cancer Res* **54**, 3396-3397.

Morii K, Tanaka R, Takahashi Y, Minoshima S, Fukuyama R, Shimizu N, Kuwano R (1991). Structure and chromosome assignment of human S100 alpha and beta subunit genes. *Biochem Biophys Res Commun* **175**, 185-191.

Morimoto R, Fodor E (1984). Cell specific expression of heat shock proteins in chicken reticulocytes and lymphocytes. *J Cell Biol* **99**, 1316-1323.

Morisset M, Capony F, Rochefort H (1986). The 52-kDa estrogen-induced protein secreted by MCF7 cells is a lysosomal acidic protease. *Biochem Biophys Res Commun* **138**, 102-109.

Morosetti R, Kawamata N, Gombart AF, Miller CW, Hatta Y, Hirama T, Said JW, Tomonaga M, Koeffler HP (1995). Alterations of the p27 (kip1) gene in non-Hodgkin's lymphoma and adult T-cell leukaemia/lymphoma. *Blood* **86**, 1924-1930.

Morris VL, Koop S, MacDonald IC, Schmidt EE, Grattan M, Percy D, Chambers AF, Groom AC (1994). Mammary carcinoma cell lines of high and low metastatic potential differ not in extravasation but in subsequent migration and growth. *Clin Exp Metastasis* **12**, 357-367.

Mort JS, Recklies AD (1986). Interrelationship of active and latent secreted human cathepsin B precursors. *Biochem J* **233**, 57-63.

Moscatelli D (1992). Basic fibroblast growth factor (bFGF) dissociates rapidly from heparan sulphates but slowly from receptors. Implications for mechanisms of bFGF release from pericellular matrix. *J Biol Chem* **267**, 25803-25809.

Moscatelli D, Flaumenhaft R, Saksela O (1991). Interaction of basic fibroblast growth factor with extracellular matrix and receptors. *Ann NY Acad Sci* **638**, 177-181.

Moscatelli D, Presta M, Rifkin DB (1986). Purification of a factor from human placenta that stimulates capillary endothelial cell protease production, DNA synthesis, and migration. *Proc Natl Acad Sci USA* **83**, 2091-2095

Mosner J, Deppert W (1994). P53 and mdm2 are expressed independently during cellular proliferation. *Oncogene* **9**, 3321-3328.

Motokura T, Bloom T, Kim HG, Juppner H, Ruderman JV, Kronenberg HM, Arnold A (1991). A novel cyclin encoded by a *bcl1*-linked candidate oncogene. *Nature* **350**, 512-515.

Moyzis RK, Buckingham J, Cram LS, Dani M, Deaven LL, Jones MD, Meyne J, Ratliff RL, Wu JR (1988). A highly conserved repetitive DNA sequence, (TTA GGG)n, present at the telomere of human chromosomes. *Proc Natl Acad Sci USA* **85**, 6622-6626.

Mueller BM, Yu YB, Llaug WE (1995). Over-expression of plasminogen activator inhibitor-2 in human melanoma cells inhibits spontaneous metastasis in SCID/SCID mice. *Proc Natl Acad Sci USA* **92**, 205-209.

Mukhopadhyay D, Tsiokas L, Zhou XM, Foster D, Brugge JS, Sukhatme VP (1995). Hypoxic induction of human vascular endothelial growth factor expression through c-src activation. *Nature* **375**, 577-581.

Mulder JWR, Kruyt PM, Sewnath M, Oosting J, Seldenrijk CA, Weidema WF, Offerhaus GJA, Pals ST (1994). Colorectal cancer prognosis and expression of exon-V6-containing CD44 proteins. *Lancet* **344**, 1470-1472.

Mulder JWR, Wielenga JVM, Polak MM, Vandenberg FM, Adolf GR, Herrlich P, Pals ST, Offerhaus GJA (1995). Expression of mutant p53 protein and CD44 variant proteins in colorectal tumorigenesis. *Gut* **36**, 76-80.

Muller D, Wolf C, Abecassis J, Millon R, Engelmann A, Bronner G, Rouyer N, Rio MC, Eber M, Methlin G, Chambon P, Basset P (1993). Increased stromelysin 3 gene expression is associated with increased local invasiveness in head and neck squamous cell carcinomas. *Cancer Res* **53**, 165-169.

Muller D, Millon R, Eber M, Methlin G, Abecassis J (1995). Alteration of the c-met oncogene locus in human head and neck carcinoma. *Oncol Rep* **2**, 847-850.

Munck-Wikland E, Edstrom S, Jungmark E, Kuylenstierna R, Lindholm J, Auer G (1994). Nuclear DNA content, proliferating cell nuclear antigen (PCNA) and p53 immunostaining in predicting progression of laryngeal cancer *in situ* lesions. *Int J Cancer* **56**, 95-99.

Munemitsu S, Souza B, Muller O, Albert I, Rubinfeld B, Polakis P (1994). The APC gene product associates with microtubules *in vivo* and promotes their assembly *in vitro*. *Cancer Res* **54**, 3676-3681.

Munemitsu S, Albert I, Souza B, Rubinfeld B, Polakis P (1995). Regulation of intracellular beta catelin levels by the adenomatous polyposis coli (APC) tumour suppressor protein. *Proc Natl Acad Sci USA* **92**, 3046-3050.

Munger K, Werness BA, Dyson N, Phelsps WC, Harlow E, Howley PM (1989). Complex formation of human papillomavirus E7 proteins with the retinoblastoma suppressor gene product. *EMBO J* **8**, 4099-4105.

Munro S, Pelham HRB (1984). Use of peptide tagging to detect proteins expressed from cloned genes: deletion mapping and functional domains of *Drosophila* hsp70. *EMBO J* **3**, 3087-3093.

Murnane JP, Young BR (1989). Nucleotide sequence analysis of novel junctions near an unstable integrated plasmid in human cells. *Gene* **84**, 201-205.

Murphy G, Reynolds JJ, Werb Z (1985). Biosynthesis of tissue inhibitor of metalloproteinases by human fibroblasts in culture. Stimulation by 12-O-tetradecanoylphorbol 13-acetate and interleukin-1 in parallel with collagenase. *J Biol Chem* **260**, 3079-3083.

Murphy G, Reynolds JJ, Hembry RM (1989). Metalloproteinases and cancer invasion and metastasis. *Int J Cancer* **44**, 757-760.

Murphy G, Willenbrock F, Ward RV, Cockett MI, Eaton D, Docherty AJ (1992). The C-terminal domain of 72 kDa gelatinase A is not required for catalysis, but is essential for membrane activation and modulates interaction with tissue inhibitors of metalloproteinases. *Biochem J* **283**, 637-641.

Murphy LC, Murphy LJ, Tsuyuki D, Duckworth ML, Shiu RP (1988). Cloning and characterisation of a cDNA encoding a highly conserved, putative calcium-binding protein, identified by an anti-prolactin receptor serum. *J Biol Chem* **263**, 2397-2401.

Murphy LJ (1994). Growth factors and steroid hormone action in endometrial cancer. *J Steroid Biochem Molec Biol* **48**, 419-423,

Murray AW (1992). Creative blocks: cell cycle checkpoints and feedback control. *Nature* **359**, 599-604.

Murty VVVS, Li RG, Houldsworth J, Bronson DL, Reuter VE, Bosl GJ, Chaganti RSK (1994).

Frequent allelic deletions and loss of expression characterise the DCC gene in male germ cell tumours. *Oncogene* **9**, 3227-3231.

Musgrove EA, Lee CSL, Buckley MF, Sutherland RL (1994). Cyclin D1 induction in breast cancer cells shorten G(1) and is sufficient for cells arrested in G(1) to complete the cell cycle. *Proc Natl Acad Sci USA* **91**, 8022-8026.

Muta H, Iguchi H, Kono A, Sep Y, Tomoda H, Nawata H (1994). NM23 expression in human gastric cancers. Possible correlation of NM23 with lymph node metastasis. *Int J Oncol* **5**, 93-96.

Muta H, Noguchi M, Perucho M, Ushio K, Sugihara K, Ochiai A, Nawata H, Hirohashi S (1996). Clinical implications of microsatellite instability in colorectal cancers. *Cancer* **77**, 265-270.

Myeroff LL, Markowitz SD (1993). Increased nm23-H1 and nm23-H2 messenger RNA expression and absence of mutations in colon carcinomas of low and high metastatic potential. *J Natl Cancer Inst* **85**, 147-152.

Myeroff LL, Parsons R, Kim SJ, Hedrick L, Cho KR, Orth K, Mathis M, Kinzler KW, Lutterbaugh J, Park K, Bang YJ, Lee HY, Park JB, Lynch HT, Roberts AB, Vogelstein B, Markowitz SD (1995). A transforming growth factor β receptor type II gene mutation common in colon and gastric but rare in endometrial cancers with microsatellite instability. *Cancer Res* **55**, 5545-5547.

Myers CE, La Rocca RV, Cooper MR, Danesi R, Jamis-Dow CA, Stein CA, Linehan WM (1991). Role of suramin in cancer biology and treatment. In: *Molecular Foundations of Oncology*, Broder S (ed.). Williams & Wilkins, Baltimore, pp. 419-431.

Nagafuchi A, Takeichi M, Tsukita S (1991). The 102 kDa cadherin-associated protein: Similarity to vinculin and posttranscriptional regulation of expression. *Cell* **65**, 849-857.

Nagasaka S, Tanabe KK, Bruner JM, Saya H, Sawaya RE, Morrison RS (1995). Alternative RNA splicing of the hyaluronic acid receptor CD44 in the normal human brain and in brain tumours. *J Neurosurg* **82**, 858-863.

Nagase H, Enghild JJ, Suzuki K, Salvesen G (1990). Stepwise activation mechanisms of the precursor of matrix metalloproteinase 3 (stromelysin) by proteinases and (4-aminophenyl) mercuric acetate. *Biochemistry* **29**, 5783-5789.

Nagayama K, Watatani M (1993). Analysis of genetic alterations related to the development and progression of breast carcinoma. *Jap J Cancer Res* **84**, 1159-1164.

Nagy J, Clark JS, Cooke A, Campbell AM, Connor JM, Purushotham AD, George WD (1995). Expression and loss of heterozygosity of c-*met* proto-oncogene in primary breast cancer. *J Surg Oncol* **60**, 95-99.

Nagy J, Curry GW, Hillan KJ, Mallon E, Purushotham AD, George WD (1996). Hepatocyte growth factor scatter factor, angiogenesis and tumour cell proliferation in primary breast cancer. *Breast* **5**, 105-109.

Nakagawa H, Heinrich G, Pelletier J, Housman DE (1995). Sequence and structural requirements for high affinity DNA binding by the *wt* gene product. *Mol Cell Biol* **15**, 1489-1498.

Nakai M, Takeda A, Cleary ML, Endo T (1993). The bcl-2 protein is inserted into the outer membrane but not into the inner membrane of rat liver mitochondria *in vitro*. *Biochem Biophys Res Commun* **196**, 233-239.

Nakajima M, Welch DR, Belloni PN, Nicolson GL (1987). Degradation of basement membrane type IV collagen and lung subendothelial matrix by rat mammary adenocarcinoma cell clones of differing metastatic potentials. *Cancer Res* **47**, 4869-4876.

Nakamori S, Ishikawa O, Ohigashi H, Kameyama M, Furukawa H, Sasaki Y, Inaji H, Higashiyama M, Imaoka S, Iwanaga T, Funai H, Wada A, Kimura N (1993). Expression of nucleoside diphosphate kinase/*nm23* gene product in human pancreatic cancer: an association with lymph node metastasis and tumour invasion. *Clin Exp Metastasis* **11**, 151-158.

Nakanishi M, Robetorye RE, Pereira-Smith OM, Smith JR (1995a). The C-terminal region of p21 (Sdi1/waf1/cip1) is involved in proliferating cell nuclear antigen binding but does not appear to be required for growth inhibition. *J Biol Chem* **270**, 17060-17063.

Nakanishi M, Robetorye RE, Adami GR, Pereira-Smith OM, Smith JR (1995b). Identification of the active region of the DNA synthesis inhibitory gene p21 (Sdi1/cip1/waf1). *EMBO J* **14**, 555-563.

Nakashima H, Inoue H, Mori M, Ueo H, Ikeda M, Akiyoshi T (1995). Microsatellite instability in Japanese gastric cancer. *Cancer* **75**, 1503-1507.

Nakata B, Appert HE, Lei SZ, Yamashita Y, Chung YS, Sowa M, Myles JL, Mao CA, Howard JM (1994). Immunohistochemical study of cathepsin B and cathepsin D in pancreatic cancer. *Oncol Res* **1**, 543-546.

Nakayama H, Yasui W, Yokozaki H, Tahara E (1993). Reduced expression of nm23 is associated with metastasis of gastric carcinomas. *Jap J Cancer Res* **84**, 184-190.

Nakayama T, Ohtsuru A, Nakao K, Shima M, Nakata K, Watanabe K, Ishii N, Kimura N, Nagataki S (1992). Expression in hepatocellular carcinoma of nucleoside diphosphate kinase, a homologue of the nm23 gene product. *J Natl Cancer Inst* **84**, 1349-1354.

Nakayama T, Toguchida J, Wadayama BI, Kanoe H, Kotoura Y, Sasaki MS (1995). Mdm2 gene amplification in bone and soft tissue tumours. Association with tumour progression in differentiated adipose tissue tumours. *Int J Cancer* **64**, 342-346.

Narita T, Kawakami-Kimura N, Matsuura N, Hosono J, Kannagi R (1995). Corticosteroids and medroxyprogesterone acetate inhibit the induction of E-selectin on the vascular endothelium by MDA-MB-231 breast cancer cells. *Anticancer Res* **15**, 2523-2527.

Natali PG, Nicotra MR, Cavaliere R, Giannarelli D, Bigotti A (1991). Tumour progression in human malignant melanoma is associated with changes in $\alpha 6/\beta 1$ laminin receptor. *Int J Cancer* **49**, 168-172.

Nazeer T, Church K, Amato C, Ambros RA, Rosano TG, Malfetano JH, Ross JS (1994). Methods in pathology. Comparative quantitative immunohistochemical and immunoradiometric determinations of cathepsin D in endometrial adenocarcinoma. Predictors of tumour aggressiveness. *Modern Pathol* **7**, 469-474.

Neame SJ, Isacke CM (1992). Phosphorylation of CD44 *in vivo* requires both ser323 and ser325 but does not regulate membrane localisation or cytoskeletal interaction in epithelial cells. *EMBO J* **11**, 4733-4738.

Needham GK, Sherbet GV, Farndon JR, Harris AL (1987). Binding of urokinase to specific receptor sites on human breast cancer membranes. *Br J Cancer* **55**, 13-16.

Neri A, Baldini L, Trecca D, Cro L, Polli E, Maido AT (1993). p53 gene mutations in multiple myeloma are associated with advanced forms of malignancy. *Blood* **81**, 128-135.

Neubauer A, Brendel C, Vogel D, Schmidt CA, Heide I, Huhn D (1993). Detection of p53 mutations using non-radioactive SSCP analysis. p53 is not frequently mutated in myelodysplatic syndrome (MDS). *Amer Haematol* **67**, 223-226.

Newcomb EW, Madonia WJ, Pisharody S, Lang FF, Koslow M, Miller DC (1993). A correlative study of p53 protein alterations and p53 gene mutation in glioblastoma multiforme. *Brain Pathol* **3**, 229-225.

Nguyen M, Millar DG, Yong VW, Korsmeyer SJ, Shore GC (1993a). Targeting of Bcl-2 to the mitochondrial outer membrane by a COOH-terminal signal anchor sequence. *J Biol Chem* **268**, 25265-25268.

Nguyen M, Strubel NA, Bischoff U (1993b). A role for sialyl Lewis-X/A glycoconjugates in capillary morphogenesis. *Nature* **365**, 267-269.

Nichols KE, Re GG, Yan YX, Garvin AJ, Haber DA (1995). Wt1 induces expression of insulin-like growth factor 2 in Wilms tumour cells. *Cancer Res* **55**, 4540-4543.

Nicholson RC, Mader S, Nagpal S, Leid M, Rochette-Egly C, Chambon P (1990). Negative regulation of the rat stromelysin gene promoter by retinoic acid is mediated by an AP1 binding site. *EMBO J* **9**, 4443-4454.

Nicholson S, Sainsbury RJC, Halcrow P, Kelly P, Angus B, Wright B, Henry J, Farndon JR, Harris AL (1991). Epidermal growth factor (EGFr): results of a 6 year follow up study in operable breast cancer with emphasis on the node negative subgroup. *Br J Cancer* **63**, 146-150.

Nickells RW, Browder LW (1985). Region-specific heat shock protein synthesis correlates with a biphasic acquisition of thermotolerance in *Xenopus laevis* embryos. *Develop Biol* **112**, 391-395.

Nickerson J, Wells W (1988). The microtubule associated nucleoside diphophasphate kinase. *J Biol Chem* **259**, 11297-11304.

Nicolaides NC, Papadopoulos N, Liu B, Wel YF, Carter KC, Ruben SM, Rosen CA, Haseltine WA, Fleishmann RD, Fraser CM, Adams MA, Venter JC, Dunlop MG, Hamilton SR, Peterson GM, de la Chapelle A, Vogelstein B, Kinzler KW (1994). Mutations of two PMS homologues in hereditary non-polyposis colon cancer. *Nature* **371**, 75-80.

Nicolson GL (1987). Tumour cell instability, diversification and progression to the metastatic phenotype. *Cancer Res* **47**, 1473-1487.

Nicolson GL (1988). Cancer metastasis: Tumour cell and host organ properties important in metastasis to specific secondary sites. *Biochim Biophys Acta* **948**, 175-224.

Nicolson GL, Babiche RA, Frazier ML, Blick M, Tressler RJ, Reading CL, Irimura T, Rotter V (1986). Differential expression of metastasis-associated cell surface glycoproteins and mRNA in a murine large cell lymphoma. *J Cell Biochem* **31**, 305-312.

Nielsen AL, Nyholm HCJ (1995). Endometrial adenocarcinoma of endometrioid subtype with squamous differentiation. An immunohistochemical study of MIB 1 (Ki-67 paraffin), cathepsin D, and c-erbB2 protein (p185). *Int J Gynaec Pathol* **14**, 230-234.

Nigro JM, Baker SJ, Preisinger AC, Jessup JM, Hostetter R, Cleary K, Bigner SH, Davidson N, Baylin S, Devilee P, Glover T, Collins FS, Weston A, Modali R, Harris CC, Vogelstein B (1989). Mutations in the p53 gene occur in diverse human tumour types. *Nature* **342**, 705-708.

Nihei T, Sato N, Takahashi S, Ishikawa M, Sagae S, Kudo R, Kikuchi K, Inoue A (1993). Demonstration of selective protein complexes of p53 with 73-kDa heat shock cognate protein, but not with 72-kDa heat shock protein in human tumour cells. *Cancer Lett* **73**, 181-189.

Nilbert M, Rydholm A, Mitelman F, Meltzer PS, Mandahl N (1995). Characterisation of the 12q13-15 amplicon in soft tissue tumours. *Cancer Genet Cytogent* **83**, 32-36.

Nilsson P, Mehle C, Remes K, Roos G (1994). Telomerase activity *in vivo* in human malignant haematopoietic cells. *Oncogene* **41**, 908-912.

Nishida N, Fukuda Y, Komeda T, Kita R, Sando T, Furukawa M, Amenomori M, Shibagaki, I, Nakao K, Ikenaga M, Ishizaki K (1994). Amplification and over-expression of the cyclin D1 gene in aggressive human hepatocellular carcinoma. *Cancer Res* **54**, 3107-3110.

Nishisho I, Nakamura Y, Miyoshi Y, Miki Y, Ando H, Horii A, Koyama K (1991). Mutations of chromosome 5q21 genes in FAP and colorectal cancer patients. *Science* **253**, 665-669.

Nobori T, Miura K, Wu D, Lois A, Takabayashi K, Carson DA (1994). Deletion of the cyclin-dependent kinase-4 inhibitor gene in multiple human cancers. *Nature* **368**, 753-756.

Noda A, Ning Y, Venable SF, Pereira-Smith OM, Smith JR (1994). Cloning of senescent cell derived inhibitors of DNA synthesis using an expression screen. *Exp Cell Res* **211**, 90-98.

North G (1991). Cell cycle - Starting and stopping. *Nature* **351**, 604-605.

Nourse J, Firpo E, Glanagan WM, Coats S, Polyak K, Lee MH, Massague J, Crabtree GR, Roberts JM (1994). Interleukin-2 mediated elimination of the p27 (kip1) cyclin dependent kinase inhibitor prevented by rapamycin. *Nature* **372**, 570-573.

Nowell PC (1976). The clonal evolution of tumour cell populations. Acquired genetic lability permits stepwise selection of variant sublines and underlies tumour progression. *Science* **194**, 23-28.

Nowell PC, Hungerford DA (1960). A minute chromosome in human granulocytic leukaemia. *Science* **132**, 1497.

Nunez G, London L, Hockenbery D, Alexander M, McKearn JP, Korsmeyer SJ (1990). Deregulated *bcl-2* gene expression selectively prolongs survival of growth factor-deprived haemopoietic cell lines. *J Immunol* **144**, 3602-3610.

Nunez G, Hockenbery D, McDonnell TJ, Sorensen CM, Korsmeyer SJ (1991). Bcl-2 maintains B-cell memory. *Nature* **353**, 71-73.

Ogasawara S, Maesawa C, Tamura G, Satodate R (1994). Lack of mutations of the adenomatous polyposis coli gene in oesophageal and gastric carcinomas. *Virchows Arch Pathol* **424**, 607-611.

Ogawa Y, Chung YS, Nakata B, Takatsuka S, Maeda K, Sawada T, Kato Y, Yoshikawa K, Sakurai M, Sowa M (1995). Microvessel quantitation in invasive breast cancer by staining for factor VIII-related antigen. *Br J Cancer* **71**, 1297-1301.

Ogden GR, Kiddie RA, Lunny DP, Lane DP (1992). Assessment of p53 protein expression in normal, benign and malignant oral mucosa. *J Pathol* **166**, 389-394.

Ohta T, Terada T, Nagakawa T, Tajima H, Itoh H, Fonseca L, Miyazaki I (1994). Pancreatic trypsinogen and cathepsin B in human pancreatic carcinoma and associated metastatic lesions. *Br J Cancer* **69**, 152-156.

Okada T, Okuno H, Mitsui Y (1994). A novel *in vitro* assay system for transendothelial tumour cell invasion. Significance of E-selectin and alpha (3) integrin in the transendothelial invasion by HT1080 fibrosarcoma cells. *Clin Exp Metastasis* **12**, 305-314.

Okamoto A, Sameshima Y, Yokoyama S, Terashima Y, Sugimura T, Terada M, Yokota J (1991a). Frequent allelic losses and mutations of the *p53* gene in human ovarian cancer. *Cancer Res* **51**, 5171-5176.

Okamoto A, Sameshima Y, Yamada Y, Teshima Y, Terashima Y, Terada M, Yokota J (1991b). Allelic loss on chromosome 17p and *p53* mutations in human endometrial carcinoma of the uterus. *Cancer Res* **51**, 5632-5636.

Okamura K, Sato Y, Matsuda T, Hamanaka R, Ono M, Kohno K, Kuwano M (1991). Endogenous basic fibroblast growth factor-dependent induction of collagenase and interleukin-6 in tumour necrosis factor-treated human microvascular endothelial cells. *J Biol Chem* **266**, 19162-19165.

Okuda T, Valentine MB, Shurtleff SA, Hulshof MG, Komuro H, Raimondi SC, Pui CH, Beach D, Sherr CJ, Look AT, Downing JR (1994). Frequent deletion of *INK4a/MTS1* in paediatric acute lymphoblastic leukaemia. *Blood* **84** (Suppl. 1), 298a.

Oliner JD, Kinzler KW, Meltzer PS, George DL, Vogelstein B (1992). Amplification of a gene encoding a p53 associated protein in human sarcomas. *Nature* **358**, 80-83.

Olovnikov AM (1996). Telomeres, telomerase, and ageing. Origin of the theory. *Exp Gerontol* **31**, 443-448.

Olson DJ, Papkoff J (1994). Regulated expression of wnt family members during proliferation of C57MG mammary cells. *Cell Growth Diff* **5**, 197-206.

Oltvai ZN, Milliman CL, Korsmeyer SJ (1993). Bcl-2 heterodimerises *in vivo* with a conserved homologue, bax, that accelerates programmed cell death. *Cell* **74**, 609-619.

Onishi Y, Azuma Y, Sato Y, Mizuno Y, Tadakuma T, Kizaki H (1993). Topoisomerase inhibitors induce apoptosis in thymocytes. *Biochim Biophys Acta* **1175**, 147-154.

Oren M, Maltzman W, Levine AJ (1981). Post-translational regulation of the 54K cellular antigen in normal and transformed cells. *Mol Cell Biol* **8**, 101-110.

Orkins SH, Goldman DS, Sallan SE (1984). Development of homozygosity for chromosome 11p marker in Wilms tumour. *Nature* **309**, 172-174.

Osaki A, Toi M, Yamada H, Kawami H, Kuroi K, Toge T (1992). Prognostic significance of co-expression of c-erbB2 oncoprotein and epidermal growth factor receptor in breast cancer patients. *Amer J Surg* 323-326.

Oshima M, Sugiyama H, Kitagawa K, Taketo M (1993). APC gene messenger RNA. Novel isoforms that lack exon 7. *Cancer Res* **53**, 5589-5591.

Oshima M, Oshima H, Kobayashi M, Tsutsumi M, Taketo MM (1995). Evidence against dominant negative mechanisms of intestinal polyp formation by APC gene mutations. *Cancer Res* **55**, 2719-2722.

Osifchin NE, Jiang D, Ohtani-Fujita N, Fujita T, Carroza M, Kim SJ, Sakai T, Robbins PD (1994). Identification of a p53 binding site in the human retinoblastoma susceptibility gene promoter. *J Biol Chem* **269**, 6383-6389.

Ostrowski LE, Finch J, Krieg P, Matrisian L, Patskan G, O'Connell JF, Philips J, Slaga TJ, Breathnach R, Bowden GT (1988). Expression pattern of a gene for a secreted metallopro-teinase during late stages of tumour progression. *Molec Carcinogen* **1**, 13-19.

Otto A, Deppert W (1993). Upregulation of mdm-2 expression in Meth a tumour cells tolerating wild type p53. *Oncogene* **8**, 2591-2603.

Otto T, Birchmeier W, Schmidt U, Hinke A, Schipper J, Rubben H, Raz A (1994). Inverse relation of E-cadherin and autocrine motility factor receptor expression as a prognostic factor in patients with bladder cancer. *Cancer Res* **54**, 3120-3123.

Ovens GP, Hahn WE, Cohen JJ (1991). Identification of mRNAs associated with programmed cell death. *Mol Cell Biol* **11**, 4177-4188.

Overall CM, Wrana JL, Sodek J (1989a). Transforming growth factor-β regulation of collagenase, 72 kDa progelatinase, TIMP and PAI-1 expression in rat bone cell populations and human fibroblasts. *Connect Tiss Res* **20**, 289-294.

Overall CM, Wrana JL, Sodek J (1989b). Independent regulation of collagenase, 72 kDa progelatinase and metallo-endoproteinase inhibitor expression in human fibroblasts by transforming growth factor-β. *J Biol Chem* **264**, 1860-1969.

Owens OJ, Stewart C, Leake RE (1991). Growth factors in ovarian cancer. *Br J Cancer* **64**, 1177-1181.

Ozawa M, Baribault M, Kemler R (1989). The cytoplasmic domain of the cell adhesion molecule uvomorulin associates with three independent proteins structurally related in different species. *EMBO J* **8**, 1711-1717.

Ozkaynak E, Finley D, Solomon MJ, Varshavsky A (1987). The yeast ubiquitin genes: a family of natural gene fusions. *EMBO J* **6**, 1429-1439.

Paciucci R (1994). Role of 300-kDa complexes as intermediates in tubulin folding and dimerisation. Characterisation of a 25-kDa cytosolic protein involved in the GTP-dependent release of monomeric tubulin. *Biochem J* **301**, 105-110.

Padhy LC, Shih C, Cowing D, Finkelstein R, Weinberg RA (1982). Identification of a phosphoprotein specifically induced by the transforming DNA of rat neuroblastoma. *Cell* **28**, 865-871.

Painter RB, Young BR (1980). Radiosensitivity in ataxia telangiectasia. *Proc Natl Acad Sci USA* **77**, 7315-7317.

Pajusola K, Aprelikova O, Pelicci G, Weich H, Claesson-Welsh L, Alitalo K (1994). Signalling properties of flt4, a proteolytically processed receptor tyrosine kinase related to two VEGF receptors. *Oncogene* **9**, 3545-3555.

Palacios J, Benito N, Pizarro A, Limeres MA, Suarez A, Cano A, Gamallo C (1995a). Relationship between erbB2 and E-cadherin expression in human breast cancer. *Virchows Arch* **427**, 259-263.

Palacios J, Benito N, Pizarro A, Suarez A, Espada J, Cano A, Gamallo C (1995b). Anomalous expression of P-cadherin in breast carcinoma. Correlation with E-cadherin expression and pathological features. *Amer J Pathol* **146**, 605-612.

Palter KB, Watanabe M, Stinson L, Mahowald AP, Craig EA (1986). Expression and localisation of *Drosophila melanogaster* hsp70 cognate protein. *Mol Cell Biol* **6**, 1187-1203.

Pandey S, Wang E (1995). Cell en route to apoptosis are characterised by up-regulation of c-fos, c-myc, c-jun, cdc2 and rb phosphorylation, resembling events of early cell cycle traverse. *J Cell Biochem* **58**, 135-150.

Pantel K, Schlimok G, Braun S, Kutter D, Lindemann F, Schaller G, Funke I, Izbicki JR, Riethmuller G (1993). Differential expression of proliferation-associated molecules in individual micrometastatic carcinoma cells. *J Natl Cancer Inst* **85**, 1419-1424.

Papadopoulos N, Nicolaides NC, Wei Y, Ruben SM, Carter KC, Rosen CA, Haseltine WA, Fleischmann RD, Fraser CM, Adams MD, Venter C, Hamilton SR, Petersen GM, Watson P, Lynch HT, Peltomaki P, Mecklin J, de La Chapelle A, Kinzler KW, Vogelstein B (1994). Mutation of a *mutL* homologue in hereditary colon cancer. *Science* **263**, 1625-1629.

Papkoff J (1994). Identification and biochemical characterisation of secreted wnt-1 protein from P19 embryonal carcinoma cells induced to differentiate along the neuroectodermal lineage. *Oncogene* **9**, 313-317.

Pardee AB (1989). G1 events and regulation of cell proliferation. *Science* **246**, 603-608.

Park DJ, Wilczynski SP, Paquette RL, Miller CW, Koeffler PH (1994). *p53* mutations in HPV-negative cervical carcinoma. *Oncogene* **9**, 205-210.

Park S, Bernard A, Bove KE, Sens DA, Hazenmartin DJ, Garvin AJ, Haber DA (1993). Inactivation of wt1 in nephrogenic rests, genetic precursors to Wilms tumour. *Nature Genet* **5**, 363-367.

Parker C, Sherbet GV (1992a). Modulation of gene function by retinoic acid. *Pathobiology* **60**, 278-283.

Parker C, Sherbet GV (1992b). Modulators of intracellular Ca^{2+} and the calmodulin inhibitor W-7 alter the expression of metastasis associated genes *mts1* and *nm23* in metastatic variants of the B16 murine melanoma. *Melanoma Res* **2**, 337-343.

Parker C, Sherbet GV (1993). The Ca^{2+} channel blocker verapamil enhances melanogenesis without altering metastatic potential in the B16 murine melanoma. *Melanoma Res* **3**, 347-350.

Parker C, Whittaker, PA, Weeks RJ, Thody AJ, Sherbet GV (1991). Modulators of metastatic behaviour alter the expression of metastasis-associated genes *mts1* and *nm23* in metastatic variants of the B16 murine melanoma. *Clin Biotech* **3**, 217-222.

Parker C, Usmani BA, Draper S, Sherbet GV (1992). Metastasis associated gene *mts1* but not *nm23* expression correlates with epidermal growth factor receptor status in human breast cancer. *J Expt Clin Cancer Res* **11**, 58.

Parker C, Lakshmi MS, Piura B, Sherbet GV (1994a). Metastasis associated *mts1* gene expression correlates with increased p53 protein expression. *DNA Cell Biol* **13**, 343-351.

Parker C, Whittaker PA, Usmani BA, Lakshmi MS, Sherbet GV (1994b). Induction of *18A2/mts1* gene expression and its effects on metastasis and cell cycle control. *DNA Cell Biol* **13**, 1021-1028.

Parker SB, Eichele G, Zhang PM, Rawls A, Sands AT, Bradley A, Olson EN, Harper JW, Elledge SJ (1995). P53-independent expresion of *p21* (Cip1) in muscle and other terminally differentiating cells. *Science* **267**, 1024-1027.

Parkin NT, Kitajewski J, Varmus HE (1993). Activity of wnt-1 as a transmembrane protein. *Genes Develop* **7**, 2181-2193.

Parr BA, Shea MJ, Vassileva G, McMahon AP (1993). Mouse *wnt* genes exhibit discrete domains of expression in the early embryonic CNS and limb buds. *Development* **119**, 247-261.

Pasini F, Pelosi G, Mostacci R, Santo A, Masotti A, Spangnolli P, Recaldin E, Cetto GL (1995). Detection at diagnosis of tumour cells in bone marrow aspirates of patients with small cell lung cancer (SCLC) and clinical correlations. *Ann Oncol* **6**, 86-88.

Patel DD, Hale LP, Whichard LP, Radcliff G, Mackay CR, Haynes BF (1995). Expression of CD44 molecules and CD44 ligands during human thymic foetal development. Expression of CD44 isoforms is developmentally regulated. *Int Immunol* **7**, 277-286.

Patel U, Chen HC, Banerjee S (1994). Dinucleotide repeat polymorphism at 9 loci in sporadic colorectal cancer. *Cell Mol Biol Res* **40**, 683-691.

Pathak S, Risin S, Brown NW, Berry K (1994). Telomeric association of chromosomes is an early manifestation of programmed cell death. *Int J Oncol* **4**, 323-328.

Patterson C, Prelella MA, Endege WO, Yoshizumi M, Lee ME, Haber E (1996). Down-regulation of vascular endothelial growth factor receptors by tumour necrosis factor α in cultured human vasacular endothelial cells. *J Clin Invest* **98**, 490-496.

Patterson H, Gill S, Fisher C, Law MG, Jayatilake H, Fletcher CDM, Thomas M, Grimer R, Gusterson BA, Cooper CS (1994). Abnormalities of the *p53*, *mdm2* and *DCC* genes in human leiomyosarcomas. *Br J Cancer* **69**, 1052-1058.

Pauley RJ, Gimotty PA, Paine TJ, Dawson PJ, Wolman SR (1996). *Int2* and *erbB2* amplification and *erbB2* expression in breast tumours from patients with different outcomes. *Breast Cancer Res Treat* **37**, 65-76.

Paulus W, Tonn JC (1994). Basement membrane invasion of glioma cells mediated by integrin receptors. *J Neurosurg* **80**, 515-519.

Pavelic J, Galltroselj K, Hlavka V, Pavelic ZP, Gluckman JL, Stambrook PJ, Pavalic K (1994). NM23-H1 protein in oligodendrogliomas. *Int J Oncol* **4**, 1399-1403.

Pavletich N, Chambers KA, Pabo CO (1993). The DNA-binding domain of p53 contains the four conserved regions and the major mutation hot spots. *Genes Develop* **7**, 2556-2564.

Pavloff N, Staskus PW, Kishnani NS, Hawkes SP (1992). A new inhibitor of metalloproteinase from chicken: ChIMP03. A third member of the TIMP family. *J Biol Chem* **267**, 17321-17326.

Pawson T, Schlessinger J (1993). SH2 and SH3 domains. *Curr Biol* **3**, 434-442.

Pechan PM (1991). Heat shock proteins and cell proliferation. *FEBS Lett* **280**, 1-4.

Pedrocchi M, Schafer BW, Mueller H, Eppenberger U, Heizmann CW (1994). Expression of Ca^{2+} binding proteins of the S100 family in malignant human breast cancer cell lines and biopsy samples. *Int J Cancer* **57**, 684-690.

Peifer M (1995). Cell adhesion and signal transduction. The armadillo connection. *Trends Cell Biol* **5**, 224-229.

Peifer M, Rauskolb C, Williams M, Riggleman B, Wieschaus E (1991). The segment polarity gene armadillo interacts with the wingless signalling pathway in both embryonic and adult pattern formation. *Development* **111**, 1029-1043.

Peles E, Levy RB, Or E, Ullrich A, Yarden Y (1991). Oncogenic forms of the neu/Her2 tyrosine kinase are permanently coupled to phospholipase c-gamma. *EMBO J* **10**, 2077-2086.

Pellegata NS, Cajot JF, Stanbridge EJ (1995). The basic carboxy terminal domain of human p53 is indispensable for both transcriptional regulation and inhibition of tumour cell growth. *Oncogene* **11**, 337-349.

Pellegata NS, Antoniono RJ, Redpath JL, Stanbridge EJ (1996). DNA damage and p53-mediated cell cycle arrest: a re-evaluation. *Proc 9th Int Conf Soc Diff*, Pisa, Italy, p. 104.

Peltomaki P, Lothe RA, Aaltonen LA, Pylkkanen L, Nystrom-Lahti M, Seruca R, David L, Holm R, Ryberg D, Haugen A, Brogger A, Borresen AL, de la Chapelle A (1993). Microsatellite instability is associated with tumours that characterise the hereditary non-polyposis colorectal carcinoma syndrome. *Cancer Res* **53**, 5853-5855.

Peringa J, Molenaar WM, Timens W (1994). Integrins and extracellular matrix proteins in the different components of the Wilms tumour. *Virchows Arch Int J Pathol* **425**, 113-119.

Perschl A, Lesley J, English N, Trowbridge I, Hyman R (1995a). Role of CD44 cytoplasmic domain in hyaluronan binding. *Eur J Immnol* **25**, 495-501.

Perschl A, Lesley J, English N, Hyman R, Trowbridge IS (1995b). Transmembrane domain of CD44 is required for its detergent insolubility in fibroblasts. *J Cell Sci* **108**, 1033-1041.

Pertovaara L, Kaipainen A, Mustonen T, Orpana A, Ferrara N, Saksela O, Alitalo K (1994). Vascular endothelial growth factor is induced in response to transforming growth factor β in fibroblastic and epithelial cells. *J Biol Chem* **269**, 6271-6274.

Peters G, Brookes S, Smith R, Dickson C (1983). Tumorigenesis by mouse mammary tumour virus: evidence for a common region for provirus integration in mammary tumours. *Cell* **33**, 369-377.

Pezzella F, Tse AG, Cordell JL, Pulford KA, Gatter KC, Mason DY (1990). Expression of the *bcl-2* oncogene protein is not specific for the 14;18 chromosomal translocation. *Amer J Pathol* **137**, 225-232.

Pezzella F, Morrison H, Jones M, Gatter KC, Lane D, Harris AL, Mason DY (1993a). Immunohistochemical detection of p53 proteins and bcl-2 proteins in non-Hodgkin's lymphoma. *Histopathol* **22**, 39-44.

Pezzella F, Turley H, Kuzu I, Tungekar MF, Dunnil MS, Pierce CB, Harris A, Gatter KG, Mason DY (1993b). Bcl-2 protein in non-small cell lung carcinoma. *N Engl J Med* **329**, 690-694.

Philip EA, Stephenson TJ, Reed MWR (1996). Prognostic significance of angiogenesis in transitional cell carcinoma of the human urinary bladder. *Br J Urol* **77**, 352-357.

Phillips ML, Nudelman E, Gaeta FCA, Perez M, Singhal AK, Hakamori S, Paulson JC (1990). ELAM-1 mediates cell adhesion by recognition of a carbohydrate ligand, sialyl-Le^x. *Science* **250**, 1130-1132.

Picksley SM, Vojtesek B, Sparks A, Lane DP (1994). Immunochemical analysis of the interaction of p53 with mdm2. Fine mapping of the mdm2 binding site on p53 using synthetic peptides. *Oncogene* **9**, 2523-2529.

Pierce JH, Arnstein P, Di Marco E, Artrip J, Kraus MH, Lonardo F, Di Fiore PP, Aaronson SA (1991). Oncogenic potential of erbB2 in human mammary epithelial cells. *Oncogene* **6**, 1189-1194.

Pierceall WE, Cho KR, Getzenberg RH, Reale MA, Hendrick L, Vogelstein B, Fearon ER (1994a). NIH 3T3 cells expressing the deletion in colorectal cancer tumour suppressor gene product stimulate neurite outgrowth in rat PC12 pheochromocytoma cells. *J Cell Biol* **124**, 1017-1027.

Pierceall WE, Reale MA, Candia AF, Wright CVE, Cho KR, Fearon ER (1994b). Expression of a homologue of the deleted in colorectal cancer (DCC) gene in the nervous system of developing *Xenopus* embryos. *Develop Biol* **166**, 654-665.

Pierceall WE, Woodard AS, Morrow JS, Rimm D, Fearon ER (1995). Frequent alterations in

E-cadherin and α-catenin and β-catenin expression in breast cancer cell lines. *Oncogene* **11**, 1319-1326.

Pietenpol JA, Bohlander SK, Sato Y, Papadopoulos N, Liu B, Friedman C, Trask BJ, Roberts JM, Kinzler KW, Rowley JD, Vogelstein B (1995). Assignment of the human *p27 (kip1)* gene to 12p13 and its analysis in leukaemias. *Cancer Res* **55**, 1206-1210.

Pim D, Collins M, Banks L (1992). Human papillomavirus type 16 E5 gene stimulates the transforming activity of the epidermal growth factor receptor. *Oncogene* **7**, 27-32.

Pimentel E (1987). *Hormones, Growth Factor and Oncogenes*. CRC Press, Boca Raton, Florida, pp. 111-140.

Pinhasi-Kimhi O, Michalovitz D, Ben-Zeev A, Oren M (1986). Specific interaction between the p53 cellular tumour antigen and major heat shock proteins. *Nature* **320**, 182-185.

Pipili-Synetos E, Papageorgiou A, Sakkoua E, Sotiropoulou G, Fotsis T, Andriopoulou P, Haralabopoulos G, Peristeris P, Karakiulakis G, Maragoudakis ME (1995). Nitric oxide (NO) as a suppressor of angiogenesis. *Proc 2nd Xenobiotic Metals Toxicity Workshop of Balkan Countries*, Ioannina, Greece, p. 13.

Piris MA, Pezella F, Martinez-Montero JC, Orradre JL, Villuendas R, Sanchez-Beato M, Cuena R, Cruz MA, Martinez B, Garrido MC, Gatter K, Aiello A, Delia D, Giardini R, Rilke F (1994). P53 and *bcl-2* expression in high grade B-cell lymphomas: correlation with survival time. *Br J Cancer* **69**, 337-341.

Pisters LL, Troncoso P, Zhau HE, Li W, von Eschenbach AC, Chung LWK (1995). C-met proto-oncogene expression in benign and malignant human prostate tissues. *J Urol* **154**, 293-298.

Pizaro A, Benito N, Navarro P, Palacios J, Cano A, Quintanilla M, Contreras F, Gamallo C (1994). E-cadherin expression in basal cell carcinoma. *Br J Cancer* **69**, 157-162.

Plate KH, Breier G, Weich HA, Mennel HD, Risau W (1994). Vascular endothelial growth factor and glioma angiogenesis. Co-ordinate induction of VEGF receptors, distribution of VEGF protein and possible *in vivo* regulatory mechanisms. *Int J Cancer* **59**, 520-529.

Plebani M, Herszenyi L, Cardin R, Roveroni G, Carraro P, Paoli MD, Rugge M, Grigioni WF, Nitti D, Naccarato R, Farinati F (1995). Cysteine and serine proteinases in gastric cancer. *Cancer* **76**, 367-375.

Polans AS, Palczewski K, Assonbatres MA, Ohguro H, Witkowska D, Haley TL, Baizer L, Crabb JW (1994).Purification and primary structure of CAPL, an S-100-related calcium-binding protein isolated from bovine retina. *J Biol Chem* **269**, 6233-6240.

Pollanen R, Pyykkonene K, Jarvinen M, Rinne A, Laara E, Lehto VP, Rasanen O (1995). Immunolocalisation of cystatin A in condylomatous and dysplastic lesions of the human uterine cervix. Correlation with the presence and type of human papilloma virus infection. *Int J Gynaecol Pathol* **14**, 217-222.

Poller DN, Galea M, Pearson D, Bell J, Gullick WJ, Elston CW, Blamey RV, Ellis IO (1991). Nuclear and flow cytometric characteristics associated with over-expression of c-erbB2 oncoprotein in breast carcinoma. *Breast Cancer Res Treat* **20**, 3-10.

Polyak K, Lee MH, Erdjumentbromage H, Koff A, Roberts JM, Tempst P, Massague J (1994a). Cloning of p27 (kip1), a cyclin dependent kinase inhibitor and a potential mediator of extracellular antimitogenic signals. *Cell* **78**, 59-66.

Polyak K, Kato JY, Solomon MJ, Sherr CJ, Massague J, Roberts JM, Koff A (1994b). P27 (kip1), a cyclin cdk inhibitor, links transforming growth factor beta and contact inhibition to cell cycle arrest. *Genes Develop* **8**, 9-22.

Poncecastaneda MV, Lee MH, Latres E, Polyak K, Lacombe L, Montgomery K, Mathew S, Krauter K, Sheinfeld J, Massague J, Cordoncardo C (1995). P27 (kip1) - chromosomal mapping to 12p12-12p-13.1 and absence of mutations in human tumours. *Cancer Res* **55**, 1211-1214.

Ponta H, Sleeman J, Herrlich P (1994). Tumour metastasis formation: cell surface proteins confer metastasis-promoting or suppressing properties. *Biochim Biophys Acta* **1198**, 1-10.

Ponton A, Coulombe B, Skup D (1991). Decreased expression of tissue inhibitor of metallo-proteinases in metastatic tumour cells leading to increased levels of collagenase activity. *Cancer Res* **51**, 2138-2143.

Porschen R, Remy U, Bevers G, Schauseil S, Hengels KJ, Borchard F (1993). Prognostic significance of DNA ploidy in adenocarcinoma of the pancreas. *Cancer* **71**, 3846-3850.

Porteous D, Bickmore W, Christie S, Boyd PA, Cranston G, Fletcher JM, Gosden JR, Rout D, Seawright A, Simda OJ, van Heynigen V, Hastie ND (1987). H-ras1-selected chromosome transfer generates markers that co-localise aniridia- and genitourinary dysplasia-associated translocation break points and the Wilms tumour gene within band 11p13. *Proc Natl Acad Sci USA* **84**, 5355-5359.

Porter PL, Garcia R, Moe R, Corwin D, Gown AM (1991). C-erbB2 oncogene protein in *in situ* and invasive lobular breast neoplasia. *Cancer* **68**, 331-334.

Poste G, Doll J, Fidler IJ (1981). Interaction between clonal sub-populations affect the stability of the metastatic phenotype in polyclonal populations of B16 melanoma cells. *Proc Natl Acad Sci USA* **78**, 6226-6230.

Poste G, Tzeng J, Doll J, Grieg R, Rieman D, Zeidman I (1982). Evolution of tumour cell heterogeneity during progressive growth of individual lung metastases. *Proc Natl Acad Sci USA* **79**, 6574-6578.

Postel EH, Berberich SJ, Flint SJ, Ferrone CA (1993). Human c-myc transcription factor puf identified as nm23-H2 nucleoside diphospate kinase, a candidate suppressor of tumour metastasis. *Science* **261**, 478-480.

Postigo AA, Garcia-Vicuna R, Laffon A, Sanchez-Madrid F (1993). The role of adhesion molecules in the pathogenesis of rheumatoid arthritis. *Autoimmunity* **16**, 69-76.

Powell SM, Papadopoulos N, Kinzler KW, Smolinski KN, Meltzer SJ (1994). APC gene mutations in the mutation cluster region are rare in oesophageal cancers. *Gastroenterol* **107**, 1759-1763.

Pozzati R, Muschel R, Williams J, Padmanabhan R, Howard B, Liotta L, Khoury G (1986). Primary rat embryo cells transformed by one or two oncogenes show different metastatic potential. *Science* **232**, 223-227.

Presti JC, Jr, Rao PH, Chen Q, Reuter VE, Li FP, Fair WR, Jhanwar SC (1991). Histopathological, cytogenetic and molecular characterisation of renal cortical tumours. *Cancer Res* **51**, 1544-1552.

Preston SF, Volpi M, Pearson CM, Berlin RD (1987). Regulation of cell shape in the Cloudman melanoma cell line. *Proc Natl Acad Sci USA* **84**, 5247-5251.

Preud'homme JL, Seligman M (1972). Surface bound immunoglobulins as a cell marker in human lymphoproliferative diseases. *Blood* **40**, 777-794.

Priest JH, Phillips CN, Wang Y, Richmond A (1988). Chromosome and growth factor abnormalities in melanoma. *Cancer Genet Cytogenet* **35**, 253-262.

Pritchard-Jones K, Fleming S, Davidson D, Bickmore W, Porteous D, Gosden C, Bard J, Buckler A, Pelletier J, Housman D, van Heyningen V, Hastie N (1990). The candidate Wilms tumour gene is involved in genitourinary development. *Nature* **346**, 194-197.

Pujol JL, Simony J, Demoly P, Charpentier R, Laurent JC, Daures JP, Lehmann M, Guyot T, Godard P, Michel FB (1993). Neural cell adhesion molecule and prognosis of surgically resected lung cancer. *Amer Rev Resp Dis* **148**, 1071-1075.

Pullman WE, Bodmer WF (1992). Cloning and characterisation of a gene that regulates cell adhesion. *Nature* **356**, 529-532.

Pure E, Camp RL, Peritt D, Panettieri RA, Lazaar AL, Nayak S (1995). Defective phosphorylation and hyaluronate binding of CD44 with point mutations in the cytoplasmic domain. *J Exp Med* **181**, 55-62

Qian F, Bajkowski AS, Steiner DF, Chan SJ, Frankfater A (1989). Expression of five cathepsins in murine melanomas of varying metastatic potential and normal tisues. *Cancer Res* **49**, 4870-4875.

Qin XQ, Livingston DM, Kaelin WG, Adams PD (1994). Deregulated transcription factor E2F-1 expression leads to S-phase entry and p53-mediated apoptosis. *Proc Natl Acad Sci USA* **91**, 10918-10922.

Quantin B, Breathnach R (1988). Epidermal growth factor stimulates transcription of the c-*jun* proto-oncogene in rat fibroblasts. *Nature* **334**, 538-542.

Quenel N, Wafflart J, Bonichon F, De Mascarel I, Trojani M, Durand M, Avril A, Coindre JM (1995). The prognostic value of c-erbB2 in primary breast carcinomas. A study on 942 cases. *Breast Cancer Res Treat* **35**, 283-291.

Quesnel B, Preudhomme C, Oscier D, Lepelley P, Collyndhooghe M, Facon T, Zandecki M, Fenaux P (1994a). Over-expression of the mdm2 gene is found in some cases of haematological malignancies. *Br J Cancer* **88**, 415-418.

Quesnel B, Preudhomme C, Fournier J, Fenaux P, Peyrat JP (1994b). Mdm2 gene amplification in human breast cancer. *Eur J Cancer* **30A**, 982-984.

Radinsky R, Risin S, Fan D, Dong Z, Bielenberg D, Bucana CD, Fidler IJ (1995). Level and function of epidermal growth factor receptor predict the metastatic potential of human colon carcinoma cells. *Clin Cancer Res* **1**, 19-31.

Radotra B, McCormick D, Crockard A (1994). CD44 plays a role in adhesive interactions between glioma cells and extracellular matrix components. *Neuropath App Neurobiol* **20**, 399-405.

Rainov NG, Lubbe J, Renshaw J, Pritchard-Jones K, Luthy AR, Aguzzi A (1995). Association of Wilms tumour with primary brain tumour in siblings. *J Neuropath Exp Neurol* **54**, 214-223.

Rak J, Mitsuhashi Y, Bayko L, Filmus J, Shirasawa S, Sasazuki T, Kerbel RS (1995). Mutant *ras* oncogenes upregulate VEGF/VPF expression. Implications for induction and inhibition of tumour angiogenesis. *Cancer Res* **55**, 4575-4580.

Ramakrishna NR, Brown AMC (1993). Wingless, the *Drosophila* homologue of the proto-oncogene wnt-1 can transform mouse mammary epithelial cells. *Development* (Sp. Suppl.), 95-103.

Ranasinghe A, Warnakulasuriya KAAS, Johnson NW (1993a). Low prevalence of expression of p53 oncoprotein in oral carcinomas from Sri Lanka associated with betel and tobacco chewing. *Oral Oncol Eur J Cancer* **29B**, 147-150.

Ranasinghe A, Macgeoch C, Dyer S, Spurr N, Johnson NW (1993b). Some oral carcinomas from Sri Lanka betel/tobacco chewers overexpress p53 oncoprotein but lack mutations in exons 5-9. *Anticancer Res* **13**, 2065-2068.

Randerson J, Cawkwell L, Jack A, Child JA, Lewis F, Hall N, Johnson P, Evans P, Barrans S, Morgan GJ (1996). Microsatellite instability in follicle centre cell lymphoma. *Br J Haematol* **93**, 160-162.

Rao KV (1994). *Developmental Biology, a Modern Synthesis*. Oxford & IBH Publishing Co Pvt Ltd, Delhi.

Rao L, Debbas M, Sabbatini P, Hockenbery D, Korsmeyer S, White E (1992). The adenovirus E1A proteins induce apoptosis, which is inhibited by E1B 19-kDa and Bcl-2 proteins. *Proc Natl Acad Sci USA* **89**, 7742-7746.

Rao VN, Shao NS, Ahmad M, Reddy ESP (1996). Antisense RNA to the putative tumour suppressor gene BRCA1 transforms mouse fibroblasts. *Oncogene* 12, 523-528.

Rauscher FJ, III, Cohen DR, Curran T, Bos TJ, Vogt PK, Bohman D, Tjian, Franza R (1988). Fos-associated protein p39 is the product of the *jun* proto-oncogene. *Science* 240 1010-1016.

Rauscher FJ, III, Morris OE, Tournay DM, Curran T (1990). Binding of the Wilms tumour locus zinc finger protein to the EGR-1 consensus sequence. *Science* 250, 1259-1262.

Reale MA, Hu G, Zafar AI, Getzenberg RH, Levine SM, Fearon ER (1994). Expression of alternative splicing of the deleted in colorectal cancer (DCC) gene in normal and malignant tissues. *Cancer Res* 54, 4493-4501.

Reddy EP, Shalka AM, Curran T (1988). *The Oncogene Handbook*. Elsevier, Amsterdam.

Reddy JC, Morris JC, Wang J, English MA, Haber DA, Shi Y, Licht JD (1995). Wt1-mediated transcriptional activation is inhibited by dominant negative mutant proteins. *J Biol Chem* 270, 10878-10884.

Redwood SM, Liu BCS, Weiss RE, Hodge DE, Droller MJ (1992). Abrogation of the invasion of human bladder tumour cells by using protease inhibitor(s). *Cancer* 69, 1212-1219.

Reed JC, Tanaka S (1993). Somatic point mutations in the translocated *bcl-2* genes of non-Hodgkin's lymphomas and lymphocytic leukaemias. Implications for mechanisms of tumour progression. *Leukaemia Lymphoma* 10, 157-163.

Reed SI, Bailly E, Dulic V, Hengst L, Resnitzky D, Slingerland J (1994). G(1) control in mammalian cells. *J Cell Sci* S18, 69-73.

Reeve AE, Housiaux PJ, Gardner RJM, Chewings WE, Grindley RM, Millow LJ (1984). Loss of a Harvey ras allele in sporadic Wilms' tumour. *Nature* 309, 174-176.

Reeve AE, Eccles MR, Wilkins RJ, Bell GI, Millow LJ (1985). Expression of insulin-like growth factor II transcript in Wilms tumour. *Nature* 317, 258-260.

Reeve AE, Sih SA, Raizis AM, Feinberg AP (1989). Loss of allelic heterozygosity at a second locus on chromosome 11 in sporadic Wilms tumour cells. *Mol Cell Biol* 9, 1799-1803.

Reeve JG, Xiong J, Morgan J, Bleehan NM (1996). Expression of apoptosis regulatory genes in lung tumour cell lines. Relationship to p53 expression and relevance to acquired drug resistance. *Br J Cancer* 73, 1193-1200.

Reifenberger G, Liu L, Ichimura K, Schmidt EE, Collins VP (1993). Amplification and over-expression of the mdm2 gene in a subset of human malignant gliomas without p53 mutations. *Cancer Res* 53, 2736-2739.

Reich NC, Oren M, Levine AJ (1983). Two distinct mechanisms regulate the levels of cellular antigen p53. *Mol Cell Biol* 3, 2143-2150.

Reich R, Thompson EW, Iwamoto Y, Martin GR, Deason JR, Fuller GC, Miskin R (1988). Effects of inhibitors of plasminogen activator, serine proteinases and collagenase IV on the invasion of basement membrane by metastatic cells. *Cancer Res* 48, 3307-3312.

Reinhardt KM, Steiner M, Zillig D, Nagel HR, Blann AD, Brinckmann W (1996). Soluble intercellular adhesion molecule-1 in colorectal cancer and its relationship to acute phase proteins. *Neoplasma* 43, 65-67.

Reisman D, Greenberg M, Rotter V (1988). Human p53 oncogene contains one promoter upstream of exon 1 and a second stronger promoter within intron 1. *Proc Natl Acad Sci USA* 85, 5146-5150.

Rempel SA, Rosenblum ML, Mikkelsen T, Yan PS, Ellis KD, Golembieski WA, Sameni M, Rozhin J, Ziegler G, Sloane BF (1994). Cathepsin B expression and localisation in glioma progression and invasion. *Cancer Res* 54, 6027-6031.

Remvikos Y, Laurent-Puig P, Salmon RJ, Frelat G, Dutrillaux B, Thomas G (1990). Simultaneous monitoring of p53 protein and DNA content of colorectal adenocarcinomas by flow cytometry. *Int J Cancer* **45**, 450-456.

Remvikos Y, Tominaga O, Hammel P, Laurent-Puig P, Salmon RJ, Dutrillaux B, Thomas G (1992). Increased p53 protein content of colorectal tumours correlates with poor survival. *Br J Cancer* **66**, 758-764.

Represa J, Leon Y, Miner C, Giraldez F (1991). The int-2 proto-oncogene is responsible for induction of the inner ear. *Nature* **353**, 561-563.

Reynisdottir I, Polyak K, Iavarone A, Massague J (1995). Kip1/cip1 and ink4 cdk inhibitors cooperate to induce cell cycle arrest in response to TGF beta. *Genes Develop* **9**, 1831-1845.

Ricardi VM, Sujansky E, Smith AC, Francke U (1978). Chromosomal imbalance in the aniridia-Wilms tumour association: 11p interstitial deletion. *Paediatrics* **61**, 604-610.

Ricardi VM, Hittner HM, Francke U, Yunis JJ, Ledbetter D, Borges W (1980). The aniridia-Wilms tumour association: the critical role of chromosome band 11p13. *Cancer Genet Cytogenet* **2**, 131-137.

Rice GE, Bevilacqua MP (1981). An inducible endothelial cell surface glycoprotein mediates melanoma adhesion. *Science* **246**, 1303-1306.

Rifkin DB, Moscatelli D (1989). Recent developments in the cell biology of basic fibroblast growth factor. *J Cell Biol* **25**, 1-6.

Riggleman B, Schedl P, Wieschaus E (1990). Spatial expression of the *Drosophila* segment polarity gene armadillo is post-transcriptionally regulated by wingless. *Cell* **63**, 549-560.

Rimm DL, Sinard JH, Morrow JS (1995). Reduced α-catenin and E-cadherin expression in breast cancer. *Lab Invest* **72**, 506-512.

Riou G, Le MG, Favre M, Jeannel D, Bourhis J, Orth G (1992). Human papillomavirus-negative status and c-*myc* gene overexpression: independent prognostic indicators of distant metastasis for early stage invasive cervical cancers. *J Natl Cancer Inst* **84**, 1525-1526.

Risinger JI, Berchuck A, Kohler MF, Watson P, Lynch HT, Boyd J (1993). Genetic instability of microsatellites in endometrial carcinomas. *Cancer Res* **53**, 5100-5103.

Risinger JI, Berchuck A, Kohler MF, Boyd J (1994). Mutations of the E-cadherin gene in human gynecologic cancers. *Nature Genet* **7**, 98-102.

Risinger JI, Umar A, Boyer JC, Evans AC, Berchuck A, Kunkel TA, Barrett JC (1995). Microsatellite instability in gynaecological sarcomas and in *hMSH2* mutant uterine sarcoma cell lines defective in mismatch repair activity. *Cancer Res* **55**, 5664-5669.

Ro J, El-Naggar A, Ro JY, Blick M, Frye D, Fraschini G, Fritsche H, Hortobagyi G (1989). C-erbB2 amplification in node negative human breast cancer. *Cancer Res* **49**, 6941-6944.

Roberts AB, Sporn MB (1990). The transforming growth factor betas. In: *Peptide Growth Factors and their Receptors: Handbook of Experimental Pharmacology*, Sporn MB, Roberts AB, (eds). Springer Verlag, New York, pp. 419-472.

Roberts AB, Sporn MB, Assoian RK, Smith JM, Roche NS, Wakefield LM, Heine U, Liotta LA, Falanga V, Kehri JH, Fauci AS (1986). Transforming growth factor type *β*: Rapid induction of fibrosis and angiogenesis in vivo and stimulation of collagen formation in vitro. *Proc Natl Acad Sci USA* **83**, 4167-4171.

Roberts DD (1996). Regulation of tumour growth and metastasis by thrombospondin-1. *FASEB J* **10**, 1183-1191.

Rochefort H (1994). Estrogens, protease and breast cancer. From cell lines to clinical applications. *Eur J Cancer* **30A**, 1583-1586.

Rochefort H, Capony F, Garcia M (1990). Cathepsin D: A protease involved in breast cancer metastasis. *Cancer Metastasis Rev* **9**, 321-331.

Rochester DE, Winer JA, Shah DM (1986). The structure and expression of maize genes encoding the major heat shock protein hsp70. *EMBO J* **5**, 451-458.

Rochlitz CF, Scott GK, Dodson JM, Liu E, Dollbaum C, Smith HS, Benz CC (1989). Incidence of activating *ras* oncogene mutations associated with primary and metastatic breast cancer. *Cancer Res* **49**, 357-360.

Rodeck U, Bossler A, Kari C, Humphreys CW, Gyorfi T, Maurer J, Thiel E, Menssen HD (1994). Expression of the wt1 Wilms tumour gene by normal and malignant human melanocytes. *Int J Cancer* **59**, 78-82.

Rodenhuis S, Slebos RJC (1992). Clinical significance of *ras* oncogene activation in human lung cancer. *Cancer Res* **52**, 2665-2669.

Rodrigues NR, Rowan A, Smith MEF, Kerr IB, Bodmer WF, Gannor JV, Lane DP (1990). p53 mutations in colorectal cancer. *Proc Natl Acad Sci USA* **87**, 7555-7559.

Roelink H, Wang J, Black DM, Solomon E, Nusse R (1993). Molecular cloning and chromosomal localisation to 17q21 of the human wnt-3 gene. *Genomics* **17**, 790-792.

Roemer K, Mueller-Lantzsch N (1996). P53 transactivation domain mutant q22, s23 is impaired for repression of promoters and mediation of apoptosis. *Oncogene* **12**, 2069-2079.

Rose EA, Glaser T, Jones C, Smith CL, Lewis WH, Call KM, Minden M, Champagne E, Bonetta L, Yeger H, Housman DE (1990). Complete physical map of the WAGR region of 11p13 localises a candidate Wilms tumour gene. *Cell* **60**, 495-508.

Rosen A, Sevelda P, Klein M, Dobianer K, Hruza C, Czerwenka K, Hanak H, Vavra N, Salzer H, Leodolter S, Meld M, Spona J (1993). First experience with FGF-3 (int-2) amplification in women with epithelial ovarian cancer. *Br J Cancer* **67**, 1122-1125.

Rosenberg CL, Kim HG, Shows TB, Kronenberg HM, Arnold A (1991a). Rearrangement and over expression of D11S5287E, a candidate oncogene on chromosome 11q13 in benign parathyroid tumours. *Oncogene* **6**, 449-453.

Rosenberg CL, Wong E, Petty EM, Bale AE, Tsujimoto Y, Harris NL, Arnold A (1991b). *PRAD D1*, a candidate *BCL1* oncogene. Mapping and expression in centrocytic lymphoma. *Proc Natl Acad Sci USA* **88**, 9638-9642.

Rosenberg P, Wingren S, Simonsen E, Stal O, Risberg B, Nordenskjold B (1989). Flow cytometric measurements of DNA index and S-phase on paraffin-embedded early stage endometrial cancer. An important prognostic indicator. *Gynaecol Oncol* **35**, 50-54.

Rosenfeld MR, Meneses P, Dalmau J, Drobnjak M, Cordon-Cardo C, Kaplitt MG (1995). Gene transfer of wild type p53 results in restoration of tumour suppressor function in a medulloblastoma cell line. *Neurology* **45**, 1533-1539.

Rosengard AM, Krutsch HC, Shearn A, Biggs JR, Barker E, Margulies IMK, King CR, Liotta LA, Steeg PS (1989). Reduced nm23/awd protein in tumour metastasis and aberrant *Drosophila* development. *Nature* **342**, 177-180.

Rosenman SJ, Gangi AA, Tedder TF, Gallatin WM (1993). Syn-capping of human lymphocyte-T adhesion activation molecules and their redistribution during interaction with endothelial cells. *J Leuk Biol* **53**, 1-10.

Ross JS, Nazeer T, Figge HL, Fisher HG, Rifkin MD (1995). Quantitative immunohistochemical determination of cathepsin D levels in prostatic carcinoma biopsies. Correlation with tumour grade, stage, PSA level, and DNA ploidy status. *Amer J Clin Pathol* **104**, 36-41.

Roussel E, Gingras MC, Ro JY, Branch C, Roth JA (1994). Loss of alpha(1)beta(1) and reduced expression of other beta(1)-integrins and CAM in lung adenocarcinoma compared with pneumocytes. *J Surg Oncol* **56**, 198-208.

Rowley H, Jones AS, Field JK (1995). Chromosome 18 - A possible site for a tumour suppressor gene deletion in squamous cell carcinoma of the head and neck. *Clin Otolaryngol* **20**, 266-271.

Roy LM, Gittinger CK, Landreth GE (1989). Characterisation of epidermal growth factor receptor associated with cytoskeletons of A431 cells. *J Cell Physiol* **140**, 295-304.

Roy LM, Gittinger CK, Landreth GE (1991). Epidermal growth factor treatment of A431 cells alters the binding capacity and electrophoretic mobility of the cytoskeletally associated epidermal growth factor receptor. *J Cell Physiol* **146**, 63-72.

Roychowdhury DF, Tseng A, Fu KK, Windberg V, Weidner N (1996). New prognostic factors in nasopharyngeal carcinoma. Tumour angiogenesis and c-*erbB2* expression. *Cancer* **77**, 1419-1426.

Royds JA, Stephenson TJ, Rees RC, Shorhouse AJ, Silcocks PB (1993). NM23 protein expression in ductal *in situ* and invasive human breast carcinoma. *J Natl Cancer Inst* **85**, 727-731.

Rozhin J, Sameni M, Ziegler G, Sloane BF (1994). Pericellular pH affects distribution and secretion of cathepsin B in malignant cells. *Cancer Res* **54**, 6517-6525.

Rubin JS, Chan AML, Bottaro DP, Burgess WH, Taylor WG, Cech AC, Hirschfield DW, Wong J, Miki T, Finch FW, Aaronson SA (1991). A broad spectrum human lung fibroblast-derived mitogen is a variant of hepatocyte growth factor. *Proc Natl Acad Sci USA* **88**, 415-419.

Ruggeri BA, Bauer B, Zhang SY, Kleinszanto AJP (1994). Murine squamous cell carcinoma cell lines produced by a complete carcinogenesis protocol with benzo(a)pyrene exhibit characteristic p53 mutations and the absence of H-ras and cyl-1 cyclin D1 abnormalities. *Carcinogenesis* **15**, 1613-1619.

Ruiz P, Dunon D, Sonnenberg A, Imhof BA (1993). Suppression of mouse melanoma metastasis by EA-1, a monoclonal antibody specific for alpha(6) integrins. *Cell Adhesion Commun* **1**, 67-81.

Ruppert C, Ehrenforth S, Tutschek B, Vering A, Beckmann MW, Scharrer I, Bender HG (1994). Proteases associated with gynaecological tumours. *Int J Oncol* **4**, 717-721.

Ruppert JM, Stillman B (1993). Analysis of a protein binding domain of p53. *Mol Cell Biol* **13**, 3811-3820.

Rusch VW, Reuter VE, Kris MG, Kurie J, Miller WH, Jr, Nanus DM, Albino AP, Dmitrovsky E (1992). *Ras* oncogene point mutation: an infrequent event in bronchioalveolar cancer. *J Thoracic Cardiovasc Surg* **104**, 1465-1469.

Ryan RE, Sloane FB, Sameni M, Wood PL (1995). Microglial cathepsin B. An immunological examination of cellular and secreted species. *J Neurochem* **65**, 1035-1045.

Ryseck RP, Hirai SI, Yaniv M, Bravo R (1988). Transcriptional activation of c-*jun* during the G0/G1 transition in mouse fibroblasts. *Nature* **334**, 535-537.

Sadaie MR, Hager GL (1994). Induction of developmentally programmed cell death and activation of HIV by sodium butyrate. *Virology* **202**, 513-518.

Sadhu C, Lipsky B, Erickson HP, Hayflick J, Dick KO, Gallatin WM, Staunton DE (1994). LFA-1 binding site in ICAM-3 contains a conserved motif and non-contiguous aminoacids. *Cell Adhesion Commun* **2**, 429-440.

Sadowski I, Pawson T, Lagarde A (1988). v-*fps* protein tyrosine kinase coordinately enhances the malignancy and growth factor responsiveness of preneoplastic lung fibroblasts. *Oncogene* **2**, 241-248.

Saegusa M, Takano Y, Hashimura M, Shoji Y, Okayasu I (1995). The possible role of bcl-2 expression in the progression of tumours of the uterine cervix. *Cancer* **76**, 2297-2303.

Sager R, Gadi IK, Stephens L, Grabowy CT (1985). An example of accelerated evolution in tumorigenic cells. *Proc Natl Acad Sci USA* **82**, 7015-7019.

Sainsbury JRC, Farndon JR, Harris AL, Sherbet GV (1985a). Epidermal growth factor receptors on human breast cancers. *Br J Surg* **72**, 186-188.

Sainsbury JRC, Farndon JR, Sherbet GV, Harris AL (1985b). Epidermal growth factor receptors and oestrogen receptors in human breast cancer. *Lancet* **1**, 364-366.

Sainsbury JRC, Malcolm AJ, Appleton DR, Farndon JR, Harris AL (1985c). Presence of epidermal growth factor receptor as predictor of poor prognosis in patients with breast cancer. *J Clin Pathol* **38**, 1225-1228.

Sainsbury JRC, Needham GK, Farndon JR, Malcolm AH, Harris AL (1987). Epidermal growth factor receptor status as predictor of early recurrence and death from breast cancer. *Lancet* **1**, 1398-1402.

Saito S, Tanio Y, Tachibana I, Hayashi S, Kishimoto T, Kawase I (1994). Complementary DNA sequence encoding the major neural cell adhesion molecule isoform in a human small cell lung cancer cell line. *Lung Cancer* **10**, 307-318.

Sakakibara Y (1988). The dnaK gene of *Escherichia coli* functions in initiation of chromosome replication. *J Bacteriol* **170**, 972-979.

Sakakura C, Sweeney EA, Shirahama T, Igarashi Y, Hakamori S, Nakatani H, Tsujimoto H, Imanishi T, Ohgaki M, Ohyama T, Yamazaki J, Hagiwara A, Yamaguchi T, Sawai K, Takahashi T (1996). Over-expression of bax sensitizes human breast cancer MCF-7 cells to radiation-induced apoptosis. *Int J Cancer* **67**, 101-105.

Sakakura T, Kusakabe M (1994). Can tenascin be redundant in cancer development? *Persp Develop Neurobiol* **2**, 111-116.

Sakamoto N, Iwahana M, Tanaka NG, Osada Y (1991). Inhibition of angiogenesis and tumour growth by synthetic laminin peptide CDPYIGSR-NH$_2$. *Cancer Res* **51**, 903-906.

Sakamoto R, Watanabe T, Kito T, Yamamura Y, Kiriyama K, Kannagi R, Ueda R, Takagi H, Takahashi T (1994). Expression of neural cell adhesion molecule in normal gastric mucosa and in gastric carcinoid tumours. *Eur Surg Res* **26**, 230-239.

Salnikow K, Cosentino S, Klein C, Costa M (1994). Loss of thrombospondin transcriptional activity in nickel-transformed cells. *Mol Cell Biol* **14**, 851-858.

Salowe SP, Mary AI, Cuca GC, Smith CK, Kopka IE, Hagmann WK, Hermes JD (1992). Characterisation of the zinc binding sites in human stromelysin-1 - stoichiometry of the catalytic domain and identification of a cysteine ligand in the proenzyme. *Biochemistry* **31**, 4535-4540.

Samowitz WS, Thliveris A, Spirio LM, White R (1995). Alternatively spliced adenomatous polyposis coli (APC) gene transcripts that delete exons mutated in attenuated APC. *Cancer Res* **55**, 3732-3734.

Sanchez ER, Faber LE, Henzel WJ, Pratt WB (1990). The 56-59 kilodalton protein identified in untransformed steroid receptor complexes is a unique protein that exists in cytosol in complex with both 70 and 90 kilodalton heat shock proteins. *Biochem* **29**, 5145-5152.

Sano T, Tsujino T, Yoshida K, Nakayama H, Haruma K, Ito H, Nakamura Y, Kajiyama G, Tahara E (1991). Frequent loss of heterozygosity on chromosome 1q, 5q, and 17p in human gastric carcinomas. *Cancer Res* **51**, 2926-2931.

Santarosa M, Favaro D, Quaia M, Spada A, Sacco C, Talamini R, Galligioni E (1995). Expression and release of intercellular adhesion molecule-1 in renal cancer patients. *Int J Cancer* **62**, 271-275.

Santos A, Osorioalmeida L, Baird PN, Silva JM, Boavida MG, Cowell J (1993). Insertional inactivation of the wt1 gene in tumour cells from a patient with WAGR syndrome. *Human Genet* **92**, 83-86.

Santos CLS, Giorgi RR, Frochtengarten F, Elias MCQB, Chammas R, Brentani RR (1994).

Regulation of vitronectin receptor expression by retinoic acid on human melanoma cells. *Int J Clin Lab Res* **24**, 148-153.

Sardet C, Vidal M, Cobrinik D, Geng Y, Onufryk C, Chen A (1995). E2F-4 and E2F-5, two members of the E2F family, are expressed in the early phase of the cell cycle. *Proc Natl Acad Sci USA* **92**, 2403-2407.

Sarkar NH (1995). Clonal variations among multiple primary mammary tumours and within a tumour of individual mice. Insertional mutations of int oncogenes. *Virology* **212**, 490-499.

Sarkar NH, Haga S, Lehner AF, Zhao W, Imai S, Moriwaki K (1994). Insertional mutation of int proto-oncogenes in the mammary tumours of a new strain of mice derived from the wild in China. Normal tissue-specific and tumour tissue-specific expression of int-3 transcripts. *Virology* **203**, 52-62.

Sarnow P, Ho YS, Williams J, Levine AJ (1982). Adenovirus Elb-58kD tumour antigen and SV40 large T antigen are physically associated with the same 54 kDa cellular protein in transformed cells. *Cell* **28**, 387-394.

Sarzani R, Arnaldi G, Depirro R, Moretti P, Schiaffino S, Rappelli A (1992). A novel endothelial tyrosine kinase cDNA homologus to platelet derived growth factor receptor cDNA. *Biochem Biophys Res Commun* **186**, 706-714.

Sasaki H, Nishii H, Takahashi H, Tada A, Furusato M, Terashima Y, Siegal GP, Parker SI, Kohler MF, Berchuck A, Boyd J (1993). Mutations of the K-*ras* proto-oncogene in human endometrial hyperplasia and carcinoma. *Cancer Res* **53**, 1906-1910.

Sasano H, Date F, Imatani A, Asaki S, Nagura H (1993). Double immunostaining for c-*erb*B2 and p53 in human stomach cancer cells. *Hum Pathol* **24**, 584-589.

Sato T, Tanigami A, Yamakawa K, Akiyama F, Kasumi F, Sakamoto G, Nakamura Y (1990). Allelotype of breast cancer: cumulative allele losses promote tumour progression in primary breast cancer. *Cancer Res* **50**, 7184-7189.

Sato T, Ito A, Mori Y, Yamashita K, Hayakawa T, Nagase H (1991). Hormonal regulation of collagenolysis in uterine cervical fibroblasts. Modulation of synthesis of procollagenase, prostromelysin and tissue inhibitor of metalloproteinases (TIMP) by progesterone and estradiol-17-beta. *Biochem J* **275**, 645-650.

Sato Y, Suto Y, Pietenpol J, Golub TR, Gilliland DG, Davis EM, Lebeau MM, Roberts JM, Vogelstein B, Rowley JD, Bohlander SK (1995). Tel and kip1 define the smallest region of deletions on 12p13 in haematopoietic malignancies. *Blood* **86**, 1525-1533.

Satoh K, Narumi K, Isemura M, Sakai T, Abe T, Matsushima K, Okuda K, Motomiya M (1992). Increased expression of the 67kDa laminin receptor gene in human small cell lung cancer. *Biochem Biophys Res Commun* **182**, 746-752.

Sawada R, Tsuboi S, Fukuda M (1994). Differential E-selectin dependent adhesion efficiency in sublines of a human colon cancer exhibiting distinct metastatic potential. *J Biol Chem* **269**, 1425-1431.

Sawan A, Lascu, I, Veron M, Anderson JJ, Wright C, Horne CHW, Angus B (1994). NDP-K/nm23 expression in human breast cancer in relation to relapse, survival and other prognostic factors: An immunohistochemical study. *J Pathol* **172**, 27-34.

Sawano A, Takahashi T, Yamaguchi S, Aonuma M, Shibuya M (1996). Flt-1 but not KDR/flk-1 tyrosine kinase is a receptor for placental growth factor, which is related to vascular endothelial growth factor. *Cell Growth Diff* **7**, 213-221.

Saxena A, Clark WC, Robertson JT, Ikejiri B, Oldfield EH, Ali IU (1992). Evidence for the involvement of a potential second tumour suppressor gene on chromosome 17 distinct from p53 in malignant astrocytoma. *Cancer Res* **52**, 6716-6721.

Scambia G, Panici PB, Battaglia F, Ferrandino G, Baiocchi G, Greggi S, De Vincenzo R, Mancerso

S (1992). Significance of epidermal growth factor receptor in advanced ovarian cancer. *J Clin Oncol* **10**, 529-535.

Scambia G, Panici PB, Ferrandina G, Di Stefano M, Romanini ME, Sica G, Mancuso S (1995). Significance of cathepsin D expression in uterine tumours. *Eur J Cancer* **31A**, 1449-1454.

Schalken LM, Ebeling SB, Isaacs JT, Treiger B, Bussemakers MJB, Jong MEM, van de Ven WJM (1988). Down modulation of fibronectin mRNA in metastasizing rat prostatic cancer cells revealed by differential hybridisation analysis. *Cancer Res* **48**, 2042-2046.

Schaller MD, Borgman CA, Cobb BS, Vines RR, Reynolds AB, Parsons JT (1992). p125[FAK], a structurally distinctive protein kinase associated with focal adhesion. *Proc Natl Acad Sci USA* **89**, 5192-5196.

Schardt C, Heymanns J, Schardt C, Rotsch M, Havemann K (1993). Differential expression of the intercellular adhesion molecule-1 (ICAM-1) in lung cancer cell lines of various histological types. *Eur J Cancer* **29A**, 2250-2255.

Schauer IE, Siriwardana S, Langan TA, Sclafani RA (1994). Cyclin D1 over-expression vs retinoblastoma inactivation. Implications for growth control evasion in non-small cell and small cell lung cancer. *Proc Natl Acad Sci USA* **91**, 7827-7831.

Schechter AL, Stern DF, Vaidhyanathan L, Decker SJ, Drebin JA, Greene MI, Weinberg RA (1984). The neu oncogene: an erbB-related gene encoding a 185 000 M_r tumour antigen. *Nature* **312**, 513-516.

Schechter AL, Hung MC, Vaidyanathan L, Weinberg RA, Yang-Feng TL, Francke U, Ullrich A, Coussens L (1985). The *neu* gene: An erb*β*-homologous gene distinct from and unlinked to the gene encoding the EGF receptor. *Science* **229**, 976-978.

Scheffner M, Munger K, Byrne JC, Howley PM (1991). The state of the p53 and retinoblastoma genes in human cervical carcinoma cell lines. *Proc Natl Acad Sci USA* **88**, 5523-5527.

Scheffner M, Munger K, Huibregste JM, Howley PM (1992). Targeted degradation of the retinoblastoma protein by human papilloma virus by E7-E6 fusion proteins. *EMBO J* **11**, 2425-2431.

Scherer SJ, Welter C, Zang KD, Dooley S (1996). Specific *in vitro* binding of p53 to the promoter region of the human mismatch repair gene HMSH2. *Biochem Biophys Res Commun* **221**, 722-728.

Schimmelpenning H, Eriksson ET, Pallis L, Skoog L, Cedermark B, Auer GU (1992). Immuno-histochemical c-erbB2 proto-oncogene expression and nuclear DNA content in human mammary carcinoma *in situ. Amer J Clin Pathol* **97** (Suppl. 1), S48-S52.

Schipper JH, Frixen UH, Behrens J, Unger A, Jahnke K, Birchmeier W (1991). E-cadherin expression in squamous cell carcinomas of head and neck: Inverse correlation with tumour dedifferentiation and lymph node metastasis. *Cancer Res* **51**, 6328-6337.

Schlegel J, Bocker T, Zirngibl H, Fofstadter F, Ruschoff J (1995). Detection of microsatellite instability in human colorectal carcinomas using a non-radioactive PCR-based screening technique. *Virchows Arch Int J Path* **426**, 223-227.

Schonthal A, Herrlich P, Rahmsdorf HJ, Ponta H (1983). Requirement for fos gene expression in the transcriptional activation of collagenase by other oncogenes and phorbol esters. *Cell* **54**, 325-334.

Schottelius A, Brennscheidt U, Ludwig WD, Mertelsmann RH, Herrmann F, Lubbert M (1994). Mechanisms of p53 alteration in acute leukaemias. *Leukaemia* **8**, 1673-1681.

Schubert D, Heinemann S, Carlisle W, Tarikas H, Kimes B, Patrick J, Steinbach JH, Culp W, Brandt BL (1974). Clonal cell lines from the rat central nervous system. *Nature* **249**, 224-227.

Schutte M, da Costa LT, Hahn SA, Moskaluk C, Hoque ATMS, Rozenblum E, Weinstein CL, Bittner M, Melzer PS, Trent JM, Yeo CJ, Hruban RH, Kern SE (1995a). Identification by representational difference analysis of a homozygous deletion in pancreatic carcinoma that lies within the *BRCA2* region. *Proc Natl Acad Sci USA* **92**, 5950-5954.

Schutte M, Rozenblum E, Moskaluk CA, Guan X, Hoque ATMS, Hahn SA, da Costa LT, de Jong PJ, Kern SE (1995b). An integrated high resolution physical map of the *DPC/BRCA2* region at the chromsome 13q12. *Cancer Res* **55**, 4570-4574.

Schutte M, Hruban RH, Hendrick L, Cho KR, Nadasdy GM, Weinstein CL, Bova GS, Isaacs WB, Cairns P, Nawroz H, Sidransky D, Casero RA, Jr, Meltzer PS, Hahn SA, Kern SE (1996). *DPC4* gene in various tumour types. *Cancer Res* **56**, 2527-2530.

Schuuring E, Verhoen E, van Tinteren H, Peterse JL, Nunnink B, Thunnisswen FBJM, Devilee P, Cornelisse CJ, van de Vijver MJ, Mooi WJ, Michalides RJAM (1992). Amplification of genes within the chromosome 11q13 region is indicative of poor prognosis in patients with operable breast cancer. *Cancer Res* **52**, 5229-5234.

Scorilas A, Yotis J, Gouriotis D, Keramopoulos A, Ampela K, Trangas T, Talieri M (1993). Cathepsin D and c-erbB2 have an additive prognostic value for breast cancer patients. *Anticancer Res* **13**, 1895-1900.

Scott J, Cowell J, Robertson ME, Priestley LM, Wadey R, Hopkins B, Pritchard J, Bell GI, Rall LB, Graham CR, Knott TJ (1985). Insulin-like growth factor II gene expression in Wilms tumour and embryonic tissue. *Nature* **317**, 260-262.

Scott NP, Sagar P, Stewart J, Blair GE, Dixon MF, Quirke P (1991). p53 in colorectal cancer: clinicopathological correlations and prognosis significance. *Br J Cancer* **63**, 317-319.

Seemuller U, Arnhold M, Fritz H, Wiedenmann K, Machleidt W, Heinzel R, Appelhans H, Gassen HG, Lottspeich F (1986). The acid stable proteinase inhibitor of human mucous secretions (HUSI-I antileukoprotease) couple aminoacid sequence as revcaled by protein and cDNA sequencing and structural homology to whey proteins and Rcd sea turtle proteinase inhibitor. *FEBS Lett* **199**, 43-48.

Seftor REB, Seftor EA, Gehlsen KR, Stetler-Stevenson WG, Brown PD, Ruoslahti E, Hendrix MJC (1992). Role of the α_v/β_3 integrin in human melanoma cell invasion. *Proc Natl Acad Sci USA* **89**, 1557-1561.

Segawa Y, Ohnoshi T, Ueoka H, Kimura I (1993). Neural cell adhesion molecule expression and clinical features in small cell lung cancer. A semiquantitative immuno-histochemical approach using an immunogold-silver staining method. *Acad Med Okayama* **47**, 281-287.

Seki H, Tanaka J, Sato Y, Kato Y, Umezawa A, Koyama K (1993). Neural cell adhesion molecule (NCAM) and perineural invasion in bile duct cancer. *J Surg Oncol* **53**, 78-83.

Seki H, Koyama K, Tanaka JI, Sato Y, Umezawa A (1995). Neural cell adhesion molecule and perineural invasion in gall bladder cancer. *J Surg Oncol* **58**, 97-100.

Selinfreund RH, Barger SW, Welsh MJ, van Eldik LJ (1990). Antisense inhibition of glial S100 beta production results in alterations in cell morphology, cytoskeletal organisation, and cell proliferation. *J Cell Biol* **111**, 2021-2028.

Sellins KS, Cohen JJ (1987). Gene induction by gamma irradiation leads to DNA fragmentation in lymphocytes. *J Immunol* **139**, 3199-3206.

Sellins KS, Cohen JJ (1991a). Hyperthermia induces apoptosis in thymocytes. *Radiation Res* **126**, 88-95.

Sellins KS, Cohen JJ (1991b). Cytotoxic T-lymphocytes induce different types of DNA damage in target cells of different origin. *J Immunol* **147**, 795-803.

Selvakumaran M, Lin HK, Miyashita T, Wang HG, Krajewsky S, Reed JC, Hoffman B, Liebermann D (1994a). Immediate early up-regulation of *bax* expression by p53 but not TGFβ1: a paradigm for distinct apoptotic pathways. *Oncogene* **9**, 1791-1798.

Selvakumaran M, Lin HK, Tjin Tham Sjin R, Reed JC, Liebermann DA, Hoffman B (1994b). The novel primary response gene MyoD 118 and the proto-oncogene myb, and bcl-2 modulate transforming growth factor β-1 induced apoptosis of myeloid leukaemia cells. *Mol Cell Biol* **14**, 2352-2360.

Semba S, Yokozaki H, Yamamoto S, Yasui W, Tahara E (1996). Microsatellite instability in precancerous lesions and adenocarcinomas of the stomach. *Cancer* **77**, 1620-1627.

Senger DR, Galli SJ, Dvorak AM, Perruzzi CA, Harvey VS, Dvorak HF (1983). Tumour cells secrete a vascular permeability factor that promotes accumulation of ascites fluid. *Science* **219**, 983-985.

Serrano M, Hannon GJ, Beach D (1993). A new regulatory motif in cell cycle control causing specific inhibition of cyclinD/CDK4. *Nature* **366**, 704-707.

Sers C, Riethmuller G, Johnson JP (1994). MUC18, a melanoma-progression associated molelcule, and its potential role in tumour vascularisation and hematogenous spread. *Cancer Res* **54**, 5689-5694.

Seruca R, Santos NR, David L, Constancia M, Barroca H, Carneiro F, Seixas M, Peltomaki P, Lothe R, Sobrinho-Simoes M (1995). Sporadic gastric carcinomas with microsatellite instability display a particular clinocopathologic profile. *Int J Cancer* **64**, 32-36.

Seshadri R, Kutlaca RJ, Trainor K, Matthews C (1987). Mutation rate of normal and malignant human lymphocytes. *Cancer Res* **47**, 407-409.

Seto M, Jaeger U, Kockett RD, Graninger W, Bennett SC, Goldman P, Korsmeyer SJ (1988). Alternative promoters and exons, somatic mutation and transcriptional deregulation of the bcl-2-Ig fusion gene in lymphoma. *EMBO J* **7**, 123-131.

Shackleford GM, Willert K, Wang JW, Varmus HE (1993a). The wnt-1 proto-oncogene induces changes in morphology, gene expression and growth factor responsiveness in PC12 cells. *Neuron* **11**, 865-875.

Shackleford GM, MacArthur CA, Kwan HC, Varmus HE (1993b). Mouse mammary tumour virus infection accelerates mammary carcinogenesis in wnt-1 transgenic mice by insertional activation of int-2/fgf3 and hst/fgf-4. *Proc Natl Acad Sci USA* **90**, 740-744.

Shan B, Zhu X, Chen PL, Furfee T, Yang Y, Sharp D, Lee WH (1992). Molecular cloning of cellular genes encoding retinoblastoma-associated proteins. Identification of a gene with properties of the transcription factor E2F. *Mol Cell Biol* **12**, 5620-5631.

Shapiro SD, Campbell EJ, Kobayashi DK, Welgus HG (1991). Dexamethasone selectively modulates basal and lipopolysaccharide-induced metalloproteinase and tissue inhibitor of metalloproteinase production by human alveolar macrophages. *J Immunol* **146**, 2724-2729.

Sharma HW, Sokoloski JA, Perez JR, Maltese JY, Sartorelli AC, Stein CA, Nichols G, Khaled Z, Telang NT, Narayanan R (1995). Differentiation of immortal cells inhibits telomerase activity. *Proc Natl Acad Sci USA* **92**, 12343-12346.

Shattuck-Eidens D, McClure M, Simard J, Labrie F, Narod S, Couch F, Hoskins K, Weber B, Castilla L, Erdos M, Brody L, Friedman L, Ostermeyer E, Szabo C, King MC, Jhanwar S, Offit K, Norton L, Gilewski T, Lubin M, Osborne M, Black D, Boyd M, Steel M, Ingles S, Haile R, Linblom A, Olsson H, Borg A, Bishop DT, Solomon E, Radice P, Spatti G, Gayther S, Ponder B, Warren W, Stratton M, Liu QY, Fujimura F, Lewis C, Skolnick MH, Goldgar DE (1995). A collaborative survey of 80 mutations in the BRCA1 breast cancer and ovarian cancer susceptibility gene. Implications for presymptomatic testing and screening. *J Amer Med Assoc* **273**, 535-541.

Shaulian E, Zauberman A, Ginsberg D, Oren M (1992). Identification of a minimal transforming domain of p53: negative dominance through abrogation of sequence-specific DNA binding. *Mol Cell Biol* **12**, 5581-5592.

Shaulsky G, Goldfinger N, Ben-Zeev A, Rotter V (1990). Nuclear accumulation of p53 protein is mediated by several nuclear localisation signals and plays a role in tumorigenesis. *Mol Cell Biol* **10**, 6565-6577.

Shaw P, Bovey R, Tardy S, Sahli R, Sordat B, Costa J (1992). Induction of apoptosis by wild type p53 in a human colon tumour-derived cell line. *Proc Natl Acad Sci USA* **89**, 4495-4499.

Sheikh MS, Li XS, Chen JC, Shao ZM, Ordones JV, Fontana JA (1994). Mechanisms of regulation of waf1/cip1 gene expression in human breast carcinoma: role of p53-dependent and independent signal transduction pathways. *Oncogene* **9**, 3407-3415.

Sheng M, Thompson, MA, Greenberg ME (1991). A Ca^{2+}-regulated transcription factor phosphorylated by calmodulin-dependent kinases. *Science* **252**, 1427-1430.

Sheppard JR, Koestler TP, Corwin SP, Buscarino C, Doll J, Lester B, Grieg RG, Poste G (1984). Experimental metastasis correlates with cyclic AMP accumulation in B16 melanoma clones. *Nature* **308**, 544-547.

Sherbet GV (1970). Epigenetic processes and their relevance to the study of neoplasia. *Adv Cancer Res* **13**, 97-167.

Sherbet GV (1974). Epigenetic mechanisms and paraneoplastic phenomena. *Ann NY Acad Sci* **230**, 516-532.

Sherbet GV (1982). *The Biology of Tumour Malignancy*. Academic Press, London.

Sherbet GV (1987). *The Metastatic Spread of Cancer*. Macmillan, Basingstoke & London.

Sherbet GV, Lakshmi MS (1995). Expression of the transmembrane glycoprotein CD44 and the metastasis-associated gene *18A2/mts1* in B16 murine melanoma. *Anticancer Res* **15** (5A), 1679.

Sherbet GV, Lakshmi MS (1997). Retinoids and growth factor signal transduction. In: *Retinoids in Biology & Medicine*, Sherbet GV (ed.). JAI Press Inc., Greenwich, CT.

Sherbet GV, Parker C, Usmani BA, Lakshmi MS (1995). Epidermal growth factor receptor status correlates with cell proliferation related *18A2/mts1* gene expression in human carcinoma cell lines. *Ann NY Acad Sci* **768**, 272-275.

Sherbet GV, Cajone F, Albertazzi E, Lakshmi MS (1996). Induction of heat shock protein HSP28 and down regulation of 18A2/mts1 gene are associated with inhibition of proliferation of B16 murine melanoma cell lines. *Proc Amer Assoc Cancer Res* **37**, 74.

Sherr CJ (1993). Mammalian G1 cyclins. *Cell* **73**, 1059-1065.

Shew JY, Ling N, Yang X, Fodstad O, Lee WH (1989). Antibodies detecting abnormalities of the retinoblastoma susceptibility gene product (pp110RB) in osterosarcomas and synovial sarcomas. *Oncogene Res* **1**, 205-214.

Shi DR, He GP, Cao SL, Pan WS, Zhang HZ, Yu DH, Hung MC (1992). Over-expression of the c-erbB2 neu encoded p185 protein in primary lung cancer. *Mol Carcinogen* **5**, 213-218.

Shibagaki I, Shimada Y, Wagata T, Ikenaga M, Imamura M, Ishizaki K (1994). Allelotype analysis of oesophageal squamous cell carcinoma. *Cancer Res* **54**, 2996-3000.

Shibanuma M, Karoki T, Nose K (1992). Cell cycle dependent phosphorylation of HSP28 by $TGF\beta$-1 and H_2O_2 in normal mouse osteoblastic cells (MC3T3-E1) but not in their ras-transformants. *Biochem Biophys Res Commun* **187**, 1418-1425.

Shibata D, Peinado MA, Ionov Y, Malkhosyan S, Perucho M (1994). Genomic instability in repeated sequences is an early somatic event in colorectal tumorigenesis that persists after transformation. *Nature Genet* **6**, 273-281.

Shibuya K, Kaji H, Itoh T, Ohyama Y, Tsujikami A, Tate S, Takeda A, Kumagai I, Hirao I, Miura K, Inagaki F, Samejima T (1995a). Human cystatin A is inactivated by engineered truncation. The NH_2 terminal region of the cysteine proteinase inhibitor is essential for expression of its inhibitory activity. *Biochemistry* **34**, 12185-12192.

Shibuya K, Kaji H, Ohyama Y, Tate S, Kainosho M, Inagaki F, Samejima T (1995b). Significance of the highly conserved gly-4 residue in human cystatin A. *J Biochem* **118**, 635-642.

Shibuya M, Yamaguchi S, Yamane A, Ikeda T, Tojo A, Matsushime H, Sato M (1990). Nucleotide sequence and expression of a novel human receptor type tyrosine kinase gene (flt) closely related to the fms family. *Oncogene* **5**, 519-524.

Shih C, Padhy LC, Murray M, Weinberg RA (1981). Transforming genes of carcinomas and neuroblastomas introduced into mouse fibroblasts. *Nature* **290**, 261-264.

Shih IM, Wang TL, Westra WH (1996). Diagnostic and biological implications of Mel-CAM expression in mesenchymal neoplasms. *Clin Cancer Res* **2**, 569-575.

Shimoyama Y, Hirohashi S (1991a). Cadherin intercellular adhesion molecule in hepatocellular carcinomas: loss of E-cadherin expression in an undifferentiated carcinoma. *Cancer Lett* **57**, 131-135.

Shimoyama Y, Hirohashi S (1991b). Expression of E- and P-cadherin in gastric carcinomas. *Cancer Res* **51**, 2185-2192.

Shin DM, Kim, J, Ro JY, Hittelman J, Roth JA, Hong WK, Hittelman WN (1994). Activation of *p53* gene expression in premalignant lesions during head and neck tumorigenesis. *Cancer Res* **54**, 321-326.

Shinamura K, Hirano S, McMahon AP, Takeichi M (1994). Wnt-1-dependent regulation of local E-cadherin and alpha-N-catenin expression in the mouse brain. *Development* **120**, 2225-2234.

Shing Y, Folkman J, Sullivan R, Butterfield C, Murray J, Klagsbrun M (1984). Heparin affinity: purification of a tumour-derived capillary endothelial cell growth factor. *Science* **223**, 1296-1299.

Shing Y, Folkman J, Haudenschild C, Lund D, Crum R, Klagsbrun M (1985). Angiogenesis is stimulated by a tumour-derived endothelial cell growth factor. *J Cell Biochem* **29**, 275-287.

Shiozaki H, Kadowsaki T, Doki Y, Inoue M, Tamura S, Oka H, Iwagawa T, Matsui S, Shimaya K, Takeichi M, Mori T (1995). Effect of epidermal growth factor on cadherin-mediated adhesion in human oesophageal cancer cell line. *Br J Cancer* **71**, 250-258.

Shipman R, Schraml P, Colombi M, Raefle G, Ludwig CU (1993). Loss of heterozygosity on chromosome 11p13 in primary bladder carcinoma. *Human Genet* **91**, 455-458.

Shirasawa S, Urabe K, Yanagawa Y, Toshitani K, Iwama T, Sasazuki T (1991). p53 gene mutations in colorectal tumours from patients with familial polyposis coli. *Cancer Res* **51**, 2874-2878.

Shirodkar S, Ewen M, DeCaprio JA, Morgan J, Livingston DM, Chittenden T (1992). The transcription factor E2F interacts with the retinoblastoma product and a p107-cyclin A complex in a cell cycle-regulated manner. *Cell* **68**, 157-166.

Sidebottom E, Clark SR (1983). Cell fusion regulates progressive growth from metastasis. *Br J Cancer* **47**, 399-406.

Sidky YA, Borden EC (1987). Inhibition of angiogenesis by interferons: Effects on tumour and lymphocyte-induced vascular responses. *Cancer Res* **47**, 5155-5161.

Sidky YA, Borden EC (1989). Action of interferons on the tumour-induced angiogenesis model *in vitro*. *J Invest Dermatol* **93**, 578.

Sidransky D, Mikkelsen T, Schwechheimer K, Rosenblum ML, Cavanee W, Vogelstein B (1992). Clonal expansion of p53 mutant cells is associated with brain tumour progression. *Nature* **355**, 846-848.

Sierra A, Lloveras B, Castellague X, Moreno L, Garcia-Ramirez M, Fabra A (1995). Bcl-2 expression is associated with lymph node metastasis in human ductal breast carcinoma. *Int J Cancer* **60**, 54-60.

Sigurdsson H, Baldetorp B, Borg A, Dalberg M, Ferno M, Killander D, Olsson H (1990). Indicators of prognosis in node negative breast cancer. *N Engl J Med* **322**, 1045-1053.

Siitonen SM, Kononen JT, Helin JH, Rantala IS, Holli KA, Isola JJ (1996). Reduced E-cadherin expression is associated with invasiveness and unfavourable prognosis in breast cancer. *Amer J Clin Pathol* **105**, 394-402.

Silagi S, Bruce SA (1970). Suppression of malignancy and differentiation in melanotic melanoma. *Proc Natl Acad Sci USA* **66**, 72-78.

Silly H, Goldman JM, Cross NCP (1994). The mutiple tumour suppressor 1 (p16) gene in acute myeloid leukaemia and chronic myeloid leukaemia. *Blood* **83** (Suppl. 1), 297a.

Simms LA, Algar EM, Smith PJ (1995). Splicing of exon-5 in the wt1 gene disrupted in Wilms' tumour. *Eur J Cancer* **31A**, 2270-2276.

Simon M, Grone HJ, Johren O, Kullmer J, Plate KH, Risau W, Fuchs E (1995). Expression of vascular endothelial growth factor and its receptors in human renal ontogeny and in adult kidney. *Amer J Physiol* **37**, F240-F250.

Sinadinovic J, Cvejic D, Savin S, Micic JV, Jancic-Zguricas M (1989). Enhanced acid protease activity lysosomes from papillary thyroid carcinoma. *Cancer* **63**, 1179-1182.

Sinha AA, Gleason DF, Stanley NA, Wilson MJ, Sameli M, Sloane BF (1995). Cathepsin B in angiogenesis of human prostate. An immunohistochemical and immunoelectron microscopic analysis. *Anat Rec* **241**, 353-362.

Sistonen L, Keski-Oja J, Ulmanen I, Holtta E, Wikgren B, Alitalo K (1987). Dose effects of transfected c-Ha-ras (val 12) oncogene in transformed cell clones. *Exp Cell Res* **168**, 518-530.

Sivaparvathi M, Sawaya R, Wang SW, Rayford A, Yamamoto M, Liotta LA, Nicolson GL, Rao JS (1995). Over-expression and localisation of cathepsin B during the progression of human gliomas. *Clin Exp Metastasis* **13**, 49-56.

Sivaparvathi M, Yamamoto M, Nicoson GL, Gokaslan ZL, Fuller GN, Liotta LA, Sawaya R, Rao JS (1996a). Expression and immunohistochemical localisation of cathepsin L during the progression of human gliomas. *Clin Exp Metastasis* **14**, 27-34.

Sivaparvathi M, Sawaya R, Gokaslan ZL, Chintala KS, Roa JS (1996b). Expression and the role of cathepsin H in human glioma progression and invasion. *Cancer Lett* **104**, 121-126.

Slamon DJ, deKernion JB, Verma IM, Cline MJ (1984). Expression of cellular oncogenes in human malignancies. *Science* **224**, 256-262.

Slamon DJ, Clark GM, Wong S, Levin WJ, Ullrich A, McGuire WL (1987). Human breast cancer: correlation of relapse and survival with amplification of the HER-2/neu oncogene. *Science* **235**, 177-182.

Slamon DJ, Godolphin W, Jones LA, Holt JA, Wong SG, Keith DE, Levin WJ, Stuart SG, Udove J, Ullrich A, Press MT (1989). Studies of the HER-2/neu proto-oncogene in human breast and ovarian cancer. *Science* **244**, 707-712.

Slebos RJC, Lee MH, Plunkett BS, Kessis TD, Williams BO, Jacks T, Hendrick L, Kastan MB, Cho KR (1994). P53-dependent G(1) arrest involved pRB-related proteins and is disrupted by the human papillomavirus 16-E7 oncoprotein. *Proc Natl Acad Sci USA* **91**, 5320-5324.

Sloane BF (1990). Cathepsin B and cystatins. Evidence for a role in cancer progression. *Semin Cancer Biol* **1**, 137-152.

Sloane BF, Dunn JR, Honn KV (1981). Lysosomal cathepsin B: correlation with metastatic potential. *Science* **212**, 1151-1153.

Sloane BF, Honn KV, Sadler JG, Turner WA, Kimpson JJ, Taylor JD (1982). Cathepsin B activity in B16 melanoma cells. A possible marker for metastatic potential. *Cancer Res* **42**, 980-986.

Sloane BF, Moin K, Krekpela E, Rozhin J (1990). Cathepsin B and its endogenous inhibitors: the role in tumour malignancy. *Cancer Metastasis Rev* **9**, 333-352.

Smith ML, Chen IT, Zhan QM, Bae IS, Chen CY, Gilmer TM, Kastan MB, O'Connor PM, Fornace AJ (1994). Interaction of the p53-regulated protein GADD45 with proliferating cell nuclear antigen. *Science* **266**, 1376-1380.

Smolich BD, Papkoff J (1994). Regulated expression of wnt family members during neuroectodermal differentiation of P19 embryonal carcinoma cells. Overexpression of wnt-1 perturbs normal differentiation-specific properties. *Develop Biol* **166**, 300-310.

Smolich BD, McMahon JA, McMahon AP, Papkoff J (1993). Wnt family proteins are secreted and associated with the cell surface. *Mol Biol Cell* **4**, 1267-1275.

Smolle J, Soyer HP, Smollenjuettner FM, Stettner H, Kerl H (1991). Computer simulation analysis of morphological patterns in human melanocytic skin tumours. *Path Res Pract* **187**, 986-992.

Soini Y, Paakko P, Nuorva K, Kamel D, Linnala A, Virtanen I, Lehto VP (1993). Tenascin in immunoreactivity in lung tumours. *Amer J Clin Pathol* **100**, 145-150.

Soini Y, Niemela A, Kamel D, Herva R, Bloigu R, Paakko P, Vahakangas K (1994). p53 immunohistochemical positivity as a prognostic marker in intracranial tumours. *APMIS* **102**, 786-792.

Sokol SY (1993). Mesoderm formation in *Xenopus* ectodermal explants over-expressing Xwnt-8. Evidence for a co-operating signal reaching the animal pole by gastrulation. *Development* **118**, 1335-1342.

Sommerfield JH, Meeker AK, Piatyszek MA, Bova GS, Shay JW, Coffey DS (1996). Telomerase activity. A prevalent marker of malignant human prostate tissue. *Cancer Res* **56**, 218-222.

Sommers CL, Gelmann EP, Kemler R, Cowin P, Byers SW (1994). Alterations in β-catenin phosphorylation and plakoglobin expression in human breast cancer cells. *Cancer Res* **54**, 3544-3552.

Songyang Z, Shoelson SE, Chaudhuri M, Gish G, Pawson T, Haser WG, King F, Roberts T, Ratnofsky S, Lechleider RJ, Neel BG, Birge RB, Fajardo JE, Chou MM, Hanafusa H, Schaffhausen B, Cantley LC (1993). SH2 domains recognise specific phosphopeptidase sequences. *Cell* **72**, 767-778.

Sonnenberg A, Modderman PW, Hogervorst F (1988). Laminin receptor on platelets is the integrin VLA-6. *Nature* **336** 487-489.

Soussi T, Caron de Fromentel C, May P (1990). Structural aspects of the p53 protein in relation to gene evolution. *Oncogene* **5**, 945-952.

Southgate R, Ayme A, Voellmy R (1983). Nucleotide sequence analysis of the *Drosophila* small heat shock gene cluster at locus 67B. *J Mol Biol* **165**, 35-37.

Sozzi G, Miozzo M, Donbhi R, Pilotti S, Cariani CT, Pastorino U, Dellaporta G, Pierotii MA (1992). Deletions of 17p and p53 mutations in preneoplastic lesions of the lung. *Cancer Res* **52**, 6079-6082.

Spafford MF, Koeppe J, Pan ZX, Archer PG, Meyers AD, Franklin WA (1996). Correlation of tumour markers p53, blc-2, CD34, CD44-H, CD44V6, and Ki-67 with survival and metastasis in laryngeal squamous cell carcinoma. *Arch Otolaryngol* **122**, 627-632.

Spandidos DA, Agnantis NJ (1984). Human malignant tumours of the breast, as compared to their respective normal tissue, have elevated expression of Harvey *ras* oncogene. *Anticancer Res* **4**, 269-272.

Spandidos DA, Wilkie NM (1984). Malignant transformation of early passage rodent cells by a single mutated human oncogene. *Nature* **310**, 469-475.

Spector NL, Samson W, Ryan C, Gribben J, Urba W, Welch WJ, Nadler LM (1992). Growth arrest of human lymphocytes B is accompanied by induction of the low molecular weight mammalian heat shock protein (HSP28). *J Immunol* **148**, 1668-1673.

Spector NL, Ryan C, Samson W, Levine H, Nadler LM, Arrigo AP (1993). Heat shock protein is a unique marker of growth arrest during macrophage differentiation of HL-60 cells. *J Cell Physiol* **156**, 619-625.

Spector NL, Mehlen P, Ryan C, Hardy L, Samson W, Levine H, Nadler LM, Fabre N, Arrigo AP (1994). Regulation of the 28 kDa heat shock protein by retinoic acid during differentiation of human leukaemic HL-60 cells. *FEBS Lett* **337**, 184-188.

Sporn MB, Roberts AB (1987). Peptide growth factors: current status and therapeutic opportunities. In: *Important Advances in Oncology*, De Vita V, Jr, Hellman S, Rosenberg SA (eds). Lippincott, Philadelphia PA, pp. 75-86.

Sporn MB, Roberts AB (1988). Peptide growth factors are multi-functional. *Nature* **332**, 217-219.

Sporn MB, Roberts AB, Wakefield LM, de Cromburgghe B (1987). Some recent advances in the chemistry and biology of transforming growth factor beta. *J Cell Biol* **105**, 1039-1045.

Springer TA (1990). Adhesion receptors of the immune systems. *Nature* **346**, 425-434.

Springman EB, Angleton EL, Birkedal-Hansen H, van Wart HE (1990). Multiple modes of activation of latent human fibroblast collagenase. Evidence for the role of a cys-73 active site zinc complex in latency and a cysteine switch mechanism for activation. *Proc Natl Acad Sci USA* **87** 364-368.

Spyratos F, Delarue JC, Andrieu C, Lidereau R, Champeme MH, Hacene K, Brunet M (1990). Epidermal growth factor receptors and prognosis in primary breast cancer. *Breast Cancer Res Treat* **17**, 83-89.

Sreenath T, Matrisian LM, Stetler-Stevenson WG, Gattoni-Celli S, Pozzatti RO (1992). Expression of matrix metalloproteinase genes in transformed rat cell lines of high and low metastatic potential. *Cancer Res* **52**, 4942-4947.

Stal O, Hatschek T, Carstensen J, Nordenskjold B (1991). DNA analysis in the management of breast cancer. *Diagnostic Oncol* **1**, 140-154.

Stahl JA, Leone A, Rosengard AM, Porter L, Richter-King C, Steeg PS (1991). Identification of a second human nm23 gene, nm23-H2. *Cancer Res* **51**, 445-449.

Starnaud R, Moir JM (1993). Wnt-1 inducing factor-1. A novel G/C box-binding transcription factor regulating the expression of wnt-1 during neuroectodermal differentiation. *Mol Cell Biol* **13**, 1590-1598.

Starzynska T, Bromley M, Ghosh A, Stern PL (1992). Prognostic significance of p53 over-expression in gastric and colorectal cancer. *Br J Cancer* **66**, 558-562.

Staunton DE, Marlin SD, Stratowa C (1994). Primary structure of intercellular adhesion molecule (ICAM-1) demonstrates interaction between members of the immunoglobulin and integrin supergene families. *Cell* **56**, 849-853.

Steeg PS, Bevilacqua G, Kopper L, Thorgierson VP, Talmadge JE, Liotta LA, Sobel ME (1988a). Evidence for a novel gene associated with low tumour metastatic potential. *J Natl Cancer Inst* **80**, 200-204.

Steeg PS, Bevilacqua G, Pozzatti R, Liotta LA, Sobel ME (1988b). Altered expression of nm23, a gene associated with low tumour metastatic potential, during adenovirus 2 EIA inhibition of experimental metastasis. *Cancer Res* **48**, 6550-6554.

Steeg PS, Leone A, Rosengard A, King CR, Stahl J, Flatow U, Liotta LA (1990). A novel gene nm23 is associated with low tumour metastatic potential. *Clin Exp Metastasis* **8** (Suppl. 1), 16.

Stegmaier K, Pendse S, Barker GF, Brayward P, Ward DC (1995). Frequent loss of heterozygosity at the *tel* gene locus in acute lymphoblastic leukaemia of childhood. *Blood* **86**, 38-44.

Steinbach F, Tanabe K, Alexander J, Edinger M, Tubbs R, Brenner W, Stockle M, Novick AC, Klein EA (1996). The influence of cytokines on the adhesion of renal cancer cells to endothelium. *J Urol* **155**, 743-748.

Steinman HM (1995). The bcl-2 oncoprotein functions as a pro-oxidant. *J Biol Chem* **270**, 3487–3490.

Steinman RA, Hoffman B, Iro A, Guillouf C, Liebermann DA, El Houseine ME (1994). Induction of p21 (WAF1/CIP1) during differentiation. *Oncogene* **9**, 3389–3396.

Stenger J, Mayr GA, Mann K, Tegtmeyer P (1992). Formation of stable p53 homotetramers and multiples of tetramers. *Mol Carcinogen* **5**, 102–106.

Stenmark-Askmalm M, Stal O, Sullivan S, Ferraud L, Sun XF, Carstensen J, Nordenskjold B (1994). Cellular accumulation of p53 protein: an independent prognostic factor in stage II breast cancer. *Eur J Cancer* **30A**, 175–180.

Stern DF, Heffernan PA, Weinberg RA (1986). P185, a product of the neu proto-oncogene, is a receptor-like protein associated with tyrosine kinase activity. *Mol Cell Biol* **6**, 1729–1740.

Stetler-Stevenson WG, Krutzsch HC, Liotta LA (1989a). Tissue specific inhibitor of metalloproteinase (TIMP-2): a new member of the metalloproteinase family. *J Biol Chem* **264**, 17374–17378.

Stetler-Stevenson WG, Krutzsch HC, Wacher MP, Margulies IMK, Liotta LA (1989b). The activation of type IV collagenase proenzyme: sequence identification of the major conversion product following organomercurial activation. *J Biol Chem* **264**, 1353–1356.

Stetler-Stevenson WG, Liotta LA, Kleiner DE, Jr (1993). Extracellular matrix 6: Role of matrix metalloproteinases in tumour invasion and metastasis. *FASEB J* **7**, 1434–1441.

Stevenson MA, Calderwood SK (1990). Members of the 70 kilodalton heat shock protein family contain a highly conserved calmodulin binding domain. *Mol Cell Biol* **10**, 1234–1238.

Stewart N, Hicks GG, Paraskevas F, Mowat M (1995). Evidence for a second cell cycle block at G2/M by p53. *Oncogene* **10**, 109–115.

Stoolman LM (1989). Adhesion molecules controlling lymphocyte migration. *Cell* **56**, 907–910.

Stoppelli M, Tacchertti C, Cubellis M, Corti A, Hearing V, Cassani G, Appella E, Blasi F (1986). Autocrine saturation of pro-urokinase receptors on human A431 cells. *Cell* **45**, 675–684.

Stralfors P, Hiraga A, Cohen P (1985). The protein phophatases involved in cellular regulation. *Eur J Biochem* **149**, 295–303.

Strasser A, Whittingham S, Vaux DL, Bath ML, Adams JM, Cory S, Harris AW (1991). Enforced bcl-2 expression in B-lymphoid cells prolongs antibody responses and elicits autoimmune disease. *Proc Natl Acad Sci USA* **88**, 8661–8665.

Stratton MR, Williams S, Fisher C, Ball A, Westbury G, Gusterson BA, Fletcher CDM, Knight JC, Fung YK, Reeves BR, Cooper CS (1989). Structural alterations of the RB1 gene in human soft tissue tumours. *Br J Cancer* **60**, 202–205.

Stretch JR, Gatter KC, Ralfkiaer E, Lane DP, Harris AL (1991). Expression of mutant p53 in melanoma. *Cancer Res* **51**, 5976–5979.

Strickler JG, Zheng J, Shu QP, Burgart LJ, Alberts SR, Shibata D (1994). P53 mutations and microsatellite instability in sporadic gastric cancer. When guardians fail. *Cancer Res* **54**, 4750–4755.

Stricklin GP, Welgus HG (1983). Human skin fibroblast collagenase inhibitor. Purification and biochemical characterisation. *J Biol Chem* **258**, 2252–2258.

Strohmeyer T, Reissmann P, Cordon-Cardo C, Hartmann M, Ackermann RM, Slamon D (1991). Correlation between retinoblastoma gene expression and differentiation in human testicular tumours. *Proc Natl Acad Sci USA* **88**, 6662–6666.

Stubblefield E, Sanford J (1987). A general survey of genetics and cancer. *Anticancer Res* **7**, 1132–1104.

Sturzbecher HW, Chumakov P, Welch WJ, Jenkins JR (1987). Mutant p53 proteins bind hsp72/73 cellular heat shock related proteins in SV40-transformed monkey cells. *Oncogene* **1**, 201-211.

Sturzbecher HW, Addison C, Jenkins JR (1988). Characterisation of mutant p53-hsp 72/73 protein-protein complexes by transient expression in monkey COS cells. *Mol Cell Biol* **8**, 3740-3747.

Sturzbecher HW, Maimets T, Chumakov P, Brain R, Addison C, Simanin V, Rudge K, Philip R, Grimaldi M, Court W, Jenkins JR (1990). p53 interacts with p34^{cdc2} in mammalian cells: Implications for cell cycle control and oncogenesis. *Oncogene* **5**, 795-801.

Su LK, Burrell M, Hill DE, Gyuris J, Brent R, Wiltshire R, Trent J, Vogelstein B, Kinzler KW (1995). APC binds to the novel protein EB1. *Cancer Res* **55**, 2972-2977.

Subler MA, Martin DW, Deb S (1992). Inhibition of viral and cellular promoters by human wild type p53. *J Virol* **66**, 4757-4762.

Sueyoshi T, Uwani M, Itoh N, Okamoto H, Muta T, Tokunaga F, Takada K, Iwanaga S (1990). Cysteine proteinase inhibitor in the ascitic fluid of sarcoma 180 tumour-bearing mice is a low molecular weight kininogen. *J Biol Chem* **265**, 10030-10035.

Sugarbaker EV (1979). Cancer metastasis. A product of tumour host interactions. *Curr Prob Cancer* **3**, 1-59.

Sugerman PB, Savage NW, Xu LJ, Walsh LJ, Seymour GJ (1995). Heat shock protein expression in oral epithelial dysplasia and squamous cell carcinoma. *Oral Oncol Eur J Cancer B* **31B**, 63-67.

Sukoh N, Abe S, Nakajima I, Ogura S, Isobe H, Inoue K, Kawakami Y (1994). Immunohistochemical distributions of cathepsin B and basement membrane antigens in human lung adenodarcinoma. Association with invasion and metastasis. *Virchows Arch Pathol* **424**, 33-38.

Sulekova Z, Reinasanchez J, Ballhausen WG (1995). Multiple APC messenger RNA isoforms encoding exon-15 sort open reading frames are expressed in the context of a novel exon-10A-derived sequence. *Int J Cancer* **63**, 435-441.

Sun XF, Carstensen JM, Zhang H, Stal O, Wingren S, Haschek T, Nordenskjold B (1992). Prognostic significance of cytoplasmic p53 oncoprotein in colorectal adenocarcinoma. *Lancet* **340**, 1369-1373.

Sun XF, Carstensen JM, Stal O, Zhang H, Nilsson E, Sjodahl R, Nordenskjold B (1993). Prognostic significance of p53 expression in relation to DNA ploidy in colorectal adenocarcinoma. *Virchows Arch B* **423**, 443-448.

Sunderkotter C, Goebeler M, Schulze-Osthoff K, Bhardway R, Sorg C (1991). Macrophage derived angiogenesis factors. *Pharmacol Ther* **51**, 195-216.

Sutherland GR (1979). Heritable fragile sites on human chromosomes. I. Factors affecting expression in lymphocyte culture. *Amer J Human Genet* **31**, 125-135.

Suzuki H, Sugihira N (1993). Prognostic value of DNA ploidy in primary gastric leiomyosarcoma. *Br J Surg* **80**, 1549-1550.

Suzuki H, Harpaz N, Tarmin L, Yin J, Jiang HY, Bell JD, Hontanosas M, Groisman GM, Abraham JM, Meltzer SJ (1994). Microsatellite instability in ulcerative colitis-associated colorectal dysplasias and cancers. *Cancer Res* **54**, 4841-4844.

Suzuki S, Sano K, Tanihara H (1991). Diversity of the cadherin family: evidence for eight new cadherins in nervous tissue. *Cell Regulation* **2**, 261-270.

Swift M, Morrell D, Massey RB, Chase CL (1991). Incidence of cancer in 161 families affected by ataxia telangiectasia. *N Engl J Med* **325**, 1831-1836.

Sy MS, Guo YJ, Stamenkovic I (1991). Distinct effects of two CD44 isoforms on tumour growth *in vivo*. *J Exp Med* **174**, 859-866.

Syrigos KN, Krausz T, Waxman J, Pandha H, Rowlinson-Busza G, Verne J, Epenetos AA, Pignatelli M (1995). E-cadherin expression in bladder cancer using formalin fixed paraffin embedded tissues. Correlation with histopathological, grade tumour size and survival. *Int J Cancer* **64**, 367-370.

Szabo CI, King MC (1995). Inherited breast and ovarian cancer. *Human Mol Genet* **4**, 1811-1817.

Szekanecz Z, Haines GK, Lin TR, Harlow LA, Goerdt S, Rayan G, Koch AE (1994). Differential distribution of intercellular adhesion molecules (ICAM-1, ICAM-2, and ICAM-3) and the MS-1 antigen in normal and diseased human synovia. Their possible pathogenetic and clinical significance in rheumatoid arthritis. *Arthritis Rheumatism* **37**, 221-231.

Takada A, Ohmori K, Takahashi N, Tsuyuoka Y, Yago A, Zenita K, Hasegawa A, Kannagi R (1991). Adhesion of human cancer cells to vascular endothelium mediated by a carbohydrate antigen, sialyl Lewis A. *Biochem Biophys Res Commun* **179**, 713-719.

Takada A, Ohmori K, Yoneda T, Tsuyuoka K, Kasegawa A, Kiso M, Kannagi R (1993). Contribution of carbohydrate antigens sialyl Lewis-A and sialyl Lewis-X to adhesion of human cancer cells to vascular endothelium. *Cancer Res* **53**, 354-361.

Takahashi K, Isobe T, Ohtsuki Y, Akagi T, Sonobe H, Okuyama T (1984). Immunohistochemical study on the distribution of α and β subunits of S100 protein in human neoplasms and normal tissues. *Virchows Arch Cell Pathol* **45**, 385-396.

Takahashi S, Mikami T, Watanabe Y, Okazaki M, Okazaki Y, Okazaki A, Sato T, Asaishi K, Hirata K, Narimatusu E, Mori M, Sato N, Kikuchi I (1994). Correlation of heat shock protein 70 expression with oestrogen receptor levels in invasive human breast cancer. *Amer J Clin Pathol* **101**, 519-525.

Takamatsu K, Auerbach LB, Gerardyschahn R, Eckhardt M, Jaques G, Madry N (1994). Characterisation of tumour associated neural cell adhesion molecule in human serum. *Cancer Res* **54**, 2598-2603.

Takano S, Gately S, Neville ME, Herblin WF, Gross JL (1994). Suramin, an anticancer and angiosuppressive agent, inhibits endothelial cell binding of basic fibroblast growth factor, migration, proliferation and induction of urokinase-type plasminogen activator. *Cancer Res* **54**, 2654-2660.

Takayama T, Shiozaki H, Inoue M, Tamura S, Oka H, Kadowaki T, Takatsuka V, Nagafuchi A, Tsukita S, Mori T (1994). Expression of E-cadherin and α-catenin molecules in human breast cancer tissues and association with clinicopathological features. *Int J Oncol* **5**, 775-780.

Takeda M, Yamamoto M, Hasegawa Y, Saitoh Y (1995). Endothelial leukocyte adhesion molecule-1 mediated vasoinvasion of human pancreatic adenocarcinoma. *J Surg Res* **59**, 653-657.

Takeichi M (1988). The cadherins: Cell-cell adhesion molecules controlling animal morphogenesis. *Development* **102**, 639-655.

Takeichi M (1990). Cadherins: a molecular family important in selective cell-cell adhesion. *Annu Rev Biochem* **59**, 237-252.

Takeichi M (1991). Cadherin cell adhesion receptors as a morphogenetic regulator. *Science* **251**, 1451-1455.

Takemura H, Hughes AR, Thastrup O, Putney JW (1989). Activation of calcium entry by the tumour promoter thapsigargin in parotid acinar cells. *J Biol Chem* **264**, 12266-12271.

Takenaga K, Nakamura Y, Sakiyama S, Hasegawa Y, Sato K, Endo H (1994a). Binding of pEL98 protein, an S100-related protein, to nonmuscle tropomyosin. *J Cell Biol* **124**, 757-768.

Takenaga K, Nakamura Y, Sakiyama S (1994b). Expression of a calcium-binding protein pEL98 (mts1) during differentiation of human promyelocytic leukaemia HL-60 cells. *Biochem Biophys Res Commun* **202**, 94-101.

Takenaga K, Nakamura Y, Endo H, Sakiyama S (1994c). Involvement of S100-related calcium binding protein pEL98 (mts1) in cell motility and tumour cell invasion. *Jap J Cancer Res* **85**, 831-839.

Takeuchi K, Yamaguchi A, Urano T, Goi T, Nakagawara G, Shiku M (1995). Expression of CD44 variant exons 8-10 in colorectal cancer and its relationship to metastasis. *Jpn J Cancer Res* **86**, 292-297.

Takeuchi S, Bartram CR, Wada DM, Reiter A, Hatta Y, Seriu T, Lee E, Miller CW, Miyoshi I, Koeffler HP (1995). Allelotype analysis of childhood acute lymphoblastic leukaemia. *Cancer Res* **55**, 5377-5382.

Takigawa M, Nishida Y, Suzuki F, Kishi JI, Yamashita K, Hayakawa T (1990a). Induction of angiogenesis in chick yolk sac membrane by polyamines and its inhibition by tissue inhibitors of metalloproteinases (TIMP-1 and TIMP-2). *Biochem Biophys Res Commun* **171**, 1264-1271.

Takigawa M, Enomoto M, Nishida Y, Pan HO, Kinoshita A, Suzuki F (1990b). Tumour angiogenesis and polyamines: α-difluoromethylornithine, an irreversible inhibitor of orthinine decarboxylase, inhibits B16 melanoma-induced angiogenesis *in ovo* and the proliferation of vascular endothelial cells *in vitro*. *Cancer Res* **50**, 4131-4138.

Talmadge JE, Benedict K, Madsen J, Fidler IJ (1984). Development of biological diversity and susceptibility to chemotherapy in murine cancer metastasis. *Cancer Res* **41**, 3801-3805.

Tamura G, Maesawa C, Suzuki Y, Tamada H, Satoh M, Ogasawara S, Kashiwaba M, Satodate R (1994). Mutations of the APC gene occur during early stages of gastric adenoma development. *Cancer Res* **54**, 1149-1151.

Tanabe KK, Ellis LM, Saya H (1993). Expression of CD44R1 adhesion molecule in colon carcinomas and metastases. *Lancet* **341**, 725-726.

Tanaka N, Ishihara M, Kitagawa M, Harada H, Kimura T, Matsuyama T, Lamphier MS, Aizawa S, Mak TW, Taniguchi T (1994). Cellular commitment to oncogene-induced transformation or apoptosis is dependent on the transcription factor IRF-1. *Cell* **77**, 829-839.

Tanda N, Kawakami Y, Saito T, Noji S, Nohno T (1995). Cloning and characterisation of wnt-4 and wnt-11 cDNAs from chick embryo. *DNA Seq* **5**, 277-281.

T'Ang A, Varley JM, Chakraborty S, Murphree AL, Fung YKT (1988). Structural rearrangement of the retinoblastoma gene in human breast carcinoma. *Science* **242**, 263-266.

Tangir J, Muto MG, Berkowitz RS, Welch WR, Bell DA, Mok SC (1996). A 400 kb novel deletion unit centromeric to the BRCA1 gene in sporadic epithelial ovarian cancer. *Oncogene* **12**, 735-740.

Tarabykina S, Ambartsumian N, Grigorian M, Gerogiev G, Lukanidin EM (1996). Activation of *mts1* transcription by insertion of a retrovirus-like IAP element. *Gene* **168**, 151-155.

Tay JSH (1995). Molecular genetics of Wilms tumour. *J Paediat Child Health* **31**, 379-383.

Taylor RS, Ramirez RD, Ogoshi M, Chaffins M, Piatyszek MA, Shay JW (1996). Detection of telomerase activity in malignant and non-malignant skin conditions. *J Invest Dermatol* **106**, 759-765.

Templeton DJ, Parks SH, Lanier L, Weinberg RA (1991). Non-functional mutants of retinoblastoma protein are characterised by defects in phosphorylation, viral oncoprotein association and nuclear tethering. *Proc Natl Acad Sci USA* **88**, 3033-3037.

Teramoto T, Satonaka K, Kitazawa S, Fujimori T, Hayashi K, Maeda S (1994). *p53* gene abnormalities are closely related to hepatoviral infections and occur at a late stage of hepatocarcinogenesis. *Cancer Res* **54**, 231-235.

Terman BI, Carrion ME, Kovacs E, Rasmussen BA, Eddy RL, Shows TB (1991). Identification of a new endothelial cell growth factor receptor tyrosine kinase. *Oncogene* **6**, 1677-1683.

Terman BI, Dougher-Vermazen M, Carrion ME, Dimitrov D, Armellino DC, Gospodarowicz D, Bohlen P (1992). Identification of the KDR tyrosine kinase as a receptor for vascular endothelial cell growth factor. *Biochem Biophys Res Commun* **187**, 1579-1586.

Tervahauta A, Eskelinen M, Syrjanen S, Lipponen P, Pajarinen P, Syrjanen K (1991). Immuno-histochemical demonstration of c-erbB2 oncoprotein expression in female breast cancer and its prognostic significance. *Anticancer Res* **11**, 1677-1682.

Tetu B, Brisson J, Cote C, Brisson S, Potvin D, Roberge N (1993). Prognostic significance of cathepsin D in node-positive breast carcinoma. An immunohistochemical study. *Int J Cancer* **55**, 429-435.

Thastrup O, Cullen PJ, Drobak BK, Hanley MR, Dawson AP (1989). Thapsigargin, a tumour promoter, discharges intracellular Ca^{2+} stores by specific inhibition of the endoplasmic reticulum Ca^{2+}-ATPase. *Proc Natl Acad Sci USA* **87**, 2466-2470.

Theile M, Hartmann S, Scherthan H, Arnold W, Deppert W, Frege R, Glaab F, Haensch W, Scherneck S (1995). Suppression of tumorigenicity of breast cancer cells by transfer of human chromosome 17 does not require transferred BRCA1 and p53 genes. *Oncogene* **10**, 439-447.

Thibodeau SN, Bren G, Schaid D (1993). Microsatellite instability in cancer of the proximal colon. *Science* **260**, 816-819.

Thliveris A, Samowitz W, Matsunami N, Groden J, White R (1994). Demonstration of promoter activity and alternative splicing in the region 5' to exon-1 of the APC gene. *Cancer Res* **54**, 2991-2995.

Thomas KA, Gimenez-Gallego G (1986). Fibroblast growth factors: Broad spectrum mitogens with potent angiogenic activity. *Trends Biochem Sci* **11**, 81-84.

Thomas WS, Oltvai ZN, Yang E, Wang K, Boise LH, Thompson CB, Korsmeyer SJ (1995). Multiple bcl-2 family members demonstrate selective dimerisations with bax. *Proc Natl Acad Sci USA* **92**, 7834-7838.

Thompson EW, Reich R, Shima TB, Albini A, Graf G, Martin GR, Dickson RB, Lippman ME (1988). Differential regulation of growth and invasiveness of MCF7 breast cancer cells by antiestrogens. *Cancer Res* **48**, 6764-6788.

Thompson EW, Katz D, Shima TB, Wakeling AE, Lippman ME, Dickson RB (1989). ICI 164,384 a pure antagonist of estrogen-stimulated MCF7 cell proliferation and invasiveness. *Cancer Res* **49**, 6929-6939.

Thompson EW, Nakamura S, Shima TB, Melchiori A, Martin GR, Salahuddin SZ, Gallo RC, Albini A (1991). Supernatants of acquired immunodeficiency syndrome-related Kaposi's sarcoma cells induce endothelial cell chemotaxis and invasiveness. *Cancer Res* **51**, 2670-2676.

Thompson EW, Brunner N, Torri J, Johnson MD, Boulay V, Wright A, Lippman ME, Steeg PS, Clarke R (1993). The invasive and metastatic properties of hormone-independent but hormone responsive variants of MCF-7 human breast cancer cells. *Clin Exp Metastasis* **11**, 15-26.

Thompson ME, Zimmer WE, Haynes AL, Valentine DL, Forss-Petter S, Scammell JG (1992). Prolactin granulogenesis is associated with increased secretogranin and aggregation in the golgi apparatus of GH4C1 cells. *Endocrinol* **131**, 318-326

Thompson ME, Jensen RA, Obermiller PS, Page DL, Holt JT (1995). Decreased expression of BRCA1 accelerates growth and is often present during sporadic breast cancer progression. *Nature Genet* **9**, 444-450.

Thomssen C, Schmitt M, Goretzki L, Oppelt P, Pache L, Dettmar P, Janicke F, Graeff H (1995).

Prognostic value of the cysteine proteases cathepsin B and cathepsin L in human breast cancer. *Clin Cancer Res* **1**, 741-746.

Thorlacius S, Jonasdottir O, Eyfjord JE (1991). Loss of heterozygosity at selective sites on chromosomes 13 and 17 in human breast carcinoma. *Anticancer Res* **11**, 1501-1508.

Tiemeyer M, Swiesler SJ, Ishihara M, Moreland M, Schweingruber H, Hirtzer P, Brandley BK (1991). Carbohydrate ligands for endothelial-leukocyte adhesion molecule-1. *Proc Natl Acad Sci USA* **88**, 1138-1142,

Timpl R (1989). Structure and biological activity of basement membrane proteins. *Eur J Biochem* **180**, 487-502.

Tischer E, Mitchell R, Hartman T, Silva M, Gospodarowicz D, Fiddes JC, Abraham JA (1991). The human gene for vascular endothelial growth factor. Multiple protein forms are encoded through alternative exon splicing. *J Biol Chem* **266**, 11947-11954.

Tissieres A, Mitchell HK, Tracy UM (1974). Protein synthesis in salivary gland of *Drosophila melanogaster*: relation to chromosome puffs. *J Mol Biol* **85**, 389-398.

Tiwari RK, Borgen PI, Wong GY, Cordon-Cardo C, Osborne MP (1992). HER-2/neu amplification and over-expression in primary human breast cancer is associated with early metastasis. *Anticancer Res* **12**, 419-426.

Tlsty TD (1990). Normal diploid human and rodent cells lack a detectable frequency of gene amplification. *Proc Natl Acad Sci USA* **86**, 3231-3236.

Tlsty TD, Margolin BH, Lum K (1989). Differences in the rates of gene amplification in nontumorigenic and tumorigenic cell lines as measured by Luria-Delbruck fluctuation analysis. *Proc Natl Acad Sci USA* **86**, 9441-9445.

Toguchida J, Ishizaki K, Sasaki MS, Ikenaga M, Suginoto M, Kotoura Y, Yamamuro T (1988). Chromosomal reorganisation for the expression of recessive mutation of retinoblastoma susceptibility gene in the development of osteosarcoma. *Cancer Res* **48**, 3939-3943.

Toguchida J, Yamaguchi T, Ritchie B, Beauchamp RL, Dayton SH, Herrera GE, Yamamuro T, Kotoura Y, Sasaki MS, Little JB, Weichselbaum RR, Ishizaki K, Yandell DW (1992). Mutation spectrum of the p53 gene in bone and soft tissue sarcoma. *Cancer Res* **52**, 6194-6199.

Toh Y, Pencil SD, Nicolson GL (1994). A novel candidate metastasis-associated gene, mta1, differentially expressed in highly metastatic mammary adenocarcinoma cell lines: cDNA cloning, expression, and protein analysis. *J Biol Chem* **269**, 22958-22963.

Toh Y, Pencil SD, Nicolson GL (1995). Analysis of the complete sequence of the novel metastasis-associated candidate gene, *mta1*, differentially expressed in mammary adeno-carcinoma and breast cancer cell lines. *Gene* **159**, 97-104.

Toi M, Nakamura T, Mukaida H, Wada T, Osaki A, Yamada H, Toge T, Nimoto M, Hattori T (1990). Relationship between epidermal growth factor receptor status and various prognostic factors in human breast cancer. *Cancer* **65**, 1980-1984.

Tommasi S, Pardiso A, Mangia A, Barletta A, Simone G, Slamon DJ, De Lena M (1991). Biological correlation between HER-2/neu and proliferative activity of human breast cancer. *Anticancer Res* **11**, 1395-1400.

Tonini GP, Casalaro A, Cara A, Dimartino D (1991). Inducible expression of calcyclin, a gene with strong homology to S-100 protein, during neuroblastoma cell differentiation and its prevalent expression in Schwann-like cell lines. *Cancer Res* **51**, 1733-1737.

Touitou I, Cavailles V, Garcia M, Defrenne A, Rochefort H (1988). Differential regulation of cathepsin D by sex steroids in mammary cancer and uterine cells. *Mol Cell Endocrinol* **66**, 231-238.

Tozawa K, Sakurada S, Kohri K, Okamoto T (1995). Effects of antinuclear factor Kappa B reagents in blocking adhesion of human cancer cells to vascular endothelial cells. *Cancer Res* **55**, 4162-4167.

Tozeren A, Kleinman HK, Grant DS, Morales D, Mercurio AM, Byers SW (1995). E-selectin mediated dynamic interactions of breast cancer and colon cancer cells with endothelial cell monolayers. *Int J Cancer* **60**, 426-431.

Trent JM (1985). Cytogenetic and molecular biologic alterations in human breast cancer: review. *Breast Cancer Res Treat* **5**, 221-229.

Trent JM, Wiltshire R, Su LK, Nicolaides NC, Vogelstein B, Kinzler KW (1995). The gene for the APC-binding protein β-catenin (CTNNB1) maps to chromosome 3p22, a region frequently altered in human malignancies. *Cytogenet Cell Genet* **71**, 343-344.

Tsang TC (1993). New model for 7 kDa heat shock proteins potential mechanism of action. *FEBS Lett* **323**, 1-3.

Tsuda H, Hirohashi S, Shimosato Y, Hirota T, Tsugane S, Yamamoto H, Miyajima N, Toyoshima K, Yamamoto T, Yokota J, Yoshida T, Sakamoto H, Terada M, Sugimura T (1989). Correlation between long term survival in breast cancer patients and amplification of two putative oncogene co-amplification units hst1/int-2 and c-erbB2/ear-1. *Cancer Res* **49**, 3104-3108.

Tsuda H, Iwaya K, Fukutomi T, Hirohashi S (1993). p53 mutations and c-*erb*B2 amplification in intraductal and invasive breast carcinomas of high histologic grade. *Jpn J Cancer Res* **84**, 394-401.

Tsuda T, Tahara E, Kajiyama G, Sakamoto H, Terada M, Sugimura T (1989). High incidence of co-amplification of hst-1 and int-2 genes in human oesophageal carcinomas. *Cancer Res* **49**, 5505-5508.

Tsujimoto Y, Cossman J, Jaffe E, Croce CM (1985a). Involvement of the bcl-2 gene in human follicular lymphoma. *Science* **228**, 1440-1443.

Tsujimoto Y, Gorham J, Cossman J, Jaffe E, Croce CM (1985b). The t(14;18) chromosome translocation involved in B-cell neoplasms result from mistakes in VDJ joining. *Science* **229**, 1390-1393.

Tsujimoto Y, Bashir MM, Givol I, Cossman J, Jaffe E, Croce CM (1987). DNA rearrangements in human follicular lymphoma can involve the 5' or the 3' region of the bcl-2 gene. *Proc Natl Acad Sci USA* **84**, 1329-1331.

Tsushima H, Sumi H, Ikeda R, Mihara H, Hopsu-Havu VK (1989). Purification and characterisation of a cathepsin D-like enzyme from human melanoma tissue and its action on fibrinogen. *Eur Rev Med Pharmacol Sci* **11**, 451-461.

Tsutsumiishii Y, Tadokoro K, Hanaoka F, Tsuchida N (1995). Response of heat shock element within the human HSP70 promoter to mutated p53 genes. *Cell Growth Differen* **6**, 1-8.

Tuck SP, Crawford L (1989). Characterisation of the human p53 gene promoter. *Mol Cell Biol* **9**, 2163-2172.

Tulchinsky E, Grigorian MS, Ebralidze AK, Milshina NI, Lukanidin EM (1990). Structure of gene *mts1*, transcribed in metastatic tumour cells. *Gene* **87**, 219-223,

Tulchinsky E, Ford HL, Kramerov D, Reshetnyak E, Grigorian M, Zain S, Lukanidin E (1992). Transcriptional analysis of the *mts1* gene with specific references to 5' flanking sequences. *Proc Natl Acad Sci USA* **89**, 9146-9150.

Tulchinsky E, Kramerov D, Ford HL, Reshetnyak E, Lukanidin E, Zain S (1993). Characterisation of a positive regulatory element in the *mts1* gene. *Oncogene* **8**, 79-86.

Tulchinsky E, Grigorian M, Tkatch T, Georgiev G, Lukanidin E (1995). Transcriptional regulation of the *mts1* gene in human lymphoma cells: the role of DNA methylation. *Biochim Biophys Acta* **1261**, 243-248.

Turleau C, De Grouchy J, Chavin-Colin F, Martelli H, Voyer M, Charlas R (1984). Trisomy 11p15 and Beckwith-Wiedemann syndrome. A report of two cases. *Human Genet* **67**, 219-221.

Turley EA, Tretiak M (1985). Glycosaminoglycan production by murine melanoma variants *in vivo* and *in vitro*. *Cancer Res* **45**, 5098-5105.

Turley H, Pezzella F, Kocialkowski S, Comley M, Kaklamanis L, Fawcet J, Simmons D, Harris AL, Gatter KC (1995). The distribution of the deleted in colon cancer (DCC) protein in human tissues. *Cancer Res* **55**, 5628-5631.

Turpeenniemi-Hujanen T, Thorgeirsson UP, Hart IR, Grant SS, Liotta LA (1985). Expression of collagenase IV (basement membrane collagenase) activity in murine tumour cell hybrids that differ in metastatic potential. *J Natl Cancer Inst* **75**, 99-103.

Uchida T, Wada LC, Wang CX, Egawa S, Ohtani H, Koshiba K (1994). Genomic instability of microsatellite repeats and mutations of H-, K-, and N-ras and p53 genes in renal cell carcinoma. *Cancer Res* **54**, 3682-3685.

Ueki K, Rubio MP, Ramesh V, Correa KM, Rutter JL, Vondeimling A, Buckler AJ, Gusella JF, Louis DN (1994). MTS1/CDKN2 gene mutations are rare in primary human astrocytomas with allelic loss of chromosome 9p. *Human Mol Genet* **3**, 1841-1845.

Ueki N, Nakazato M, Ohkawa T, Ikeda T, Amluro Y, Hada T, Higashino K (1992). Excessive production of transforming growth factor $\beta 1$ can play an important role in the development of tumorigenesis by its action for angiogenesis: validity of neutralising antibodies to block tumour growth. *Biochim Biophys Acta* **1137**, 189-196.

Ueki T, Koji T, Tamiya S, Nakane PK, Tsuneyoshi M (1995). Expression of basic fibroblast growth factor and fibroblast growth factor receptors in advanced gastric carcinoma. *J Pathol* **177**, 353-361.

Uff CR, Neame SJ and Isacke CM (1995). Hyaluronan binding by CD44 is regulated by a phosphorylation-independent mechanism. *Eur J Immunol* **25**, 1883-1887.

Uhlsteidl M, Mullerholzner E, Zeimet AG, Adolf GR, Daxenbichler G, Marth C, Daput O (1995). Prognostic value of CD44 splice variant expression in ovarian cancer. *Oncology* **52**, 400-406.

Umar A, Boyer JC, Thomas DC, Nguyen DC, Risinger JI, Boyd J, Ionov Y, Perucho M, Kunkel TA (1994). Defective mismatch repair in extracts of colorectal and endometrial cancer cell lines exhibiting microsatellite instability. *J Biol Chem* **269**, 14367-14370.

Umesh M, Wolf D, Frossard PM (1988). *Ban*II and *Sca*I RFLPs at the human p53 gene locus. *Nucleic Acids Res* **16**, 7757.

Underwood M, Bartlett J, Reeves J, Gardiner DS, Scott R, Cooke T (1995). C-erbB2 gene amplification: a molecular marker in recurrent bladder tumours? *Cancer Res* **55**, 2422-2430.

Ura H, Denno R, Hirata K (1996). Correlation between nm23 protein and several cell adhesion molecules in human gastric carcinoma. *Jpn J Cancer Res* **87**, 512-517.

Urano T, Fushida S, Furukawa K, and Shiku H (1992). Human nm23-H1 protein and H2 protein have similar nucleoside diphosphate kinase activities. *Int J Cancer* **1**, 425-430.

Usmani BA (1993). *Genomic instability and the metastatic potential of B16 murine melanomas*, Ph.D. thesis, University of Newcastle upon Tyne, UK.

Usmani BA, Sherbet GV (1996). Homologous recombination in variants of the B16 murine melanoma with reference to their metastatic potential. *J Cell Biochem* **61**, 1-8.

Usmani BA, Lunec J, Sherbet GV (1993). DNA repair and repair fidelity in metastatic variants of the B16 murine melanoma. *J Cell Biochem* **51**, 336-344.

Vairo G, Livingston DM, Ginsberg D (1995). Functional interaction between E2F-4 and p130: evidence for distinct mechanisms underlying growth suppression by different retinoblastoma protein family members. *Genes Develop* **9**, 869-881.

Vallee BL, Auld DS (1990). Active site zinc ligands and activated H₂O of zinc enzymes. *Proc Natl Acad Sci USA* **87**, 220-224.

Valverius EM, Velu T, Shankar V, Ciardiello F, Kim C, Salomon DS (1990). Over-expression of the epidermal growth factor receptor in human breast cancer cells fails to induce estrogen-independent phenotype. *Int J Cancer* **46**, 712-718.

van Bergen en Henegouwen PMP, Defize LHK, Dekroon J, van Damme H, Verkleij AJ, Boonstra J (1989). Ligand induced association of epidermal growth factor receptor to cytoskeleton of A431 cells. *J Cell Biochem* **39**, 455-465.

van Buskirk AM, DeNagel DC, Guagliardi LE, Brodsky FM, Pierce SK (1991). Cellular and subcellular distribution of PBP 72/74 a peptide-binding protein that plays a role in antigen processing. *J Immunol* **146**, 500-506.

van den Brule FA, Engel J, Stetler-Stevenson WG, Liu FT, Sobel ME, Castronovo V (1992). Genes involved in tumour invasion and metastasis are differentially modulated by estradiol and progestin in human breast cancer cells. *Int J Cancer* **52**, 653-657.

van der Burg MEL, Henzen-Logmans SC, Foekens JA, Berns EMJJ, Rodenberg CJ, van Putten WLJ, Klijn GM (1993). The prognostic value of epidermal growth factor receptors, determined by both immunohistochemistry and ligand binding assay, in primary epithelial ovarian cancer: a pilot study. *Eur J Cancer* **29**, 1951-1957.

van der Luijt RB, Vasen HFA, Tops CMJ, Breukel C, Fodde R, Khan PM (1995). APC mutation in the alternatively spliced region of exon-9 associated with late onset familial adenomatous polyposis. *Human Genet* **96**, 705-710.

van Heyningen V, Bickmore WA, Hastie ND, Porteous DJ, Couillin P, Junien C, Boehm T, Rabbits T, Gessfler M, Bruns GAP, Yeger H, Compton DA (1989). Refined break point map of WAGR and related proteins with chromosome 11p13 markers. *Cytogenet Cell Genet* **51**, 1095.

van Meir EG, Kikuchi T, Tada M, Li H, Diserens AC, Wojcik BE, Huang HJS, Friedmann T, De Tribolet N, Cavenee WK (1994a). Analysis of the *p53* gene and its expression in human glioblastoma cells. *Cancer Res* **54**, 649-652.

van Meir EG, Polverini PJ, Chazin VR, Huang JHS, De Tribolet N, Cavenee WK (1994b). Release of an inhibitor of angiogenesis upon induction of wild-type p53 expression in gliobastoma cells. *Nature Genet* **8**, 171-176.

van Meyel DJ, Ramsay DA, Chamber AF, Macdonald DR, Cairncross JG (1994a). Absence of hereditary mutations in exons 5 through 9 of the p53 gene and exon 24 of the neurofibromin gene in families with glioma. *Ann Neurol* **35**, 120-122.

van Meyel DJ, Ramsay DA, Casson AG, Keeney M, Chambers AF, Cairncross JG (1994b). p53 mutation, expression, and DNA ploidy in evolving gliomas. Evidence for two pathways of progression. *J Natl Cancer Inst* **86**, 1011-1017.

van Roy F, Vleminckx K, Vakaet L Jr, Berx G, Fiers W, Mareel M (1992). The invasion suppressor role of E-cadherin. *Contribution Oncol* **44**, 108-126.

van Veldhuizen PJ, Sadasivan R, Garcia F, Austenfeld FMS, Stephens RL (1993). Mutant p53 expression in prostate carcinoma. *Prostate* **22**, 23-30.

Vangsted A, Drivsholm L, Andersen E, Bock E (1994). New serum markers for small cell lung cancer. 2. The neural cell adhesion molecule, NCAM. *Cancer Det Prevent* **18**, 291-298.

Varley JM, Armour J, Swallow JE, Jeffreys AJ, Ponder AJ, T'Ang A, Fung YKT, Brammar WJ, Walker RA (1989). The retinoblastoma gene is frequently altered leading to loss of expression in primary breast tumours. *Oncogene* **4**, 725-729.

Vassalli J, Baccino D, Berlin D (1985). A cellular binding site for the M_r 55,000 form of the human plasminogen activator, urokinase. *J Cell Biol* **100**, 86-92.

Viac J, Vincent C, Palacio S, Schmitt D, Claudy A (1996). Tumour necrosis factor (TNF) receptors in malignant melanoma. Correlation with soluble ICAM-1 levels. *Eur J Cancer* **32A**, 447-449.

Viel A, Giannini F, Capozzi E, Canzonieri V, Scarabelli C, Gloghini A, Boiocchi M (1994). Molecular mechanisms possibly affecting wt1 function in human ovarian tumours. *Int J Cancer* **57**, 515-521.

Verheijen RHM, Feitz WFJ, Beck JLM, Debruyne FMJ, Vooys GP, Kenemans P, Herman CJ (1985). Cell DNA content – correlation with clonogenicity in the human tumour cloning system (HTCS). *Int J Cancer* **35**, 653-657.

Verhoeven D, Vanmarck E (1993). Proliferation, basement membrane changes, metastasis and vascularization patterns in human breast cancer. *Path Res Pract* **189**, 851-861.

Vermeulen PB, Verhoeven D, Fierens H, Hubens G, Goovaerts G, van Marck E, Debruijn EA, van Oosterom AT, Dirix LY (1995). Microvessel quantification in primary colorectal carcinoma. An immunohistochemical study. *Br J Cancer* **71**, 340-343.

Vermeulen SJ, Bruyneel EA, van Roy FM, Mareel MM, Bracke ME (1995). Activation of the E-cadherin/catenin complex in human MCF-7 breast cancer cells by all-*trans* retinoic acid. *Br J Cancer* **72**, 1447-1453.

Versnel MA, Haarbrink M, Langerak AW, De Laat AAJM, Hagemeijer A, van der Kwast TH, Vandenberg-Bakker LAM, Schrier PI (1994). Human ovarian tumours of epithelial origin express PDGF *in vitro* and *in vivo*. *Cancer Genet Cytogenet* **73**, 60-64.

Vietor I, Vilcek J (1994). Pathways of heat shock protein 28 phosphorylation by TNF in human fibroblasts. *Lymphokine Cytokine Res* **13**, 315-323.

Viglietto G, Romano A, Maglione D, Rambaldi M, Paoletti I, Lago CT, Califano D, Monaco C, Mineo A, Santelli G, Manzo G, Botti G, Chiappetta G, Persico MG (1996). Neovascularisation in human germ cell tumours correlates with a marked increase in the expression of the vascular endothelial growth factor but not the placenta-derived growth factor. *Oncogene* **13**, 577-587.

Villeponteau B (1996). The RNA components of human mouse telomerases. *Sem Cell Develop Biol* **7**, 15-21.

Viola MV, Fromowitz F, Oravez S, Deb S, Schlom J (1985). *Ras* oncogene p21 expression is increased in premalignant lesions and high grade bladder carcinoma. *J Exp Med* **161**, 1213-1218.

Viola MV, Fromowit F, Oravez S, Deb S, Finkel G, Lundy J, Hand P, Thor A, Schlom J (1986). Expression of *ras* oncogene p21 in prostate cancer. *N Engl J Med* **314**, 133-137.

Visscher DW, Sarkar FH, Criss JD (1991). Correlation of DNA ploidy with c-erbB2 expression in preinvasive and invasive breast tumours. *Anal Quant Cytol Histol* **13**, 418-424.

Visscher DW, Hoyhtya M, Ottosen SK, Liang CM, Sarkar FH, Crissman JD, Fridman R (1994). Enhanced expression of tissue inhibitor of metalloproteinase-2 (TIMP-2) in the stroma of breast carcinomas correlates with tumour recurrence. *Int J Cancer* **59**, 339-344.

Vleminckx K, Mareel M, Vakaet L, Jr, Fiers W, van Roy F (1991a). Expression of E-cadherin in epithelial cell lines is negatively correlated with invasion. *Clin Exp Metastasis* **8** (Suppl. 1), 17.

Vleminckx K, Vakaet L, Jr, Mareel MM, Fiers W, van Roy FM (1991b). Genetic manipulation of E-cadherin expression by epithelial tumour cells reveals an invasion suppressor role. *Cell* **66**, 107-119.

Vlodavsky I, Eldor A, Bar-Ner M, Fridman R, Vohen IR, Klagsbrun M (1988). Heparan sulphate degradation in tumour cell invasion and angiogenesis. *Adv Exp Med Biol* **233**, 201-210.

Vlodavsky I, Bashkin P, Ishai-Michaeli R, Chajek-Shaul T, Bar-Shavit R, Haimovitz-Friedman A, Klagsbrun M, Fuks Z (1991). Sequestration and release of basic fibroblast growth factor. *Ann NY Acad Sci* **638**, 207-220.

Voeller JH, Sugars LY, Pretlow T, Gelmann E (1994). p53 oncogene mutations in human prostate cancer specimens. *J Urol* **151**, 492-495.

Voellmy R, Bromley P, Kocher HP (1982). Structural similarities between corresponding heat shock proteins from different eukaryotic cells. *J Biol Chem* **258**, 3516-3522.

Vogelstein B, Kinzler KW (1992). p53 function and dysfunction. *Cell* **70**, 523-526.

Vogelstein B, Kinzler KW (1994). Has the breast cancer gene been found? *Cell* **79**, 1-3.

Vogelstein B, Fearon ER, Hamilton SR, Kern SE, Preisinger AC, Leppert M, Nakamara Y, White R, Smits AMM, Bos JL (1988). Genetic alterations during colorectal tumour development. *N Engl J Med* **319**, 525-532.

Volpe G, Gamberi B, Pastore C, Roetto A, Pautasso M, Parvis G, Camaschella C, Mazza U, Saglio G, Gaidano G (1996). Analysis of microsatellite instability in chronic lymphoproliferative disorders. *Ann Haematol* **72**, 67-71.

Von Deimling A, Lousin DN, Von Ammon K, Petersen I, Hoell T, Chung RY, Matuza RL, Schoenfeld DA, Yasargil MG, Wiestler OD, Seizinger BR (1992). Association of growth factor receptor gene amplification with loss of chromosome 10 in human glioblastoma multiforme. *J Neurosurg* **77**, 295-301.

Vuori K, Ruoslahti E (1994). Association of insulin-receptor substrate-1 with integrins. *Science* **266**, 1576-1578.

Waber PG, Chen J, Nisen PD (1993). Infrequency of ras, p53, wt1, or rb gene alterations in Wilms tumours. *Cancer* **72**, 3732-3738.

Wada A, Sakamoto H, Katoh O, Yoshida T, Yokota J, Little PFR, Sugimura T, Terada M (1988). Two homologous oncogenes, hst1 and int-2, are closely located in human genome. *Biochem Biophys Res Commun* **157**, 828-835.

Wadey RB, Pal N, Buckle B, Yeomans E, Pritchard J, Cowell JK (1990). Loss of heterozygosity in Wilms tumour involves two distinct regions of chromosome 11. *Oncogene* **5**, 901-907.

Wagener C, Bargou RC, Daniel PT, Bommert K, Mapara MY, Royer HD, Dorken B (1996). Induction of the death promoting gene bax-α sensitizes cultured breast cancer cells to drug-induced apoptosis. *Int J Cancer* **67**, 138-141.

Wahls WP, Moore PD (1990). Relative frequencies of homologous recombination between plasmid introduced into DNA repair-deficient and other mammalian somatic cell lines. *Somatic Cell Mol Genet* **16**, 321-329.

Walker PR, Smith C, Youdale T, Leblanc J, Whitfield JF, Sikorska M (1991). Topoisomerase II-reactive chemotherapeutic drugs induce apoptosis in thymocytes. *Cancer Res* **51**, 1078-1085.

Wallet V, Mutzel R, Troll H, Barzu O, Wurster B, Vernon M, Lacombe ML (1990). *Dictyostelium* nucleoside diphosphate kinase highly homologous to nm23 and awd proteins involved in mammalian tumour metastasis and *Drosophila* development. *J Natl Cancer Inst* **82**, 1199-1202.

Waltenberger J, Mayr U, Frank H, Hombach V (1996). Suramin is a potent inhibitor of vascular endothelial growth factor. A contribution to the molecular basis of its antiangiogenic action. *J Mol Cell Cardiol* **28**, 1523-1529.

Walz G, Aruffo A, Kolanus W, Bevilacqua M, Seed B (1990). Recognition of ELAM-1 of the sialyl-Le(x) determinant on myeloid and tumour cells. *Science* **250**, 1132-1135.

Wang CY, Petryniak B, Thompson CB, Kaelin WG, Leiden JM (1993). Regulation of the Ets-related transcription factor elf-1 by binding to the retinoblastoma protein. *Science* **260**, 1330-1335.

Wang L, Patel U, Ghosh L, Chen HC, Banerjee S (1993). Mutation in the *nm23* gene is associated with metastasis in colorectal cancer. *Cancer Res* **53**, 717-720

Wang Y, Reed M, Wang P, Stenger, JE, Mayr G, Anderson ME, Schwedes JF, Tegtmeyer P (1993). p53 domains: identification and characterisation of two autonomous DNA-binding regions. *Genes Develop* **7**, 2575-2586.

Wang YS, Okan I, Pokrovskaja K, Wiman KG (1996). Abrogation of p53-induced G1 arrest by the HPV-16 E7 protein does not inhibit p53-induced apoptosis. *Oncogene* **12**, 2731-2735.

Wang ZY, Madden SL, Devel TF, Rauscher FJ, III (1992). The Wilms tumour gene product, wt1, represses transcription of the platelet-derived growth factor A chain gene. *J Biol Chem* **267**, 21999-22002.

Washington K, Gottfried MR, Telen MJ (1994). Expression of the cell adhesion molecule CD44 in gastric adenocarcinomas. *Human Pathol* **25**, 1043-1049.

Watanabe M, Takahashi Y, Ohta T, Mai M, Sasaki T, Seiki M (1996). Inhibiton of metastasis in human gastric cancer cells transfected with tissue inhibitor of metalloproteinase-1 gene in nude mice. *Cancer* **77**, 1676-1680.

Watanabe T, Hotta T, Ichikawa A, Kinoshita T, Nagai H, Uchida T, Murate T, Saito H (1994). The mdm2 oncogene over-expression in chronic lymphocytic leukaemia and low grade lymphoma of B-cell origin. *Blood* **84**, 3158-3165.

Watanabe Y, Usuda, N, Tsugane S, Kobayashi R, Hidaka H (1992). Calvasculin, an encoded protein from messenger RNA termed PEL-98, 18A2, 42A or p9Ka, is secreted by smooth muscle cells in culture and exhibits Ca^{2+}-dependent binding to 36kDa microfibril-associated glycoprotein. *J Biol Chem* **267**, 17136-17140.

Watanabe Y, Usada N, Minami H, Morita T, Tsugane S, Ishikawa R, Kohama K, Yomida Y, Hidaka H (1993). Calvasculin, as a factor affecting the microfilament assemblies in rat fibroblasts transfected by src gene. *FEBS Lett* **324**, 51-55.

Watatani M, Nagayama K, Imanishi Y, Kurooka K, Wada T, Inui H, Hirai K, Ozaki M, Yasutomi M (1993). Genetic alterations on chromosome 17 in human breast cancer. Relationship to clinical features and DNA ploidy. *Breast Cancer Res Treat* **28**, 231-239.

Watson JD (1972). Origin of concatemeric T4 DNA. *Nature New Biol* **239**, 197-201.

Watts CKW, Brady A, Sarcevic B, Defazio A, Musgrove EA, Sutherland RL (1995). Antiestrogen inhibition of cell cycle progression in breast cancer cells is associated with inhibition of cyclin dependent kinase activity and decreased retinoblastoma protein phosphorylation. *Mol Endocrinol* **9**, 1804-1813.

Waziri M, Patil SR, Hanson JW, Bartley JA (1983). Abnormality of chromosome 11 in patients with features of Beckwith–Wiedemann syndrome. *J Paediat* **102**, 873-876.

Weber E, Gunther D, Laube F, Wiederanders B, Kirschke H (1994). Hybridoma cells producing antibodies to cathepsin L have greatly reduced potential for tumour growth. *J Cancer Res Clin Oncol* **120**, 564-567.

Weghorst CM, Dragnev KH, Buzard GS, Thorne KL, Vandeborne GF, Vincent KA, Rice JM (1994). Low incidence of point mutations detected in the *p53* tumour suppressor gene from chemically induced rat renal mesenchymal tumours. *Cancer Res* **54**, 215-219.

Weinberg RA (1985). The action of oncogenes in the cytoplasm and nucleus. *Science* **230**, 770-776.

Weinberg RA (1991). Tumour suppressor genes. *Science* **254**, 1138-1146.

Weiss J, Schwechheimer K, Cavenee WK, Herlyn M, Arden KC (1993). Mutation and expression of the p53 gene in malignant melanoma cell lines. *Int J Cancer* **54**, 693-699.

Weiss L (1990). Metastatic inefficiency. *Adv Cancer Res* **54**, 159-211.

Weiss RE, Fair WR, Cordon-Cardo C (1994). Characterisation of protease expression in human prostate cancer cell lines. *Int J Oncol* **5**, 973-978.

Weitzel JN, Patel J, Smith DM, Goodman A, Safaii H, Ball HG (1994). Molecular genetic changes associated with ovarian cancer. *Gynecol Oncol* **55**, 245-252.

Welch DR (1984). *Tumour progression: analysis of the instability of the metastatic phenotype, sensitivity to radiation and chemotherapy.* Ph.D. thesis, University of Texas, Houston, TX.

Welch DR (1989). Factors involved in the development and maintenance of tumour heterogeneity. In: *Carcinogenesis and Dietary Fat*, S. Abraham (ed.). Kluwer, Boston.

Welch WJ, Suhan JP (1985). Morphological study of the mammalian stress response: characterisation of changes in cytoplasmic organelles, cytoskeleton and nucleoli and appearance of intranuclear actin filaments in rat fibroblasts after heat shock treatment. *J Cell Biol* **101**, 1198-1211.

Welsh CF, Zhu D, Bourguignon LYW (1995). Interaction of CD44 variant isoforms with hyaluronic acid and the cytoskeleton in human prostate cancer cells. *J Cell Physiol* **164**, 605-612.

Wenger CR, Beardslee S, Owens MA, Pounds G, Oldaker T, Vendely P, Pandian MR, Harrington D, Clark GM, McGuire WL (1993). DNA ploidy, S-phase, and steroid receptors in more than 127,000 breast cancer patients. *Breast Canc Res Treat* **28**, 9-20.

Werb Z, Tremble PM, Behrendtsen O, Crowley E, Damsky CH (1989). Signal transduction through the fibronectin receptors induces collagenase and stromelysin gene expression. *J Cell Biol* **109**, 877-889.

Werner H, Rauscher FJ, Sukhatme VP, Drummond IA, Roberts CT, Leroith D (1994). Transcriptional repression of the insulin-like growth factor I receptor (IGF-I-r) gene by the tumour suppressor wt1 involves binding to sequences both upstream and downstream of the IGF-Ir gene transcription start site. *J Biol Chem* **269**, 12577-12582.

Werner H, Shenorr Z, Rauscher FJ, Morris JF, Roberts CT, Leroith D (1995). Inhibition of cellular proliferation by the Wilms tumour suppressor wt1 is associated with suppression of insulin-like growth factor I receptor gene expression. *Mol Cell Biol* **15**, 3516-3522.

Werness BA, Levine AJ, Howley PM (1990). Association of human papilloma virus types 16 and 18 proteins with p53. *Science* **248**, 76-79.

Weterman MAJ, Stoopen GM, Van Muijen GNP, Kuznicki J, Ruiter DJ (1992). Expression of calcyclin in human melanoma cell lines correlates with metastatic behaviour in nude mice. *Cancer Res* **52**, 1291-1296.

Weterman MAJ, Vanmuijen GNP, Bloemers HPJ, Ruiter DJ (1993). Expression of calcyclin in human melanocytic lesions. *Cancer Res* **53**, 6061-6066.

White AE, Livanos EM, Tlsty TD (1994). Differential disruption of genomic integrity and cell cycle regulation in normal human fibroblasts by the HPV oncoproteins. *Genes Develop* **8**, 666-677.

White CW, Wolf SJ, Bowers JT, Leventhal JP, Yu A (1990). Interferon alpha therapy for pulmonary angiomatous disorders. *Amer Rev Resp Dis* **141**, A188.

Whyte MKB, Hardwick SJ, Meagher LC, Savill LJS, Haslett C (1993). Transient elevations of cytosolic free calcium retard subsequent apoptosis in neutrophils *in vitro. J Clin Invest* **92**, 446-455.

Wiegant FAC, van Bergen en Henegouwen PM, van Dongen G, Linnemans WAM (1987). Stress-induced thermotolerance of the cytoskeleton of mouse neuroblastoma cells and rat Reuber H35 hepatoma cells. *Cancer Res* **47**, 1674-1680.

Wilhelmsson A, Cuthill S, Denis M, Wikstrom AC, Gustafsson JA, Poellinger L (1990). Specific DNA binding activity of the dioxin receptor is modulated by the 90kDa heat shock protein. *EMBO J* **9**, 69-76.

Wilkinson DG, Peters G, Dickson C, McMahon AP (1988). Expression of the FGF-related proto-oncogene int-2 during gastrulation and neurulation in the mouse. *EMBO J* **7**, 691-695.

Wilkinson DG, Bhatt S, McMahon AP (1989). Expression pattern of the FGF-related proto-oncogene int-2 suggests roles in foetal development. *Development* **105**, 131-136.

Will K, Warnecke G, Bergman S, Deppert W (1995). Species-specific and tissue-specific expression of the C-terminal alternatively spliced form of the tumour suppressor p53. *Nucl Acids Res* **23**, 4023-4028.

Williamson RA, Marston FA, Angal S, Koklitis P, Panico M, Morris HR, Carne AF, Smith BJ, Harris TJ, Freedman RB (1990). Disulphide bond assignment in human tissue inhibitor of metalloproteinases (TIMP). *Biochem J* **267**, 267-274.

Willis AE, Lindahl T (1987). DNA ligase I deficiency in Bloom's syndrome. *Nature* **325**, 355-357.

Withers DA, Harvey RC, Faust JB, Melnyk O, Carey K, Meeaker TC (1991). Characterisation of a candidate *bcl-1* gene. *Mol Cell Biol* **11**, 4846-4853.

Witjes JA, Umbas R, De Bruyne FMJ, Schalken JA (1995). Expression of markers for transitional cell carcinoma in normal bladder mucosa of patients with bladder cancer. *J Urol* **154**, 2185-2189.

Wittig BM, Kaulen H, Thees R, Schmitt C, Knolle P, Stock J, Zumbuschenfelde KHM, Dippold W (1996). Elevated serum E-selectin in patients with liver metastases of colorectal cancer. *Eur J Cancer* **32A**, 1215-1218.

Wizigmannvoos S, Breier G, Risau W, Plate KH (1995). Up-regulation of vascular endothelial growth factor and its receptors in von Hippel-Lindau disease-associated and sporadic hemangioblastomas. *Cancer Res* **55**, 1358-1364.

Wolf C, Chenard MP, Grossouvre D, Bellocq JP, Chambon P, Basset P (1992). Breast cancer associated stromelysin-3-gene is expressed in basal cell carcinoma and during cutaneous wound healing. *J Invest Dermatol* **99**, 870-872.

Wolman SR, Pauley RJ, Mohammed A, Dawson PJ, Visscher DW, Sarkar FH (1992). Genetic markers as prognostic indicators in breast cancer. *Cancer* **70**, 1765-1774.

Wong GT, Gavin BJ, McMahon AP (1994). Differential transformation of mammary epithelial cells by wnt genes. *Mol Cell Biol* **14**, 6278-6286.

Wood WR, Seftor EA, Lotan D, Nakajima M, Misiorowski RL, Seftor REB, Lotan R, Hendrix MJC (1990). Retinoic acid inhibits human melanoma tumour cell invasion. *Anticancer Res* **10**, 423-432.

Wrede D, Tidy JA, Crook T, Lane D, Vousden KH (1991). Expression of RB and p53 proteins in HPV-positive and HPV-negative cervical carcinoma cell lines. *Mol Carcinogen* **4**, 171-175.

Wright C, Mellon K, Jonston P, Lane DP, Harris AL, Horne CHW, Neal DE (1991). Expression of mutant p53, c-*erb*B1 and the epidermal growth factor receptor in transitional cell carcinoma of the human urinary bladder. *Br J Cancer* **63**, 967-970.

Wright C, Thomas D, Mellon K, Neal DE, Horne CHW (1995). Expression of retinoblastoma gene product and p53 in bladder carcinoma. Correlation with Ki67 index. *Br J Urol* **75**, 173-179.

Wright WE, Brasiskyte D, Piatyszek MA, Shay JW (1996a). Experimental elongation of telomeres extends the life span of immortal cell × normal cell hybrids. *EMBO J* **15**, 1734-1741.

Wright WE, Piatyszek MA, Rainey WE, Byrd W, Shay JW (1996b). Telomerase activity in human germline and embryonic tissues and cells. *Develop Genet* **18**, 173-179.

Wu BJ, Morimoto RI (1985). Transcription of the human hsp70 gene is induced by serum stimulation. *Proc Natl Acad Sci USA* **82**, 6070-6074.

Wu BJ, Hurst HC, Jones NC, Morimoto RI (1986). The E1A 13S product of adenovirus 5-activated transcription of the cellular human HSP 70 gene. *Mol Cell Biol* **6**, 2994-2999.

Wu CL, Zukerberg LR, Ngwu C, Harlow E, Lees JA (1995). *In vivo* association of E2F and DP family proteins. *Mol Cell Biol* **15**, 2536-2546.

Wu D, Kan M, Sato GH, Okamoto T, Sato JD (1991). Characterisation and molecular cloning of a putative binding protein for heparin-binding growth factors. *J Biol Chem* **266**, 16778-16785.

Wu LT, Yee A, Liu L, Carbonaro-Hall D, Venkatesan N, Tolo V, Hall FL (1995). Early G1 induction of p21/waf1/cip1 in synchronised osteosarcoma cells is independent of p53. *Oncol Rep* **2**, 227-231.

Wu XW, Bayle JH, Olson D, Levine AJ (1993). The p53-mdm2 autoregulatory feedback loop. *Genes Develop* **7**, 1126-1132.

Wu XW, Levine AJ (1994). P53 and E2F-1 cooperate to mediate apoptosis. *Proc Natl Acad Sci USA* **91**, 3602-3606.

Wu Y, Liu YG, Lee L, Miner Z, Kulesz-Martin M (1994). Wild-type alternatively spliced p53. binding to DNA and interaction with the major p53 protein *in vitro* and in cells. *EMBO J* **13**, 4823-4830.

Wun TC, Reich E (1987). An inhibitor of plasminogen activator from human placenta. *J Biol Chem* **262**, 3646-3653.

Wyllie AH (1980). Glucocorticoid-induced thymocyte apoptosis is associated with endogenous endonuclease activation. *Nature* **284**, 555-556.

Wyllie AH (1987). Apoptosis: cell death in tissue regulation. *J Pathol* **153**, 313-316.

Wyllie AH (1993). Apoptosis. *Br J Cancer* **67**, 205-208.

Wyllie AH, Rose KA, Morris RG, Steel CM, Foster E, Spandidos DA (1987). Rodent fibroblast tumour expressing human *myc* and *ras* genes: growth, metastasis and endogenous oncogene expression. *Br J Cancer* **56**, 251-259.

Xia L, St Denis KA, Bapat B (1995). Evidence for a novel exon in the coding region of the adenomatous polyposis coli (APC) gene. *Genomics* **28**, 589-591.

Xiao ZX, Chen JD, Levine AJ, Modjtahedi H, Xing J, Sellers WR, Livingston DM (1995). Interaction between the retinoblastoma protein and the oncoprotein mdm2. *Nature* **375**, 694-698.

Xie J, Li R, Kotovuori P, Vermot Desesrochas C, Wijdenes J, Arnaout MA, Nortamo P, Gahmberg CG (1995). Intercellular adhesion molecule-2 (CD102) binds to the leukocyte integrin CD11b/CD18 through the A-domain. *J Immunol* **155**, 3619-3628.

Xiong Y, Zhang H, Beach D (1992). D-type cyclins associated with multiple protein kinases and the DNA replication and repair factor PCNA. *Cell* **71**, 505-514.

Xiong Y, Hannon G, Zhang H, Casso D, Kobayashi R, Beach D (1993a). p21 is a universal inhibitor of cyclin kinases. *Nature* **366**, 701-704.

Xiong Y, Zhang H, Beach D (1993b). Subunit rearrangement of the cyclin dependent kinases is associated with cellular transformation. *Genes Develop* **7**, 1572-1583.

Xu CF, Solomon E (1996). Mutations of the BRCA1 gene in human cancer. *Sem Cancer Biol* **7**, 33-40.

Xu CF, Brown MA, Chambers JA, Griffiths B, Nicolai H, Solomon E (1995). Distinct transcription sites generate two forms of BRCA1 messenger RNA. *Human Mol Genet* **4**, 2259-2264.

Xu D, Gruber A, Peterson C, Pisa P (1996). Suppression of telomerase activity in HL-60 cells after treatment with differentiating agents. *Leukaemia* **10**, 1354-1357.

Xu HJ, Hu SX, Hashimoto T, Takahashi R, Benedict WF (1989). The retinoblastoma susceptibility gene product: a characteristic pattern in normal cells and abnormal expression in malignant cells. *Oncogene* **4**, 807-812.

Xu HJ, Hu SX, Cagle PT, Moore GE, Benedict WF (1991). Absence of retinoblastoma protein expression in primary non-small cell lung carcinomas. *Cancer Res* **51**, 2735-2739.

Xu L, Sgroi D, Sterner CJ, Beauchamp RL, Pinney DM, Keel S, Ueki K, Rutter JL, Buckler AJ, Louis DN, Gusella JF, Ramesh V (1994). Mutational analysis of CDNK2 (MTS1/P16 INK4) in human breast carcinoma. *Cancer Res* **54**, 5262-5264.

Yagel S, Parhar RS, Jeffrey JJ, Lala PK (1988). Normal nonmetastatic human trophoblast cells share *in vitro* invasive properties of malignant cells. *J Cell Physiol* **136**, 455-462.

Yago K, Zenita K, Ginya H, Sawada M, Ohmori K, Okuma M, Kannagi R, Lowe JB (1993). Expression of alpha-(1,3)-fucosyltransferase which synthesise sialyl Le(x) and sialyl Le(a), the carbohydrate ligands for E-selectin and P-selectin, in human malignant cell lines. *Cancer Res* **53**, 5559-5565.

Yahanda AM, Bruner JM, Donehower LA, Morrison RS (1995). Astrocytes derived from p53 deficient mice provide a multistep *in vitro* model for development of malignant gliomas. *Mol Cell Biol* **15**, 4249-4259.

Yamada H, Ochi K, Nakada S, Takahara S, Nemoto T, Sekikawa T, Horiguchi-Yamada J (1995a). Interferon modulates the messenger RNA of G1-controlling genes to suppress the G1-to-S transition in Daudi cells. *Mol Cell Biochem* **152**, 149-158.

Yamada H, Sasaki M, Honda T, Wake N, Boyd J, Oshimura M, Barrett JC (1995b). Suppression of endometrial carcinoma cell tumorigenicity by human chromosome 18. *Genes Chrom Cancer* **13**, 18-24.

Yamada N, Chung YS, Sawada T, Okuno M, Sowa M (1995). Role of SPan-1 antigen in adhesion of human colon cancer cells to vascular endothelium. *Digestive Dis Sci* **40**, 1005-1012.

Yamamori T, Ito K, Nakamura Y, Yura T (1978). Transient regulation of protein synthesis in *Escherichia coli* upon up-shift of growth temperature. *J Bacteriol* **134**, 1133-1140.

Yamamoto T, Ikawa S, Akiyama T, Semba K, Nomura N, Miyajima N, Saito T, Toyoshima K (1986). Similarity of protein encoded by the human c-erbβ-2 gene to epidermal growth factor receptor. *Nature* **319**, 230-234.

Yamane A, Seetharam L, Yamaguchi S, Gotoh N, Takahashi T, Neufeld G, Shibuya M (1994). A new communication system between hepatocytes and sinusoidal endothelial cells in liver through vascular endothelial growth factor and flt tyrosine kinase receptor family (flt-1 and KDR/flk-1). *Oncogene* **9**, 2683-2690.

Yamashina K, Heppner GH (1985). Correlation of frequency of induced mutation and metastatic potential in tumour cell lines from a single mouse mammary tumour. *Cancer Res* **45**, 4015-4019.

Yan DH, Chang LS, Hung MC (1991). Repressed expression of the Her-2/c-erbB2 proto-oncogene by the adenovirus E1A gene products. *Oncogene* **6**, 1991-1996.

Yang E, Zha JP, Jockel J, Boise LH, Thompson CB, Korsmeyer SJ (1995). Bad, a heterodimeric partner for bcl-x(L) and bcl-2, displaced bax and promotes cell death. *Cell* **80**, 285-291.

Yang EV, Bryant SV (1994). Developmental regulation of a matrix metalloproteinase during regeneration of axolotl appendages. *Develop Biol* **166**, 696-703.

Yang WI, Zukerberg LR, Motokura T, Arnod A, Harris NL (1994). Cyclin D1 (BCL-1, PRAD1) protein expression in low grade B-cell lymphomas and reactive hyperplasia. *Amer J Path* **145**, 86-96.

Yang-Yen HF, Chambard JC, Sun YL, Smeal T, Schmidt TJ, Drouin J, Karin M (1990). Transcriptional interference between c-jun and the glucocorticoid receptor: Mutual inhibition of DNA binding due to direct protein–protein interaction. *Cell* **62**, 1205-1215.

Yasoshima T, Denno R, Kawaguchi S, Sato N, Okada Y, Ura H, Kikuchi K, Hirata K (1996). Establishment and characterisation of human gastric carcinoma lines with high metastatic potential in the liver. Changes in integrin expression associated with the ability to metastasise in the liver of nude mice. *Jpn J Cancer Res* **87**, 153-160.

Ye CL, Kiriyama K, Mistuoka C, Kannagi R, Ito K, Watanabe T, Kondo K, Akiyama S, Takagi H (1995). Expression of E-selectin on endothelial cells of small veins in human colorectal cancer. *Int J Cancer* **61**, 455-460.

Ye RD, Wun TC, Sadler JE (1987). cDNA cloning and expression in *Escherichia coli* of a plasminogen activator inhibitor from human placenta. *J Biol Chem* **262**, 3718-3725.

Yehiely F, Oren M (1992). The gene for the rat heat shock cognate HSP70 can suppress oncogene mediated transformation. *Cell Growth Differen* **3**, 803-809.

Yin XM, Oltvai ZN, Korsmeyer SJ (1994). BH1 and BH2 domains of bcl-2 are required for inhibition of apoptosis and heterodimersation with bax. *Nature* **369**, 321-323.

Yokozaki H, Ito R, Nakayama H, Kuniyasu H, Taniyama K, Tahara E (1994). Expression of CD44 abnormal transcripts in human gastric carcinomas. *Cancer Lett* **83**, 229-234.

Yonemura Y, Kaji M, Hirono Y, Fushida S, Tsugawa K, Fujimura T, Miyazaki I, Harada S, Yamamoto H (1996). Correlation between over-expression of c-*met* gene and the progression of gastric cancer. *Int J Oncol* **8**, 555-560.

Yonish-Rouach E, Resnitzky D, Lotem J, Sachs L, Kimchi A, Oren M (1991). Wild type p53 induces apoptosis of myeloid leukaemic cells that is inhibited by interleukin-6. *Nature* **352**, 345-347.

Yonish-Rouach E, Grunwald D, Wilder S, Kimchi A, May E, Lawrence JJ, May P, Oren M (1993). P53-mediated cell death. Relationship to cell cycle control. *Mol Cell Biol* **13**, 1415-1423.

Yoshida MC, Wada M, Satoh H, Yoshida T, Sakamoto H, Miyagawa K, Yokota J, Koda T, Kakinuma M, Sugimura T, Terada M (1988). Human hst1 (HstF1) gene maps to chromosome band 11q13 and co-amplifies with int2 gene in human cancer. *Proc Natl Acad Sci USA* **85**, 4861-4864.

Yoshida T, Schneider EL, Mdori N (1994). Cloning of the rat GADD45 cDNA and its messenger RNA expression in the brain. *Gene* **151**, 253-255.

Yoshihara Y, Oka S, Nemoto Y, Watanabe Y, Nagata S, Kagamiyama H, Mori K (1994). An ICAM-related neuronal glycoprotein, telencephalin, with brain segment-specific expression. *Neuron* **12**, 541-553.

Yoshiji H, Gomez DE, Shibuya M, Thorgeirsson UP (1996). Expression of vascular endothelial growth factor, its receptor, and other angiogenic factors in human breast cancer. *Cancer Res* **56**, 2013-2016.

Younes A, Zhao SR, Jendiroba D, Kleine HD, Cabanillas F, Andreefe M (1995). Decreased expression of the deleted in colorectal carcinoma gene in non-Hodgkin's lymphoma. *Blood* **85**, 2813-2816.

Yu D, Hung MC (1991). Expression of activated rat *neu* oncogene is sufficient to induce experimental metastasis in 3T3 cells. *Oncogene* **6**, 1991-1996.

Yu DH, Scorsone E, Hung MC (1991). Adenovirus type-5 E1A gene products act as transformation suppressors of the *neu* oncogene. *Mol Cell Biol* **11**, 1745-1750.

Yu DH, Hamada JI, Zhang H, Nicolson GL, Hung MC (1992a). Mechanisms of c-erbB2/neu oncogene-induced metastasis and repression of metastatic properties by adenovirus 5 E1A products. *Oncogene* **7**, 2263-2270.

Yu DH, Matin A, Hung MC (1992b). The retinoblastoma gene product suppresses *neu* oncogene-induced transformation via transcriptional repression of neu. *J Biol Chem* **267**, 10203-10206.

Yuan JN, Liu BH, Lee H, Shaw YT, Chiou ST, Chang WC, Lai MD (1993). Release of the p53-induced repression on thymine kinase promoter by single p53 binding sequence. *Biochem Biophys Res Commun* **191**, 662-668.

Yunis JJ, Soreng AL, Bowe AE (1987). Fragile sites are targets of diverse mutagens and carcinogens. *Oncogene* **1**, 59-69.

Yusa K, Sugimoto Y, Yamori T, Yamamoto T, Toyoshima K, Tsuro T (1990). Low metastatic potential of clone from murine colon adenocarcinoma-26 increased by transfection of activated c-*erbB2* gene. *J Natl Cancer Inst* **82**, 1633-1636.

Zachary I, Rozengurt E (1992). Focal adhesion kinase (p125^{FAK}): A point of convergence in the action of neuropeptides, integrins and oncogenes. *Cell* **71**, 891-894.

Zachary I, Sinnett-Smith, Rozengurt E (1992). Bombesin, vasopressin and endothelin stimulation of tyrosine phosphorylation in Swiss 3T3 mice. *J Biol Chem* **267**, 19031-19034.

Zamanian M, La Thangue NB (1992). Adenovirus E1A prevents the retinoblastoma gene product from repressing the activity of a cellular transcription factor. *EMBO J* **11**, 2603-2610.

Zambetti GP, Olson D, Labow M, Levine AJ (1992). A mutant p53 protein is required for the maintenance of the transformed cell phenotype in p53 plus *ras* transformed cells. *Proc Natl Acad Sci USA* **89**, 3952-3956.

Zastawny RL, Salvino R, Chen JM, Benchimol S, Ling V (1993). The core promoter region of the p-glycoprotein gene is sufficient to confer differential responsiveness to wild type and mutant p53. *Oncogene* **8**, 1529-1535.

Zauberman A, Flusberg D, Haupt Y, Barak Y, Oren M (1995). A functional p53 responsive intronic promoter is contained within the human mdm2 gene. *Nucleic Acids Res* **23**, 2584-2592.

Zhan QM, Lord KA, Alamo I, Hollander MC, Carrier F, Ron D, Kohn KW, Hoffman B, Liebermann DA, Fornace AJ (1994). The GADD and MyD genes define a novel set of mammalian genes encoding acidic proteins that synergistically suppress cell growth. *Mol Cell Biol* **14**, 2361-2371.

Zhan QM, Eldeiry W, Bae I, Alamo I, Kastan MB, Vogelstein B, Fornace AJ (1995). Similarity of the DNA damage responsive and growth suppressive properties of waf1/cip1 and GADD45. *Int J Oncol* **6**, 937-946.

Zhang H, Hannon GJ, Beach D (1994). P21-containing cyclin kinases exist in both active and inactive states. *Genes Develop* **8**, 1750-1758.

Zhang HT, Craft P, Scott PAE, Ziche M, Weich HA, Harris AL, Bicknell R (1995). Enhancement of tumour growth and vascular density by transfection of vascular endothelial cell growth factor into MCF-7 human breast carcinoma cells. *J Natl Cancer Inst* **87**, 213-219.

Zhang W, Grasso L, McClain CD, Gambel AM, Cha Y, Travali S, Deisseroth AB, Mercer WE (1995). P53-independent induction of waf1/cip1 in human leukaemia cells is correlated with growth arrest accompanying monocyte/macrophage differentiation. *Cancer Res* **55**, 668-674.

Zhang W, Piatyszek MA, Kobayashi T, Estey E, Andreeff M, Deisseroth AB, Wright WE, Shay JW (1996). Telomerase activity in human acute myelogenous leukaemia. Inhibition of telomerase activity by differentiation-inducing agents. *Clin Cancer Res* **2**, 799-803.

Zhau HYE, Zhou JX, Symmans WF, Chen BQ, Chang SM, Sikes RA, Chung LWK (1996). Transfected neu oncogene induces human prostate cancer metastasis. *Prostate* **28**, 73-83.

Zheng J, Robinson WR, Ehlen T, Yu EM, Dubeau L (1991). Distinction of low grade from high grade human ovarian carcinomas on the basis of losses of heterozygosity on chromosomes 3,6, and 11 and HER-2/*neu* gene amplification. *Cancer Res* **51**, 4045-4051.

Zhou DJ, Ahuja H, Cline MJ (1989). Proto-oncogene abnormalities in human breast cancer. C-erbB2 amplification does not correlate with recurrence of disease. *Oncogene* **4**, 105-108.

Zhou M, Shi Y, Alsediary S, Faird NR (1993). High levels of nm23 gene expresssion in advanced stage of thyroid carcinomas. *Br J Cancer* **68**, 385-388.

Zhou MX, Yeager AM, Smith SD, Findley HW (1995). Over-expression of the mdm2 gene by childhood acute lymphoblastic leukemia cells expressing the wild type p53 gene. *Blood* **85**, 1608-1614.

Zhu XL, Kumar R, Mandal M, Sharma N, Sharma HW, Dhingra U, Sokoloski JA, Hsiao RS, Narayanan R (1996). Cell cycle dependent modulation of telomerase activity in tumour cells. *Proc Natl Acad Sci USA* **93**, 6091-6095.

Ziche M, Gullino PM (1982). Angiogenesis and neoplastic progression *in vitro*. *J Natl Cancer Inst* **69**, 483-487.

Zocchi MR, Ferrero E, Toninelli E, Castellani P, Poggi A, Rugarli C (1994). Expression of NCAM by human renal cell carcinomas correlates with growth rate and adhesive properties. *Exp Cell Res* **214**, 499-509.

Zou MJ, Shi YK, Farid NR (1994). Frequent inactivation of the retinoblastoma gene in human thyroid carcinomas. *Endocrine J UK* **2**, 193-198.

Zou MJ, Shi YF, Alsedairy S, Hussain SS, Farid NR (1995). The expression of the mdm2 gene, a p53 binding protein, in thyroid carcinogenesis. *Cancer* **76**, 314-318.

Zubair A, Lakshmi MS, Sherbet GV (1992). Expression of alpha melanocyte stimulating hormone and the invasive ability of the B16 murine melanoma. *Anticancer Res* **12**, 399-402.

Zucker S, Lysik RM, Malik M, Bauer BA, Caamano J, Klein-Szanto AJP (1992). Secretion of gelatinases and tissue inhibitors of metalloproteinases by human lung cancer cell lines and revertant cell lines: not an invariant correlation with metastasis. *Int J Cancer* **52**, 366-371.

Zugmaier G, Lippman ME, Wellstein A (1992). Inhibition of pentosan polysulphate (PPS) of heparin-binding growth factors released from tumour cells and blockade by PPS of tumour growth in animals. *J Natl Cancer Inst* **84**, 1716-1724.

Zutter M, Hockenbery D, Silverman GA, Korsmeyer SJ (1991). Immunolocalisation of the bcl-2 protein within haematopoietic neoplasms. *Blood* **78**, 1062-1068.

Zylicz M, Le Bowitz JH, McMacken R, Georgopoulos C (1984). The dnaK protein of *Escherichia coli* possesses an ATPase and autophosphorylation activity and is essential in an in vitro DNA replication system. *Proc Natl Acad Sci USA* **80**, 6431-6435.

Index

Page numbers in *italic* refer to illustrations and tables; **bold** page numbers indicate a main discussion.